Handbook of Sleep Medicine

Handbook
of Sleep Medicine

Alon Y. Avidan, MD, MPH
Associate Professor
Department of Neurology
University of California, Los Angeles
Los Angeles, California

Phyllis C. Zee, MD, PhD
Professor
Department of Neurology
Northwestern University
Feinberg School of Medicine
Chicago, Illinois

. Lippincott Williams & Wilkins
a Wolters Kluwer business
Philadelphia · Baltimore · New York · London
Buenos Aires · Hong Kong · Sydney · Tokyo

Acquisitions Editor: Frances R. DeStefano
Managing Editor: Scott Scheidt
Project Manager: Jennifer Harper
Senior Manufacturing Manager: Benjamin Rivera
Marketing Manager: Adam Glazer
Design Coordinator: Terry Mallon
Production Services: Laserwords Private Limited, Chennai, India
Printer: R.R. Donnelley

Library of Congress Cataloging-in-Publication Data

Avidan, Alon.
    Handbook of sleep medicine / Alon Avidan, Phyllis Zee.
      p. ; cm.
    Includes bibliographical references and index.
    ISBN 13: 978-0-7817-6238-0 (soft cover)
    ISBN 10: 0-7817-6238-3 (soft cover)
    1. Sleep disorders—Handbooks, manuals, etc.   I. Zee, Phyllis C.
  1954-   . II. Title.
    [DNLM: 1. Sleep Disorders—physiopathology. 2. Sleep—physio-
  logy.   WM 188 A957h 2006]
    RC547.A86 2006
    616.8'498—dc22

                                                  2006001914

                                                  10 9 8 7 6 5

Contents

Contributing Authors vii

Preface ix

Acknowledgments x

Abbreviations xi

1. Populations at Risk for Sleep Disturbances 1
   Phyllis C. Zee and Alon Y. Avidan

2. Sleep-Disordered Breathing 13
   Suzette Sewell-Scheuermann and Barbara A. Phillips

3. Insomnia 36
   Ruth M. Benca

4. Hypersomnia and Narcolepsy 70
   Timothy F. Hoban and Ronald D. Chervin

5. Motor Disorders of Sleep and Parasomnias 98
   Alon Y. Avidan

6. Circadian Rhythm Sleep Disorders 137
   Brandon S. Lu, Prasanth Manthena,
   and Phyllis C. Zee

7. Sleep Disorders in Children 165
   Judith Anne Owens and Katherine Finn Davis

   Appendix A: The Epworth Sleepiness Scale 185

   Appendix B: Body Mass Index 186

   Appendix C: Interpretation of the Polysomnogram
   and the Multiple Sleep Latency Testing 187

   Appendix D: Continuous Positive Airway Pressure
   Compliance Issues Unique to Sleep Medicine 202

   Appendix E: Sleep Hygiene 205

   Appendix F: Insomnia Algorithm 208

   Appendix G: Hypersomnia Algorithm 209

   Appendix H: Stanford Sleepiness Scale 210

   Appendix I: Motor Disorders Algorithm 211

Appendix J: International Classification of Sleep
Disorders (ICSD-2)   212

Appendix K: Sleep-Stage Scoring   214

Appendix L: Valuable Resources   233

Index   235

Contributing Authors

Alon Y. Avidan, MD, MPH   *Associate Professor; Associate Director, Sleep Disorders Center, Department of Neurology, University of California, Los Angeles*

Ruth M. Benca, MD, PhD   *Professor, Department of Psychiatry, University of Wisconsin-Madison; Physician, Sleep Clinic, University of Wisconsin Hospital & Clinics, Madison, Wisconsin*

Ronald D. Chervin, MD, MS   *Associate Professor, Department of Neurology; Director, Sleep Disorders Center, University of Michigan, Ann Arbor, Michigan*

Katherine Finn Davis, PhD, RN, CPNP   *Chief Research Coordinator, Department of Pediatrics, Division of Infectious Diseases, Epidemiology & Immunology, Emory University School of Medicine, Atlanta, Georgia*

Timothy F. Hoban, MD   *Associate Professor, Departments of Pediatrics and Neurology; Director, Pediatric Sleep Medicine, Department of Pediatrics, University of Michigan, Ann Arbor, Michigan*

Brandon S. Lu, MD   *Fellow, Sleep Medicine, Department of Neurology, Northwestern University, Feinberg School of Medicine; Fellow, Sleep Medicine, Department of Neurology, Northwestern Memorial Hospital, Chicago, Illinois*

Prasanth Manthena, MD   *Instructor, Department of Neurology, Northwestern University, Chicago, Illinois*

Judith Anne Owens, MD, MPH   *Associate Professor of Pediatrics, Department of Pediatrics, Brown Medical School; Director, Pediatric Sleep Disorders Clinic, Division of Pediatric Ambulatory Medicine, Hasbro Children's Hospital, Providence, Rhode Island*

Barbara A. Phillips, MD, MSPH, FCCP   *Professor of Medicine, Pulmonary & Critical Care Division, College of Medicine, Chandler Medical Center; Director, Sleep Apnea Center, Good Samaritan Hospital, Lexington, Kentucky*

Suzette Sewell-Scheuermann, RN PhDc   *University of Kentucky, Lexington, Kentucky; Researcher, KY Research PLLC, Louisville, Kentucky*

Phyllis C. Zee, MD, PhD   *Professor, Department of Neurology; Director, Sleep Disorders Center, Northwestern University Feinberg School of Medicine, Chicago, Illinois*

Preface

The importance of the relationship between sleep and other aspects of physical and mental health is becoming increasingly apparent in primary care and in nearly every medical specialty. Sleep disturbances are common in the general population, but individuals with comorbid medical, neurologic, and psychiatric conditions are at particular risk.

Sleep affects nearly every facet of medical care. Untreated sleep apnea may exacerbate a seizure disorder, complicate pregnancy, and increase the risk of hypertension and cardiovascular events. Insomnia, the most common sleep problem, may be a precursor for depression. Circadian rhythm disturbances are least understood and vastly under-recognized. Recent advances in the pathophysiology and neurochemistry of narcolepsy has provided new tools for the treatment of sleep disorders. Pediatric sleep disorders can be associated with poor school performance and behavioral problems. Neurologic disorders often present with symptoms that result from underlying sleep disorders. Practitioners from every discipline who care for patients with sleep complaints will find the clinically based, practical approach in this book to be most useful.

The *Handbook of Sleep Disorders* offers a concise symptom-based conceptual approach to the diagnosis, evaluation, and treatment of the most common sleep disorders. The handbook offers practical algorithmic flow diagrams, which provide the flexibility of a quick, easily referenced guideline, whereas the chapters provide specific diagnostic tools and detailed reviews of treatments. Most clinicians will find this approach to be not only a practical guide but also a very important educational tool.

This handbook is not intended to be a comprehensive book of sleep medicine but rather to serve as a concise guide for the evaluation, recognition, and treatment of sleep complaints that are commonly encountered in clinical practice. Practitioners from nearly every field of medicine may therefore find this resource indispensable. The easily accessible algorithms and clinical summary could be used as a quick reference in most office or clinical settings.

Given the high prevalence of sleep disorders in nearly every medical subspecialty, this handbook will be an equally valuable resource for all clinicians coming from such fields as primary care practice, neurology, psychiatry, and pulmonary medicine.

Alon Y. Avidan, MD, MPH
Phyllis C. Zee, MD, PhD

Acknowledgments

We are fortunate to have key authors who are not only experts in their respective fields, but who have shared their wealth of knowledge and clinical experience in this book. We would like to thank all the authors for their outstanding contributions and bringing this project to a successful completion. We would like to dedicate this handbook to our teacher, **Dr. Michael S. Aldrich,** who founded the University of Michigan Sleep Disorders Center. Until his untimely death in July 2000, Dr. Aldrich was a pioneer neurologist in sleep medicine. Many of the contributors to this book have been privileged to meet and work with him in the past and remember him as a consummate mentor. Dr. Aldrich was the most influential educator in the field of sleep medicine, and his contributions and philosophy continue to inspire us.

Alon Y. Avidan, MD, MPH
Phyllis C. Zee, MD, PhD

Abbreviations

ACE	angiotensin-converting enzyme
AD	Alzheimer disease
ADHD	attention deficit–hyperactivity disorder
AED	antiepileptic drug
AHI	apnea–hypopnea index
ASPT	advanced sleep phase type
BiPAP	bilevel positive airway pressure
BMI	body mass index
BP	blood pressure
BzRA	benzodiazepine receptor agonists
CBT	cognitive behavior therapy
CHF	congestive heart failure
CNS	central nervous system
CO_2	carbon dioxide
COPD	chronic obstructive pulmonary disease
CPAP	continuous positive airway pressure
CRP	C-reactive protein
CRSD	circadian rhythm sleep disorders
CSF	cerebrospinal fluid
DSPT	delayed sleep phase type
ECG	electrocardiogram (electrocardiography)
EDS	excessive daytime sleepiness
EEG	electroencephalogram (electroencephalography)
EKG	electrokardiogram (or electrocardiogram or ECG)
EMG	electromyogram (electromyography)
EOG	electrooculogram (electrooculography)
ESRD	end-stage renal disease
FDA	Food and Drug Administration
FEV_1	forced expiratory volume over 1 second
FVC	forced vital capacity
GABA	gamma-aminobutyric acid
GERD	gastroesophageal reflux disease
GHB	gamma hydroxybutyric acid
GI	gastrointestinal
H_2O	water
HLA	human leukocyte antigen
HTN	hypertension
IRLSSG	International Restless Legs Syndrome Study Group
ICSD	International Classification of Sleep Disorders
ICSD-2	International Classification of Sleep Disorders, Second Edition

LAUP	laser-assisted uvulopalatoplasty
MS	multiple sclerosis
MSA	multiple system atrophy
MSLT	multiple sleep latency test
MVA	motor vehicle accident
MWT	maintenance of wakefulness test
NPD	nocturnal paroxysmal dystonia
NREM	nonrapid eye movement
OSA	obstructive sleep apnea
OSAHS	obstructive sleep apnea hypopnea syndrome
PEF	peak expiratory flow
PLMD	periodic limb movement disorder
PSG	polysomnogram/polysomnography
RBD	rapid eye movement behavior disorder
REM	rapid eye movement
RIP	respiratory inductive plethysmography
RLS	restless legs syndrome
RMD	rhythmic movement disorder
SaO_2	arterial oxyhemoglobin saturation
SCN	suprachiasmatic nuclei
SDB	sleep disordered breathing
SIDS	sudden infant death syndrome
SOREMP	sleep-onset rapid eye movement period
SpO_2	percutaneous saturation of oxygen
SSRI	selective serotonin reuptake inhibitor
SSS	Stanford Sleepiness Scale
TCA	tricyclic antidepressant
TST	total sleep time
UARS	upper airway resistance syndrome
UPPP	uvulopalatopharyngoplasty

Populations at Risk for Sleep Disturbances

Phyllis C. Zee and Alon Y. Avidan

Sleep disorders are common in the general population, but certain populations such as older adults, women, and patients with comorbid medical, psychiatric, and neurologic disorders are at increased risk. In this chapter, we highlight the need to identify sleep disorders in these populations and provide examples of some of the more common medical and neurologic disorders that are often associated with sleep disturbances. The association between insomnia and psychiatric disorders is covered in the chapter on insomnia (See Chapter 3).

OLDER ADULTS

The geriatric patient population is growing very fast in the United States and around the world. In the year 2000, 34 million individuals in the United States were older than 65 years. By the year 2025, this number is expected to go up to 62 million.[1] In light of this fact, geriatricians and other health care providers need to manage an increased number of conditions that increase with aging. Sleep-disordered breathing is one such condition. Elderly patients experience increased sleep fragmentation, decreased sleep efficiency, reduced quality of sleep, and decreased stages 3 and 4.[2] These changes may be related to the underlying age-related neuronal loss, as well as to a disruption of the suprachiasmatic circadian generator.

WOMEN

Complaints of sleep disturbance are more prevalent among women than men across the entire life span.[3,4] Alterations in the hormonal environment during the various phases of a woman's life, from menstruation[5] and pregnancy[6] to menopause,[7] likely contribute to insomnia in women.

Among women, there is a sharp rise of approximately 40% in the prevalence of insomnia during the period of transition to menopause and after menopause.[7,8] Although it is quite clear that sleep quality is decreased with menopause, less is known about the underlying pathophysiology of insomnia in this population. In addition to hormonal changes, hot flushes, depression, anxiety, and sleep disorders such as primary insomnia, restless legs, and sleep apnea have been proposed as causes of sleep disturbance during menopause.[3,9]

The importance of sleep-disordered breathing as an etiology of poor sleep quality in postmenopausal women is now well documented.[10–12] A recent analysis of the Wisconsin Sleep Cohort Study showed that menopause was an independent risk factor for sleep apnea–hypopnea.[12] Consideration of the many potential causes and treatments of sleep disruption provides an excellent opportunity to improve health and quality of life in this population, which is at high risk for insomnia.

SLEEP AND MEDICAL DISORDERS

Sleep disorders are often comorbid with medical conditions and negatively affect health, mood, and quality of life. Increasing evidence points to a bidirectional relationship between sleep and health, so that sleep disturbances contribute to the development or increase in severity of various medical disorders, and these same disorders result in poor sleep quality.[13,14] Patients with chronic pain (arthritis, fibromyalgia), gastrointestinal (GI) disorders (gastroesophageal reflux disease [GERD]), cardiovascular disorders (coronary heart disease, congestive heart failure [CHF], hypertension), pulmonary disorders (chronic obstructive pulmonary disease [COPD], asthma) and metabolic disorders (obesity, diabetes) are at increased risk for disturbed sleep.[15,16] Furthermore, many of the medications used to treat these conditions can also cause insomnia or daytime sleepiness.

Cardiovascular Disease

Sleep disturbance, especially chronic partial sleep loss, has been linked to problems of the cardiovascular system, including heart attack, irregular heartbeat, and stroke. Several epidemiologic surveys show a strong association between sleep complaints or shortened sleep durations and cardiovascular disease.[17–19] One study of Japanese workers found that individuals who slept for <5 hours a night had a threefold increased risk of heart attacks.[20]

Patients with coronary heart disease have more complaints of disturbed sleep than those without coronary heart disease.[21–23] Sleep-disordered breathing has been shown to increase the risk of cardiovascular disease and stroke.[24,25] Sleep-disordered breathing is associated with a wide spectrum of cardiovascular disorders, most notably, hypertension,[26] CHF, and coronary heart disease. There is some evidence to indicate that the increased vascular risk may be related to inflammation. For example, C-reactive protein (CRP) increases under both total and chronic partial sleep deprivation conditions,[27] and its level has been found to be elevated in patients with obstructive sleep apnea (OSA).[28]

Sleep disturbances are also common in patients with CHF.[16] Sleep complaints include difficulty falling asleep, as well as frequent nocturnal arousals, often associated with nocturnal dyspnea. Patients with CHF have a high prevalence of sleep-disordered breathing of the obstructive and central types.[29] It has long been recognized that Cheyne-Stokes respiration (central sleep apneas) is a common cause of nocturnal dyspnea in CHF.[30] Therefore, optimizing the treatment of CHF and sleep-disordered breathing can improve sleep in patients with CHF.[23]

Metabolic Disorders

Sleep disturbances are common among individuals with diabetes. When compared to patients without diabetes, those with diabetes reported higher rates of insomnia and excessive daytime sleepiness.[31,32] As much as 71% of this population report poor sleep quality.[33] A number of factors contribute to sleep complaints in patients with diabetes. It has also been postulated that in patients with type 1 diabetes, rapid changes in glucose levels during sleep cause awakenings and complaints of insomnia.[34] For individuals with type 2 diabetes, sleep disturbances may be related to obesity and obesity-related sleep disorders such as OSA.[35] Sleep-disordered breathing correlates highly with obesity in the population with diabetes.[35] However, independent of obesity, OSA is associated with impaired glucose tolerance, insulin resistance, and hypertension.[35–37] In addition, there is a correlation between the severity of sleep apnea and of impaired glucose metabolism, insulin resistance, and diabetes.[37,38]

Other common sources of disturbed sleep in diabetics include chronic discomfort or pain associated with diabetic peripheral neuropathy and restless legs syndrome (RLS).[39] Chronic pain, restless legs, and periodic limb movements (PLMs) can cause or exacerbate complaints of difficulty falling asleep and staying asleep.[40] A thorough assessment of sleep quality and treatment of specific sleep disorders, such as sleep apnea and restless legs, can improve the management of metabolic disorders.

Respiratory Disorders

Sleep quality is often poor in patients with COPD.[41] Impairment of pulmonary function is associated with decreased total sleep time and efficiency.[42] Sleep can have significant negative effects on respiration in patients with respiratory compromise, resulting in hypoxemia and hypercapnia,[43] which in turn can disturb sleep. Chronic dyspnea and sleep-related hypoxemia likely contribute to the disturbed sleep of patients with COPD. Therefore, therapies such as bronchodilators and nocturnal oxygen supplementation may also improve sleep quality.[29,43] In addition to lowered pulmonary function and nocturnal oxygen, OSA and other sleep disorders such as insomnia and RLS are common in older patients with COPD and likely contribute to the higher prevalence of sleep complaints in this population.[41]

Adults with asthma have more complaints of restless sleep and sleepiness than those without asthma.[44,45] Sleep can be disrupted by asthma attacks, which occur more frequently in the second half of the night, during rapid eye movement (REM) sleep.[45,46] The presence of OSA and gastroesophageal reflux should also be considered in patients with nocturnal worsening of asthma.[29] Therefore, all patients with asthma should be asked about their sleep quality and examined for symptoms of OSA, which can further disrupt sleep and cause hypoxemia during sleep.

Gastrointestinal Disorders

Patients with GI disorders have a higher prevalence of sleep disorders as compared to the general population.[47] GERD, gastritis, and peptic ulcer disease can contribute to or are associated with increased incidences of insomnia, OSA, and RLS.[48] These nocturnal symptoms are associated with decreased quality of life.[49] Furthermore, there is an association between OSA, excessive sleepiness, or insomnia and GERD, so that the odds of having GERD increase with any of these three conditions.[50] Gastric acid secretion exhibits circadian periodicity, with an increase in basal acid output in the late evening hours and decrease in the morning hours.[51] This, together with the physiologic changes associated with the sleep state, including the supine posture, mechanical effects of the abdomen, reduced arousal threshold, and delayed acid clearance by the esophagus, promotes an increase in the likelihood of acid reflux at night.[52] Seventy-four percent of individuals with chronic GERD report nocturnal heartburn,[49] which may disrupt nocturnal sleep and exacerbate bronchial asthma.[53] The occurrence of sleep-related disorders such as OSA, which is associated with the generation of negative intrathoracic pressure, may also increase acid reflux at night.[54]

Sleep complaints are also common among patients with functional dyspepsia and irritable bowel syndrome. Reported sleep disturbances include waking up repeatedly during the night and feeling tired or not adequately rested in the morning.[55] There is also evidence that in these patients, poor sleep quality may increase the severity of GI symptoms.[56,57] Therefore, treatment of sleep complaints may lead to improved management of GI disorder and vice versa.

Renal Disease

Patients with renal disease frequently complain of insomnia and excessive daytime sleepiness.[58] The etiology of sleep disturbance is often multifactorial, and may shift over time. Metabolic factors, such as uremia and mood disorders, and specific sleep disorders, such as pain, RLS, PLMs, and sleep-disordered breathing, can all contribute to poor sleep quality in this population.[59] Data indicate a higher prevalence of RLS and PLM disorder in patients with renal disease.[60] RLS is commonly seen in patients with renal insufficiency and in association with dialysis, resulting in fatigue and excessive sleepiness.[61,62] Sleep apnea is also common in patients with end-stage renal disease (ESRD), with a reported prevalence that is ten times greater than in that of the general population.[23] Therefore, it is important to recognize the impact of poor sleep quality and daytime sleepiness and the need to treat pain, depression, and specific sleep disorders, such as sleep apnea and RLS, in these patients.

SLEEP AND NEUROLOGIC DISORDERS

Epilepsy

Sleep and epilepsy have a reciprocal relationship. Sleep can affect the distribution and frequency of epileptiform discharges in humans, whereas epileptic discharges can affect sleep regulation and provoke sleep disruption. Patients with epilepsy frequently complain of symptoms such as hypersomnia, insomnia, and even greater breakthrough seizures referable to disturbed sleep. These symptoms commonly indicate an underlying sleep disorder rather than the effect of epilepsy or medication on sleep. Clinicians must be able to identify and differentiate between potential sleep disorders and sleep dysfunction related to epilepsy, and direct therapy to improve the patient's symptoms.[63] Sleep deprivation has been noted to increase interictal discharges in patients with generalized epilepsy.[64] The sleep state can promote interictal activity in as many as one third of patients with epilepsy and in up to 90% of patients with sleep state–dependent epilepsy.[63,65] Up to one third of patients with medically refractory epilepsy had evidence of OSA[66]. Treatment of OSA may reduce seizure frequency.[67,68]

Nocturnal seizures and certain types of parasomnias can have similar clinical symptoms and can become a diagnostic dilemma. The most common sleep disorders that are often confused with epilepsy include cataplexy, sleep attacks in the setting of narcolepsy, night terrors, and REM-sleep behavior disorder (RBD).[69] Some epilepsy syndromes such as benign rolandic and nocturnal frontal lobe epilepsies occur predominantly or exclusively during sleep. Hypersomnolence during the day is suggestive of an underlying sleep disorder, but frequent nocturnal seizures will also disrupt sleep and result in similar symptoms, making the distinction between sleep and seizure disorders somewhat more challenging.

Antiepileptic drugs (AEDs) also affect sleep architecture.[70] Phenytoin increases the extent of non-REM sleep, decreases sleep efficiency, and reduces sleep latency.[71] Carbamazepine increases the number of sleep-stage shifts and decreases REM sleep.[72] Benzodiazepines decrease sleep latency and reduce slow wave sleep (SWS).[70,73] Gabapentin has been shown to improve sleep efficiency and SWS and increase REM sleep.[52,74] In clinical practice, understanding the unique effects of these AEDs may offer the clinician an opportunity to improve sleep and wakefulness; medications that improve sleep disorders may require tailored dosing schedules to maximize their benefit.[63]

Multiple Sclerosis

Sleep disturbance in multiple sclerosis (MS) is common but poorly recognized, and almost half of all patients demonstrate sleep disturbances due to leg spasms, pain, immobility, nocturia, or medication.[75–77] Common sleep disorders in patients with MS include insomnia, RLS, narcolepsy, and RBD. Sleep disruption in this cohort may result in hypersomnolence, increased fatigue, and lowered pain threshold. An increased clinical awareness of sleep-related problems is therefore warranted in this patient population because these problems are extremely common and have the potential to negatively impact the overall health and quality of life.[78–83]

Dementia

Sleep disturbances are very common in patients with dementia and can cause hypersomnolence, irritability, impaired motor and cognitive skills, depression, and fatigue.[84] The underlying pathophysiologic mechanisms of sleep disturbances in patients with neurodegenerative disorders may involve direct structural alteration of the sleep-wake–generating neurons located in the suprachiasmatic nucleus or may involve external mechanisms such as insufficient light exposure.

In the early part of their disease course, patients with Alzheimer disease (AD) commonly present with disruption in sleep–wake rhythmicity, experience increased amounts and frequency of nighttime wakefulness, and have a reduction in SWS. Later on, they present with a more dramatic reduction of REM sleep, increased REM sleep latency, and alteration of the circadian rhythm, resulting in hypersomnolence.[84] In fact, sleep and cognitive dysfunction are positively correlated in AD. Patients with AD are also susceptible to "sundowning," which is described as the nocturnal exacerbation of disruptive behavior or agitation in older individuals.[85] It is frequently encountered in dementia and remains a frequent cause of institutionalization in patients with AD.

Sleep disorders are encountered in most patients with idiopathic Parkinson disease (PD), adversely affecting their quality of life.[86] As with patients with AD, the sleep problems in patients with PD also correlate with increased severity of disease. Patients with PD may experience a number of sleep disorders including insomnia, parasomnia, and daytime somnolence (including excessive daytime sleepiness and sleep attacks).[84] Excessive nocturia can disturb sleep, particularly in the severe disease group, and may be related to the natural evolution of dysautonomia in PD.[87] Parasomnias and, in particular, RBD are common in PD. Recent findings from various studies suggest the following: (i) A high percentage of patients with PD without sleep complaints may have subclinical or clinical RBD and (ii) RBD can be the heralding manifestation of PD for many years in older male patients.[88–94] In addition to its high prevalence in patients with PD, RBD is a common sleep disturbance in other neurodegenerative disorders such as multiple system atrophy (MSA) and dementia with Lewy bodies.[94–96] In a large study involving patients with MSA, RBD was diagnosed by polysomnographic (PSG) monitoring in 90% of patients; dream-enacting behaviors were reported in 69% and RBD preceded the clinical presentation of MSA in 44%.[95]

CHRONIC PAIN AND FIBROMYALGIA

Sleep and pain, the two important vital functions, interact in complex ways that ultimately impact the biologic and behavioral capacity of the individual.[97] PSG studies of patients experiencing acute pain during postoperative recovery demonstrate shortened and fragmented sleep with reduced amounts of SWS and REM sleep, and the recovery is accompanied by normalization of sleep.[97] Chronic pain conditions such as arthritis and fibromyalgia frequently coexist with insomnia. One study found that 25% of adults report that chronic pain disrupts their sleep for at least ten nights per month.[98] Chronic pain produces a vicious cycle of inactivity and fatigue during the day and sleeplessness at night. Patients with chronic pain disorders, including fibromyalgia, report significantly more sleepiness, more fatigue, and less-refreshing sleep.[99,100] Therefore, patients with chronic pain are a population at high risk for sleep disturbances. Adequate management of chronic pain requires treatment of the pain itself and of associated mood disorders, medications that can cause daytime sedation, and correction of underlying sleep disorders and poor sleep habits.

CONCLUSION

Sleep disturbances are common in the general population, but older adults, women, and individuals with comorbid medical, neurologic, and psychiatric conditions are at particular risk. For sleep disturbances that are comorbid with other conditions, treatment of the comorbid condition is always essential, but the accompanying sleep disorders must also be treated. Consequently, it is important for health care professionals to identify sleep disturbances in their patients with comorbid medical, neurologic, and psychiatric disorders. Because the etiology of poor sleep quality is often multifactorial and may shift over time, a careful evaluation for insomnia, sleep-disordered breathing, and RLS should be an integral part of the routine care of all patients.

REFERENCES

1. Census. *Population project program.* In: U.S.B.O.T., ed. Washington, DC; 2000.
2. Avidan AY. Sleep changes and disorders in the elderly patient. *Curr Neurol Neurosci Rep.* 2002;2(2):178–185.
3. Moline M, Broch L, Zak R. Sleep problems across the life cycle in women. *Curr Treat Options Neurol.* 2004;6(4):319–330.
4. Mauri M. Sleep and the reproductive cycle: A review. *Health Care Women Int.* 1990;11(4):409–421.
5. Manber R, Bootzin RR. Sleep and the menstrual cycle. *Health Psychol.* 1997;16(3):209–214.
6. Mindell JA, Jacobson BJ. Sleep disturbances during pregnancy. *J Obstet Gynecol Neonatal Nurs.* 2000;29(6):590–597.
7. Owens JF, Matthews KA. Sleep disturbance in healthy middle-aged women. *Maturitas.* 1998;30(1):41–50.
8. Bjorkelund C, Bengtsson C, Lissner L, et al. Women's sleep: Longitudinal changes and secular trends in a 24-year perspective. Results of the population study of women in Gothenburg, Sweden. *Sleep.* 2002;25(8):894–896.
9. Woodward S, Freedman RR. The thermoregulatory effects of menopausal hot flashes on sleep. *Sleep.* 1994;17(6):497–501.
10. Bixler EO, Vgontzas AN, Lin HM, et al. Prevalence of sleep-disordered breathing in women: Effects of gender. *Am J Respir Crit Care Med.* 2001;163(3 Pt 1):608–613.
11. Guilleminault C, Quera-Salva MA, Partinen M, et al. Women and the obstructive sleep apnea syndrome. *Chest.* 1988;93(1):104–109.
12. Young T, Finn L, Austin D, et al. Menopausal status and sleep-disordered breathing in the Wisconsin Sleep Cohort Study. *Am J Respir Crit Care Med.* 2003;167(9):1181–1185.
13. Boggild H, Knutsson A. Shift work, risk factors and cardiovascular disease. *Scand J Work Environ Health.* 1999;25(2):85–99.
14. Karlsson B, Knutsson A, Lindahl B. Is there an association between shift work and having a metabolic syndrome? Results from a population based study of 27,485 people. *Occup Environ Med.* 2001;58(11):747–752.
15. Klink ME, Quan SF, Kaltenborn WT, et al. Risk factors associated with complaints of insomnia in a general adult population. Influence of previous complaints of insomnia. *Arch Intern Med.* 1992;152(8):1634–1637.

16. Katz DA, McHorney CA. Clinical correlates of insomnia in patients with chronic illness. *Arch Intern Med*. 1998;158(10): 1099–1107.

17. Kripke DF, Garfinkel L, Wingard DL, et al. Mortality associated with sleep duration and insomnia. *Arch Gen Psychiatry*. 2002;59(2):131–136.

18. Newman AB, Spiekerman CF, Enright P, et al. Daytime sleepiness predicts mortality and cardiovascular disease in older adults. The Cardiovascular Health Study Research Group. *J Am Geriatr Soc*. 2000;48(2):115–123.

19. Schwartz SW, Cornoni-Huntley J, Cole SR, et al. Are sleep complaints an independent risk factor for myocardial infarction? *Ann Epidemiol*. 1998;8(6):384–392.

20. Liu Y, Tanaka H. Overtime work, insufficient sleep, and risk of non-fatal acute myocardial infarction in Japanese men. *Occup Environ Med*. 2002;59(7):447–451.

21. Schwartz S, McDowell Anderson W, Cole SR, et al. Insomnia and heart disease: A review of epidemiologic studies. *J Psychosom Res*. 1999;47(4):313–333.

22. Lukkarinen H, Hentinen M. Assessment of quality of life with the Nottingham Health Profile among patients with coronary heart disease. *J Adv Nurs*. 1997;26(1):73–84.

23. Hanly P, Zuberi-Khokhar N. Daytime sleepiness in patients with congestive heart failure and Cheyne-Stokes respiration. *Chest*. 1995;107(4):952–958.

24. Peppard PE, Young T, Palta M, et al. Prospective study of the association between sleep-disordered breathing and hypertension. *N Engl J Med*. 2000;342(19):1378–1384.

25. Shahar E, Whitney CW, Redline S, et al. Sleep-disordered breathing and cardiovascular disease: Cross-sectional results of the Sleep Heart Health Study. *Am J Respir Crit Care Med*. 2001;163(1):19–25.

26. Hamilton GS, Solin P, Naughton MT. Obstructive sleep apnoea and cardiovascular disease. *Intern Med J*. 2004;34(7):420–426.

27. Meier-Ewert HK, Ridker PM, Rifai N, et al. Effect of sleep loss on C-reactive protein, an inflammatory marker of cardiovascular risk. *J Am Coll Cardiol*. 2004;43(4):678–683.

28. Shamsuzzaman AS, Winnicki M, Lanfranchi P, et al. Elevated C-reactive protein in patients with obstructive sleep apnea. *Circulation*. 2002;105(21):2462–2464.

29. Ballard RD. Sleep and medical disorders. *Prim Care*. 2005;32(2):511–533.

30. Harrison W Jr, King C, Calhoun J, et al. Congestive heart failure: Cheyne Stokes respiration as the cause of paroxysmal dyspnea at the onset of sleep. *Arch Intern Med*. 1934;53:891.

31. Foley D, Ancoli-Israel S, Britz P, et al. Sleep disturbances and chronic disease in older adults: Results of the 2003 National Sleep Foundation Sleep in America Survey. *J Psychosom Res*. 2004;56(5):497–502.

32. Skomro RP, Ludwig S, Salamon E, et al. Sleep complaints and restless legs syndrome in adult type 2 diabetics. *Sleep Med*. 2001;2(5):417–422.

33. Vigg A. Sleep in Type 2 diabetes. *J Assoc Physicians India*. 2003;51:479–481.

34. Pillar G, Schuscheim G, Weiss R, et al. Interactions between hypoglycemia and sleep architecture in children with type 1 diabetes mellitus. *J Pediatr.* 2003;142(2):163–168.
35. Resnick HE, Redline S, Shahar E, et al. Diabetes and sleep disturbances: Findings from the Sleep Heart Health Study. *Diabetes Care.* 2003;26(3):702–709.
36. Chasens ER, Weaver TE, Umlauf MG. Insulin resistance and obstructive sleep apnea: Is increased sympathetic stimulation the link? *Biol Res Nurs.* 2003;5(2):87–96.
37. Punjabi NM, Shahar E, Redline S, et al. Sleep-disordered breathing, glucose intolerance, and insulin resistance: The Sleep Heart Health Study. *Am J Epidemiol.* 2004;160(6): 521–530.
38. Punjabi NM, Sorkin JD, Katzel LI, et al. Sleep-disordered breathing and insulin resistance in middle-aged and overweight men. *Am J Respir Crit Care Med.* 2002;165(5):677–682.
39. Walters AS, Hickey K, Maltzman J, et al. A questionnaire study of 138 patients with restless legs syndrome: The 'Night-Walkers' survey. *Neurology.* 1996;46(1):92–95.
40. Zucconi M, Ferini-Strambi L. Epidemiology and clinical findings of restless legs syndrome. *Sleep Med.* 2004;5(3):293–299.
41. Quan SF, Zee P. Evaluating the effects of medical disorders on sleep in the older patient. *Geriatrics.* 2004;59(3):37–42, quiz 45.
42. Sanders MH, Newman AB, Haggerty CL, et al. Sleep and sleep-disordered breathing in adults with predominantly mild obstructive airway disease. *Am J Respir Crit Care Med.* 2003;167(1):7–14.
43. Mohsenin V. Sleep in chronic obstructive pulmonary disease. *Semin Respir Crit Care Med.* 2005;26(1):109–116.
44. Enright PL, McClelland RL, Newman AB, et al. Underdiagnosis and undertreatment of asthma in the elderly. Cardiovascular Health Study Research Group. *Chest.* 1999;116(3):603–613.
45. Montplaisir J, Walsh J, Malo JL. Nocturnal asthma: Features of attacks, sleep and breathing patterns. *Am Rev Respir Dis.* 1982;125(1):18–22.
46. Catterall JR, Douglas NJ, Calverley PM, et al. Irregular breathing and hypoxaemia during sleep in chronic stable asthma. *Lancet.* 1982;1(8267):301–304.
47. Vege SS, Locke GR, 3rd, Weaver AL, et al. Functional gastrointestinal disorders among people with sleep disturbances: A population-based study. *Mayo Clin Proc.* 2004;79(12): 1501–1506.
48. Fass R, Quan SF, Zong A, et al. Risk factors for Nocturnal Heartburn (NH)—The Sleep Heart Health Study experience. *Gastroenterology.* 2002;122(Supp 1):T1133.
49. Farup C, Kleinman L, Sloan S, et al. The impact of nocturnal symptoms associated with gastroesophageal reflux disease on health-related quality of life. *Arch Intern Med.* 2001;161(1): 45–52.
50. Fass R, Quan SF, O'Connor GT, et al. Predictors of heartburn during sleep in a large prospective cohort study. *Chest.* 2005;127(5):1658–1666.
51. Moore JG. Circadian dynamics of gastric acid secretion and pharmacodynamics of H2 receptor blockade. *Ann N Y Acad Sci.* 1991;618:150–158.

52. Foldvary-Schaefer N, De Leon Sanchez I, Karafa M, et al. Gabapentin increases slow-wave sleep in normal adults. *Epilepsia*. 2002;43(12):1493–1497.

53. Sontag SJ, O'Connell S, Miller TQ, et al. Asthmatics have more nocturnal gasping and reflux symptoms than nonasthmatics, and they are related to bedtime eating. *Am J Gastroenterol*. 2004;99(5):789–796.

54. Graf KI, Karaus M, Heinemann S, et al. Gastroesophageal reflux in patients with sleep apnea syndrome. *Z Gastroenterol*. 1995;33(12):689–693.

55. Fass R, Fullerton S, Tung S, et al. Sleep disturbances in clinic patients with functional bowel disorders. *Am J Gastroenterol*. 2000;95(5):1195–2000.

56. Jarrett M, Heitkemper M, Cain KC, et al. Sleep disturbance influences gastrointestinal symptoms in women with irritable bowel syndrome. *Dig Dis Sci*. 2000;45(5):952–959.

57. Goldsmith G, Levin JS. Effect of sleep quality on symptoms of irritable bowel syndrome. *Dig Dis Sci*. 1993;38(10):1809–1814.

58. Iliescu EA, Coo H, McMurray MH, et al. Quality of sleep and health-related quality of life in haemodialysis patients. *Nephrol Dial Transplant*. 2003;18(1):126–132.

59. Shayamsunder AK, Patel SS, Jain V, et al. Sleepiness, sleeplessness, and pain in end-stage renal disease: Distressing symptoms for patients. *Semin Dial*. 2005;18(2):109–118.

60. Parker KP. Sleep disturbances in dialysis patients. *Sleep Med Rev*. 2003;7(2):131–143.

61. Collado-Seidel V, Kohnen R, Samtleben W, et al. Clinical and biochemical findings in uremic patients with and without restless legs syndrome. *Am J Kidney Dis*. 1998;31(2):324–328.

62. Roger SD, Harris DC, Stewart JH. Possible relation between restless legs and anaemia in renal dialysis patients. *Lancet*. 1991;337(8756):1551.

63. Vaughn BV, D'Cruz OF. Sleep and epilepsy. *Semin Neurol*. 2004;24(3):301–313.

64. Degen R, Degen HE. Sleep and sleep deprivation in epileptology. *Epilepsy Res Suppl*. 1991;2:235–260.

65. Dinner DS. Effect of sleep on epilepsy. *J Clin Neurophysiol*. 2002;19(6):504–513.

66. Malow BA, Bowes RJ, Lin X. Predictors of sleepiness in epilepsy patients. *Sleep*. 1997;20(12):1105–1110.

67. Vaughn BV, D'Cruz OF, Beach R, et al. Improvement of epileptic seizure control with treatment of obstructive sleep apnoea. *Seizure*. 1996;5(1):73–78.

68. Devinsky O, Ehrenberg B, Barthlen GM, et al. Epilepsy and sleep apnea syndrome. *Neurology*. 1994;44(11):2060–2064.

69. Bazil CW. Nocturnal seizures. *Semin Neurol*. 2004;24(3):293–300.

70. Sammaritano M, Sherwin A. Effect of anticonvulsants on sleep. *Neurology*. 2000;54(5 Suppl 1):S16–S24.

71. Wolf P, Roder-Wanner UU, Brede M. Influence of therapeutic phenobarbital and phenytoin medication on the polygraphic sleep of patients with epilepsy. *Epilepsia*. 1984;25(4):467–475.

72. Gigli GL, Placidi F, Diomedi M, et al. Nocturnal sleep and daytime somnolence in untreated patients with temporal lobe

epilepsy: Changes after treatment with controlled-release carbamazepine. *Epilepsia*. 1997;38(6):696–701.

73. Copinschi G, Van Onderbergen A, L'Hermite-Baleriaux M, et al. Effects of the short-acting benzodiazepine triazolam, taken at bedtime, on circadian and sleep-related hormonal profiles in normal men. *Sleep*. 1990;13(3):232–244.

74. Placidi F, Diomedi M, Scalise A, et al. Effect of anticonvulsants on nocturnal sleep in epilepsy. *Neurology*. 2000;54(5 Suppl 1):S25–S32.

75. Tachibana N, Howard RS, Hirsch NP, et al. Sleep problems in multiple sclerosis. *Eur Neurol*. 1994;34(6):320–323.

76. Auer RN, Rowlands CG, Perry SF, et al. Multiple sclerosis with medullary plaques and fatal sleep apnea (Ondine's curse). *Clin Neuropathol*. 1996;15(2):101–105.

77. Howard RS, Wiles CM, Hirsch NP, et al. Respiratory involvement in multiple sclerosis. *Brain*. 1992;115(Pt 2):479–494.

78. Fleming WE, Pollak CP. Sleep disorders in multiple sclerosis. *Semin Neurol*. 2005;25(1):64–68.

79. Randolph JJ, Arnett PA, Higginson CI, et al. Neurovegetative symptoms in multiple sclerosis: Relationship to depressed mood, fatigue, and physical disability. *Arch Clin Neuropsychol*. 2000;15(5):387–398.

80. Schrader H, Gotlibsen OB, Skomedal GN. Multiple sclerosis and narcolepsy/cataplexy in a monozygotic twin. *Neurology*. 1980;30(1):105–108.

81. Kato T, Kanbayashi T, Yamamoto K, et al. Hypersomnia and low CSF hypocretin-1 (orexin-A) concentration in a patient with multiple sclerosis showing bilateral hypothalamic lesions. *Intern Med*. 2003;42(8):743–745.

82. Rammohan KW, Rosenberg JH, Lynn DJ, et al. Efficacy and safety of modafinil (Provigil) for the treatment of fatigue in multiple sclerosis: A two centre phase 2 study. *J Neurol Neurosurg Psychiatry*. 2002;72(2):179–183.

83. Scammell TE, Estabrooke IV, McCarthy MT, et al. Hypothalamic arousal regions are activated during modafinil-induced wakefulness. *J Neurosci*. 2000;20(22):8620–8628.

84. Bhatt MH, Podder N, Chokroverty S. Sleep and neurodegenerative diseases. *Semin Neurol*. 2005;25(1):39–51.

85. Taylor JL, Friedman L, Sheikh J, et al. Assessment and management of "Sundowning" phenomena. *Semin Clin Neuropsychiatry*. 1997;2(2):113–122.

86. Partinen M. Sleep disorder related to Parkinson's disease. *J Neurol*. 1997;244(4 Suppl 1):S3–S6.

87. Young A, Home M, Churchward T, et al. Comparison of sleep disturbance in mild versus severe Parkinson's disease. *Sleep*. 2002;25(5):573–577.

88. Wetter TC, Trenkwalder C, Gershanik O, et al. Polysomnographic measures in Parkinson's disease: A comparison between patients with and without REM sleep disturbances. *Wien Klin Wochenschr*. 2001;113(7–8):249–253.

89. Poryazova RG, Zachariev ZI. REM sleep behavior disorder in patients with Parkinson's disease. *Folia Med (Plovdiv)*. 2005;47(1):5–10.

90. Larsen JP, Tandberg E. Sleep disorders in patients with Parkinson's disease: Epidemiology and management. *CNS Drugs*. 2001;15(4):267–275.

91. Gagnon JF, Bedard MA, Fantini ML, et al. REM sleep behavior disorder and REM sleep without atonia in Parkinson's disease. *Neurology*. 2002;59(4):585–589.

92. Boeve BF, Silber MH, Ferman TJ, et al. Association of REM sleep behavior disorder and neurodegenerative disease may reflect an underlying synucleinopathy. *Mov Disord*. 2001;16(4): 622–630.

93. Boeve BF, Silber MH, Ferman TJ. REM sleep behavior disorder in Parkinson's disease and dementia with Lewy bodies. *J Geriatr Psychiatry Neurol*. 2004;17(3):146–157.

94. Abad VC, Guilleminault C. Review of rapid eye movement behavior sleep disorders. *Curr Neurol Neurosci Rep*. 2004;4(2): 157–163.

95. Plazzi G, Corsini R, Provini F, et al. REM sleep behavior disorders in multiple system atrophy. *Neurology*. 1997;48(4): 1094–1097.

96. Iranzo A, Santamaria J, Rye DB, et al. Characteristics of idiopathic REM sleep behavior disorder and that associated with MSA and PD. *Neurology*. 2005;65(2):247–252.

97. Roehrs T, Roth T. Sleep and pain: Interaction of two vital functions. *Semin Neurol*. 2005;25(1):106–116.

98. Lamberg L. Chronic pain linked with poor sleep; exploration of causes and treatment. *JAMA*. 1999;281(8):691–692.

99. Cote KA, Moldofsky H. Sleep, daytime symptoms, and cognitive performance in patients with fibromyalgia. *J Rheumatol*. 1997;24(10):2014–2023.

100. Mahowald ML, Mahowald MW. Nighttime sleep and daytime functioning (sleepiness and fatigue) in less well-defined chronic rheumatic diseases with particular reference to the 'alpha-delta NREM sleep anomaly'. *Sleep Med*. 2000;1(3):195–207.

Sleep-Disordered Breathing

Suzette Sewell-Scheuermann and
Barbara A. Phillips

Sleep-disordered breathing (SDB) is associated with several potentially serious conditions that include the following:

1. Primary snoring
2. Upper airway resistance syndrome (UARS)
3. Obstructive sleep apnea–hypopnea syndrome (OSAHS)
4. Central sleep apnea
5. Asthma
6. Chronic obstructive pulmonary disease (COPD).

Each of these conditions has specific clinical presentations with important implications for diagnosis, treatment, morbidity, and follow-up.

PRIMARY SNORING

Primary snoring (or snoring without sleep apnea) is a complex phenomenon that occurs from an interaction between the various upper airway muscles (i.e., tongue, soft palate, and pharynx) and the airway walls. Snoring is usually an inspiratory sound, but it can also be noted on expiration. It occurs in all stages of sleep, but most frequently during stages 2 to 4. Vibration of these membranous parts of the airway creates a diffuse involvement of the airway that makes successful treatment of snoring difficult.[1]

Clinical Presentation

Patients presenting with snoring are commonly referred to an otolaryngologist usually after complaints from their bed partners about being kept awake by the loud snoring. Unlike subjective complaints of patients with OSAHS, patients with snoring do not suffer from daytime somnolence or sleepiness, insomnia, or sleep disruption.[1] However, the patient who snores may also be asymptomatic and unaware of this problem.

Classification

The second edition of the *International Classification of Sleep Disorders* (ICSD 780.53-1) defines primary snoring as a "respiratory sound generated in the upper airway during sleep that typically occurs during inspiration or expiration."[2]

Epidemiology

The Wisconsin Sleep Cohort Study reports habitual snoring in approximately 24% of adult women and 40% of adult men.[3] Snoring is the most common symptom noted in breathing disorders like OSAHS, although not all patients who snore have obstructive sleep apnea.[4] Snoring may be a precursor to the development of OSAHS, but it is not in itself a predictor of OSAHS.

Snoring occurs more often in men. This male predominance observed in epidemiologic studies remains unexplained. The prevalence of snoring appears to increase with age, although some studies have demonstrated a reduction in snoring in patients older than 60 years.[5,6] Earlier studies on snoring indicate that it may be an independent risk factor for hypertension (HTN)[5]; unfortunately, these studies did not include polysomnography (PSG) and, therefore, may include patients with frank sleep apnea. Whether snoring is a marker for sleep apnea, is a risk factor for cardiovascular and cerebrovascular disease, or results in daytime dysfunction is as yet unknown.[1] Most likely, snoring is a mild form of SDB.

Diagnostic Evaluation

There is no accepted or uniform way of evaluating snoring. When snoring is present along with symptoms of daytime sleepiness and questionable apneas, a diagnostic polysomnogram may be appropriate.

Diagnosis

Snoring is a symptom that must be explored with a review of medical history and the performance of a physical examination to determine the predisposition to sleep apnea, the need for a sleep study, and the need for more information from the patient. Snoring is no longer just considered a "noise." If snoring is causing sleep disturbances including arousals and daytime symptoms such as sleepiness, its underlying pathology should be investigated.[1]

History

Part of the assessment is to determine whether snoring is present and whether it is disrupting the patient's sleep. Table 2-1 outlines helpful hints on collecting a sleep history. Patients seek help for a variety of reasons. Daytime sleepiness is the most common complaint of patients. In some circumstances, it may be that the

Table 2-1. Essential elements of the sleep history for sleep-disordered breathing[1]

1. Obtain the history in the presence of the bed partner because the patient may not be aware of his/her snoring patterns
2. Inquire whether the snoring occurs nightly, in certain sleeping positions, or is associated with breathing pauses or gasping
3. Inquire about the risk factors including obesity, recent weight gain, use of alcohol, seasonal allergies, nasal congestion, and use of tobacco
4. Ask about daytime function; use a standard questionnaire like the Epworth Sleepiness Scale[7] (see Appendix A) to identify daytime somnolence
5. Ask about systemic diseases such as hypothyroidism or acromegaly that may increase the likelihood of snoring; inquire about any previous surgeries or trauma to the upper airways that may affect the airway function and patency

Table 2-2.   Risk factors for primary snoring

- Obesity
- Alcohol consumption before sleep
- Tobacco use
- Sedative tranquilizers or muscle relaxants
- Hypothyroidism and other medical conditions
- Supine position during sleep
- Nasal obstruction and congestion
- Abnormal upper airway anatomy

bed partner is bothered by the snoring and is experiencing sleep difficulties. This is very common.

The focus of treatment is based on whether the patient has daytime symptoms and other features associated with SDB. A thorough history should include a review of risk factors associated with primary snoring. Known risk factors are listed in Table 2-2.

Physical Examination

The presence of *obesity* (body mass index [BMI] $\geq$30 kg per m^2), *increased neck circumference* (>41 cm in women or >43 cm in men), and abnormal airway *anatomy* (i.e., enlarged tonsils and nasal–septal deviation), and the *cardiovascular status* (i.e., pulse rate, blood pressure) should be documented during physical examination. An examination of the oral pharynx is useful for the treatment of snoring if the airway is small or crowded or if inflammation is present.[1] However, a detailed examination using fiber optic nasendoscopy may be helpful in snorers presenting with these symptoms. The Mallampati classification can be very helpful in evaluating airway size (see Fig. 2-1). The classification is a relatively simple grading system that involves a preoperative ability to visualize the tonsillar pillars, soft palate, and the base of the uvula. It was designed as a means of predicting the degree of difficulty in laryngeal exposure.[8] More recently, it has been shown that a high Mallampati score and nasal obstruction are associated risk factors for obstructive sleep apnea.[9]

Differential Diagnosis

The decision to perform further assessments, including laboratory PSG, is based on whether the patient has symptoms of sleepiness or HTN. A patient who presents with simple snoring is usually a healthy individual with no other symptoms and anatomic abnormalities. The patient generally presents at the request of his/her family. When no other symptoms are present, he/she requires no further investigation, and treatment involves weight loss, avoidance of sleep in the supine position (positional therapy), or the use of an oral appliance.

A symptomatic patient presents with snoring and other complaints including:

- Unrefreshing sleep

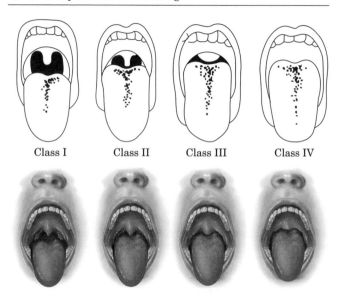

Class I   Class II   Class III   Class IV

Figure 2-1.   The Mallampati classification describes tongue size relative to oropharyngeal size. The test is conducted with the patient in the sitting position, the head held in a neutral position, the mouth wide open and relaxed, and the tongue protruding to the maximum. The subsequent classification is assigned on the basis of pharyngeal structures that are visible. Class I, visualization of the soft palate, fauces, uvula, anterior and posterior pillars; Class II, visualization of the soft palate, fauces, and uvula; Class III, visualization of the soft palate and the base of the uvula; Class IV, soft palate is not visible at all. If the patient phonates, this falsely improves the view. If the patient arches his or her tongue, the uvula is falsely obscured. The test was initially adapted to predict ease of incubation but can be used to predict the potential severity of OSA.[8,9] (From Mallampati SR, Gatt SP, Gugino LD, et al. A clinical sign to predict difficult tracheal intubation: A prospective study. *Can Anaesth Soc J.* 1985;32:429–434. With permission.)

- Excessive daytime sleepiness
- Poor or reduced performance
- Headaches
- Difficulty in concentrating or having attentional deficits.

Further examination of symptoms related to snoring is conducted in two ways: Airway assessment and nocturnal PSG. If the symptomatic patient has an abnormal airway anatomy, he/she may need additional evaluation for possible surgical intervention.

Nocturnal PSG should be considered in the following patients:

- Asymptomatic snorers contemplating a surgical treatment for snoring

- Asymptomatic snorers with known vascular disease, including HTN
- Asymptomatic snorers who may have UARS

UPPER AIRWAY RESISTANCE SYNDROME

UARS is a term used to describe patients with primary snoring who present with daytime symptoms similar to those noted in OSAHS. UARS describes an increase in airway resistance and a reduction in airflow that does not satisfy the criteria for hypopnea or apnea.[10] This syndrome is present if upper airway resistance is documented by a laboratory investigation and is associated with sleep fragmentation and daytime dysfunction. It should be noted that not every individual complaining of snoring has UARS, especially if he/she presents asymptomatically.

Management

There are various treatments for snoring, and these overlap with the treatments for OSAHS. Currently, there is no medication that consistently prevents or treats snoring in all snorers. Nonsurgical and surgical therapies for snoring are listed in Table 2-3. Most of the nonsurgical therapies include modification or elimination of risk factors related to snoring and OSAHS.

- Obesity has been consistently shown to be related to snoring and obstructive apnea.[11] Therefore, a recommendation for weight loss is a common modality in the treatment of snoring and sleep apnea. The extent of weight loss that will reduce

Table 2-3. Recommendations and treatments for snoring

Surgical Treatment for Snoring	Nonsurgical Treatment for Snoring

1. Nasal surgery
  a. Removal of nasal polyps
  b. Correction of nasal-septal deviation
2. Pharyngeal surgery
  a. UPPP
3. Laser surgery
  a. LAUP
4. Other surgical procedures currently examined in clinical trials
  a. Diathermy palatoplasty (similar to LAUP)
  b. Radiofrequency tissue volume reduction
	1. Weight loss
	2. Avoidance of alcohol
	3. Avoidance of sedatives and muscle relaxants
	4. Medications
	5. Nasal decongestants
	6. Anti-inflammatory agents
	7. Nasal lubricants
	8. Smoking cessation
	9. Sleep position modification
	10. Nasal dilators
	11. Oral appliances
	12. Nasal CPAP

UPPP, uvulopalatopharyngoplasty; LAUP, laser-assisted uvulopalatoplasty; CPAP, continuous positive airway pressure.

one's snoring is as yet unknown, but losing as little as 3 kg has been previously noted to be beneficial in reducing sleep apnea and its most common symptom—snoring.[11]

- Avoidance of alcohol, especially immediately before bedtime, may be necessary to treat snoring. Snorers are recommended to avoid drinking alcohol 3 to 5 hours before going to bed.[1]
- Various medications may be helpful, including nasal lubricants, nasal decongestants, and anti-inflammatory drugs such as inhaled steroids, if nasal obstruction or congestion is present. This is especially common with allergic rhinitis and acute episodes of snoring.
- Smoking has been linked to SDB.[1] Smoking cessation is recommended for the treatment of snoring and OSAHS.
- Sleeping in a lateral decubitus or side-lying position is recommended by most sleep experts. Although the result of such recommendations is unknown, techniques such as the sewing of tennis balls to the back of sleepwear or using a wedge-pillow to promote side-lying sleep can be instituted to prevent snoring related to a supine sleep position. (*These therapies are not recommended for the treatment of obstructive sleep apnea or hypopnea with hypoxemia.*)
- Nasal dilators are devices that are used to improve asymptomatic snoring and consist of external and internal devices placed on or in the nares. The external device is an adhesive strip that adheres to the nares and expands the nasal passage. An internal device is inserted into both nares and it splints the nasal passage open with its elastic action.
- Oral appliances are also used to improve asymptomatic snoring. Oral appliances are divided into two categories: Tongue-retaining and mandibular-advancement devices.[1] Oral appliances enlarge the oral airway by preventing the tongue from collapsing into the airway during sleep. Two types of oral appliances exist: Adjustable appliances, which allow the appliance to be titrated or advanced, and nonadjustable appliances, which are fixed.
- Nasal continuous positive airway pressure (CPAP) prevents snoring, but patients with primary snoring show poor adherence to this therapy.[1]

Surgical treatment for snoring includes nasal or pharyngeal surgery including laser and other experimental procedures.[1]

- Nasal and pharyngeal surgeries are commonly used to treat snoring when nonsurgical therapies fail. The reason why surgery is not recommended as a first-line treatment is related to the availability of nonsurgical measures and the uncertainty of the success of surgical procedures.
- Uvulopalatopharyngoplasty (UPPP) and laser-assisted uvulopalatoplasty (LAUP) procedures involve full or partial uvulectomy with reconstructive surgery of the pharynx and/or palate. The best candidates for these types of surgeries are patients with primary snoring who are not obese and have abnormal anatomy including enlarged tonsils, adenoids, and small pharyngeal inlet. Interventions such as UPPP

Table 2-4. Algorithm for approaching patients with snoring

1. Perform history and physical examination; refer for nocturnal polysomnography if risk factors or daytime symptoms exist
2. Perform thorough examination of the upper airways including the oropharynx and nasopharynx and assessment for congestion and anatomic anomalies
3. Consider the use of oral appliances
4. If clinical presentation is positive for risk factors, schedule and conduct polysomnography with follow-up
5. Review the results with the patient and referring physician
6. If moderate to severe OSAHS is present, treat with nasal CPAP
7. Encourage lifestyle modifications if risk factors exist
   a. Manage obesity
   b. Smoking cessation
   c. Refrain from alcoholic beverages for at least 3 h before bedtime
   d. Decrease use of sedatives and muscle relaxants
8. Encourage therapeutic management of comorbid conditions
9. Encourage adherence to CPAP regimen at least 4 h a night
10. Recommend that the patient notify surgeon and anesthesiologist of existing OSAHS
11. Assess for surgical intervention for refractory cases

OSAHS, obstructive sleep apnea–hypopnea syndrome; CPAP, continuous positive airway pressure.

are not generally recommended as first-line therapy for sleep apnea.[12]

Follow-up

The treatment of snoring requires that practitioners adopt a systematic approach on the basis of the risk factors. Frequently, more than one risk factor is present in snorers or the patient snores despite appropriate therapy. Follow-up is needed in these cases to identify ongoing problems. A common approach to treatment includes particular attention to lifestyle changes that are necessary to remove or modify the risk factor. If snoring is a recent occurrence, the patient should be evaluated for allergic rhinitis, nasal congestion, or other paroxysmal medical conditions. If symptoms do not resolve or worsen, then a snorer may need further evaluation in a sleep laboratory. A summary of this approach to treatment is noted in Figure 2-2 and Table 2-4.

OBSTRUCTIVE SLEEP APNEA–HYPOPNEA SYNDROME

Patients with OSAHS have brief episodes of asphyxia during which the oxygen saturation falls while carbon dioxide levels (CO_2) increase.[13] After respiration resumes, the normal oxygen and CO_2 levels are restored through several recovery breaths or "catch-up breaths." These episodes, in addition to symptoms of snoring, may be witnessed by a family member or bed partner. The patients experiencing obstructive sleep apnea may not be aware that they are apneic or may not remember waking up

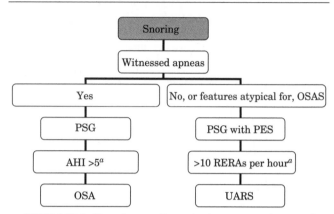

^{a}PSG/Multiple Sleep Latency Test criteria are approximate and should be considered in conjunction with a clinical history.

Figure 2-2. Algorithm for the evaluation of snoring. OSAS, obstructive sleep apnea syndrome; PSG, polysomnogram; PES, esophageal pressure; AHI, apnea–hypopnea index; RERA, respiratory effort-related arousal; OSA, obstructive sleep apnea; UARS, upper airway resistance syndrome.

to resume breathing. SDB conditions, such as obstructive apnea and hypopnea, are characterized by complete or partial obstruction of the pharynx during sleep and may result in arousal because of apnea or airflow interruption, hypoxemia, or a combination of these. This condition can be dangerous and should be investigated and treated promptly.

Clinical Presentation
Patients with OSAHS present with daytime and nocturnal symptoms. Daytime symptoms may include excessive sleepiness, headaches, poor concentration, fatigue, decreased attention, and depression. Nocturnal symptoms include snoring, witnessed apneas, choking episodes, nocturnal dyspnea, restlessness, diaphoresis, nocturia, acid reflux, and drooling.

Classification
Apnea is defined as interruption in airflow for a minimum of 10 seconds with a drop in oxygen saturation.[14] Apnea is also considered when there is a $\geq 70\%$ reduction in airflow along with these criteria. Most experts classify hypopnea as a 30% reduction in airflow for a minimum of 10 seconds with polysomnographic arousal or a reduction in oxygen saturation of at least 4%.[15]

OSAHS is defined as an apnea–hypopnea index (AHI) of at least five apneas plus hypopneas per hour of sleep, together with complaints of persistent daytime sleepiness.[14] Several medical insurance companies require an AHI of 15 or more to provide reimbursement for the patient's treatment using CPAP.

Severity of Apnea–Hypopnea Index

5 to 15 Mild
15 to 50 Moderate
>50 Severe

The severity of OSAHS should not be based on AHI alone. Consideration of the degree of hypoxemia, the level of daytime sleepiness, the degree of sleep fragmentation, and the presence of arrhythmias are also of importance. OSAHS is also associated with daytime drowsiness, which may lead to automobile accidents by the patient because of sleepiness while driving. Patients should be counseled on driving cessation through the course of the treatment of OSAHS.

Epidemiology

OSAHS was first discovered using PSG in obese patients diagnosed with Pickwickian syndrome (obesity-induced hypercarbia).[15] Later research has demonstrated sleep apnea in obese patients without hypercarbia and in nonobese patients. This has led to increased research on OSAHS and SDB. Epidemiologic studies indicate that 2% to 5% of the population meets the criteria for this syndrome.[16] Men are more likely to have sleep apnea than premenopausal women; however, the incidence in women increases after menopause. There may be differences associated with race because African Americans, Asians, and Hispanics seem to be at an increased risk for severe apnea.[17,18]

Diagnostic Evaluation

OSAHS is evaluated using historical data, physical examination, and nocturnal PSG to determine the presence of daytime symptoms, apnea or hypopnea, hypoxemia, arousals, respiratory effort, and any disturbances in sleep architecture.

History

A thorough history requires inquiry into known risk factors associated with OSAHS. Obesity and advancing age (>65 years) are primary risk factors for OSAHS. A list of the risk factors for OSAHS are listed in Table 2-5. The relationship between OSAHS and other medical diseases such as HTN, ischemic heart disease, asthma, arrhythmias, and stroke have been examined. An increase in the number of motor vehicle accidents (MVAs) related to daytime sleepiness has been noted. OSAHS has been linked to the development of these serious repercussions, especially HTN and MVA. All these factors should be evaluated in the initial examination.

Physical Examination

Vital measurements that should be performed in the assessment of OSAHS include the BMI (see Appendix B), calculated using the height and weight (kg per m²), and the neck circumference. Previous research has demonstrated that obesity is a risk factor for OSAHS, which is most likely to be noted in individuals presenting with a BMI >30 kg per m².

A measurement of the neck circumference is made in the upright position at the superior border of the cricothyroid membrane. A neck circumference of ≥17 inches in a man or ≥16

Table 2-5.   Risk factors for obstructive sleep apnea–hypopnea syndrome

- Obesity (BMI >30 kg/m^2)
- Male gender
- Family history of obstructive sleep apnea–hypopnea syndrome
- Consumption of alcohol before bedtime
- Race
- Smoking
- Drugs (growth hormone, β-blockers, testosterone, flurazepam)
- Use of sedatives
- Sleeping in a supine position
- Anatomic upper airway obstruction
- Comorbid medical conditions (coronary heart disease, stroke, endocrinopathies [i.e., hypothyroidism, acromegaly], renal failure, craniofacial anomalies [i.e., achondroplastic dwarfism], arterial hypertension, neuromuscular disorders)

BMI, body mass index.

inches in a woman is a common finding in patients with OSAHS. Research has demonstrated that the neck circumference is linked to the severity of OSAHS.[15] The review of systems should include examination of features suggesting OSAHS. In many patients, the physical examination may be normal, so a normal physical examination cannot exclude sleep apnea.

Nocturnal Polysomnography

Nocturnal PSG is a procedure carried out in a sleep laboratory. The patient having a sleep study is prepared for extensive monitoring before bedtime. Recommendations for the performance of PSG were published in 1997 by the American Sleep Disorders Association Standards of Practice Committee. Nocturnal PSG is indicated for patients who are suspected of having a SDB problem.

PROCEDURE AND ACQUISITION. When the decision is made to evaluate a patient by PSG, he/she is scheduled to return to the laboratory to prepare for the test at least 2 to 3 hours before bedtime.

PSG is used to confirm the diagnosis of OSAHS and its severity. The quality of the polygraphs depends on the techniques employed. A more thorough discussion about the standardization of techniques during PSG and sleep scoring is available in the *Manual of Standardized Terminology, Techniques, and Scoring System for Sleep Stages of Human Subjects*[19] and is discussed in Appendix C.

POLYSOMNOGRAPHIC FEATURES OF OBSTRUCTIVE APNEA. Obstructive apnea or hypopnea is noted on the polygraph when airflow is reduced or absent, but obvious chest or abdominal motion is detected, indicating an attempt by the patient to breathe. An example of these features in obstructive apnea is noted in Figure 2-3. Hypoxemia is demonstrated by a reduction in

SpO_2 (oxygen saturation as measured by pulse oximetry) during episodes of apnea or hypopnea. In this example, hypoxemia was exhibited by a 4% reduction in saturation during episodes of apnea.

Differential Diagnosis

Apnea during sleep can result from an obstruction of the upper pharynx and/or a loss of ventilatory effort. The latter condition is known as *central sleep apnea*, which is characterized by frequent episodes of decreased airflow in the absence of respiratory effort. This form of apnea is different from that associated with OSAHS. Obstructive sleep apnea is associated with obvious ventilatory effort that occurs during apnea or hypopnea. Both conditions are assessed during PSG. Most patients with apnea are usually found to have both obstructive apnea and central apnea; central apnea is seldom seen in isolation. Central apnea occurs with congestive heart failure (CHF) and/or respiratory depression.

Management

Regardless of how severe the patient's condition is, treatment should address coexisting medical and lifestyle issues that are known to increase the risk of complications associated with OSAHS. Consultation with the patient should address obesity, sleep deprivation, and the use of tobacco, alcohol, narcotics, and anesthetics. Other therapies used in the management of snoring may also be considered. If moderate to severe OSAHS exists, then nasal CPAP should be initiated.

CPAP is a noninvasive procedure that maintains the airway patency during sleep. It is now the established treatment for OSAHS. Nasal CPAP has been documented to be effective in eliminating both central and obstructive apneas. Humidifiers can be used to improve compliance and comfort. The level of pressure required by most patients is 8 to 12 cm H_2O. Although CPAP can be "titrated" in a sleep laboratory, autotitrating or "smart" CPAP machines appear to be at least as effective as in-laboratory–titrated CPAP and can save time and money.[20,21] The most common reasons cited for poor compliance with CPAP are claustrophobia, problems with the mask, and noise created by the equipment (see Appendix D).

Follow-up

It is important that the correct CPAP level be used to prevent apneas and respiratory effort-related arousals (RERAs). RERAs, the most recently described events in the spectrum of SDB, generally refers to a reduction of airflow, culminating in electroencephalogram (EEG) arousal but not meeting the criteria for apnea or hypopnea.[22]

Most patients with OSAHS are treated effectively with 9 to 11 cm H_2O of CPAP. When adequate CPAP is achieved, sleep is no longer fragmented and apneas are prevented. Most equipments also provide a method for assessment of CPAP adherence by the patient. One particular model provides a printout of compliance data.

Continued arousals or decreased compliance may indicate inadequate CPAP pressure, mask-fit problems, or other problems

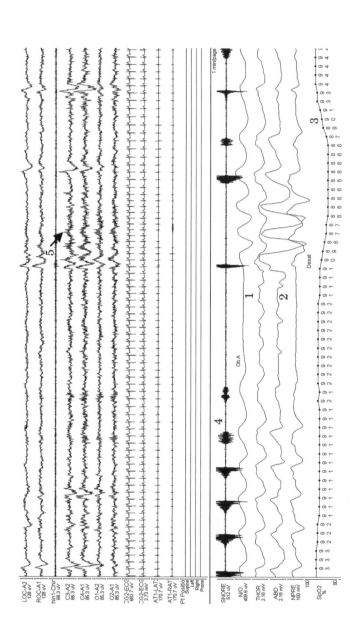

not related to the treatment. Compliance with CPAP is determined by the patient's perception of improvement, not by the severity of his/her disease. Patients may report problems associated with nasal congestion, rhinorrhea, oral dryness, abrasions, rashes, and air leaks associated with the mask. CPAP flow-related problems include chest discomfort, difficulty exhaling, and claustrophobia. The equipment can also be noisy, inconvenient, and intolerable for the patient or the bed partner. Issues and complaints like these must be dealt with seriously so that treatment is successful. Figure 2-4 is an example of a split night hypnogram from a woman with moderate to severe OSAHS. Split night studies such as that depicted in the example in the figure demonstrate the response to treatment with CPAP. The pretreatment portion of the study demonstrates hypoxemia related to SDB. Successful treatment with CPAP results in an abrupt cessation of OSAHS. However, split night procedures may underestimate the severity of the condition, because patients with SDB are usually worse in the later hours of sleep, and this severity cannot be examined if CPAP is initiated according to lab procedures for hypoxemiaIt is.

CENTRAL SLEEP APNEA

Central apnea is defined as a period of at least 10 seconds during sleep when no airflow or ventilatory effort is noted. Central apneas result from a reduced ventilatory drive, resulting in apnea or no airflow.[23] The etiology of this form of sleep apnea is unknown. Investigations have examined the ventilatory responses to hypoxia and hypercapnia during sleep. It appears that ventilatory responses to hypoxia and hypercapnia are reduced during both nonrapid eye movement (NREM) and rapid eye movement (REM) sleep. Although this has important implications, the pathogenesis of central apnea remains unknown. Central apnea may be

←

Figure 2-3. **Obstructive sleep apnea. Illustrated in this figure is a 60-second epoch from a diagnostic polysomnogram of a 73-year-old man with a history of nocturnal breathing cessation, snoring, and daytime somnolence. Obstructive sleep apnea is characterized by nasal–oral (N/O) breathing cessation(1) in the presence of persistent respiratory effort (2) and hypoxemia (3). Snoring(4) was noted electrographically and heard by the technicians monitoring the patients (snore channel, before and after the apneic event). An electroencephalographic (EEG) arousal occurred at the end of the apnea (5—arrow). The diagnosis of obstructive sleep apnea is established on the basis of a polysomnogram demonstrating an apnea–hypopnea index of more than five events per hour of sleep associated with one or more of the following: Bradytachycardia, frequent arousals from sleep, and arterial oxygen desaturation.[15] The channels are as follows: Electrooculogram (left: LOC-A2, right: ROC-A1), chin electromyogram (EMG), EEG (left central, right central, left occipital, and right occipital), electrocardiogram, limb EMG (left leg, right leg), snoring, N/O airflow, respiratory effort (thoracic and abdominal), nasal pressure, and oxygen desaturation. (From Avidan AY, Sleep apnea in the geriatric population. In: Mattson M, ed. _Sleep and aging, advances in cell aging and gerontology_, Vol. 17. Philadelphia, PA: Elsevier Inc.; 2005:79–112. With permission.)**

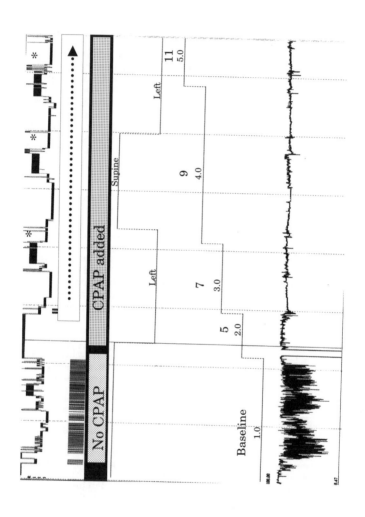

an outcome of the hypocapnia resulting from hyperventilation in response to the hypoxia.[23] Other investigations indicate that this finding may compensate for the increasing airway resistance during sleep rather than respond to the effects of hypoxia and hypercapnia.

Clinical Presentation

The patient with central apnea may present with a variable clinical picture depending on the severity of the apnea. Table 2-6 is a chart comparing the clinical presentations of central apnea with those of obstructive apnea. Patients with alveolar hypoventilation (hypercarbia and hypoxia) present with symptoms of respiratory failure. Cheyne-Stokes pattern respirations are considered a clinical manifestation of central apnea. End-stage COPD, pulmonary HTN, and CHF are the most common conditions associated with central apnea. Other patients with central apnea that is not related to alveolar hypoventilation present with symptoms that overlap with those of OSAHS.

Classification

Because of the limitations about the knowledge of central apnea and its etiology, most experts consider a frequency of more than five central apneas per hour as abnormal.

Epidemiology

SDB, either central or obstructive, is common in normal individuals. Studies have found that an incidence of disordered breathing exists in 12% to 66% of individuals, depending on the population.[23] Like OSAHS, central apnea is noted predominantly in men, although it has also been noted in postmenopausal women. Because the type of apnea was not always defined and different populations were studied, definitive conclusions about the cause of apnea are unknown. Patients with severe central apnea related to alveolar hypoventilation generally present with symptoms of CHF, cor pulmonale, polycythemia, and peripheral edema. Unfortunately, the hemodynamic effects of central apneas have not been thoroughly investigated.

Diagnostic Evaluation

Central apnea is evaluated in the sleep laboratory using the same techniques as those in OSAHS, except with additional emphasis being placed on respiratory effort. Unlike OSAHS, central

←——————————————————————————

Figure 2-4. An example of a hypnogram from a woman with obstructive sleep apnea. Continuous positive airway pressure (CPAP) was initiated at approximately 1:00 AM, which resulted in an immediate reduction in the hypoxemia noted during the baseline portion of the trial. She also managed to reach rapid eye movement (REM) sleep as a result of more fitful sleep using CPAP. Once CPAP was added, her sleep architecture improved (*dotted arrow*), and she had consolidated sleep with rebound of REM sleep (noted by **∗**). A hypnogram is a display of human sleep–wakefulness data (noted by the sleep architecture on the top of the diagram progressing from wakefulness, into light-stage, slow-wave, and REM sleep), which simultaneously records respiratory and other physiologic parameters.

Table 2-6.   Comparison of central apnea and obstructive apnea

Central Apnea	Obstructive Apnea
Clinical presentation	
Daytime sleepiness	Daytime sleepiness
Insomnia	
Mild snoring present	Prominent snoring is usually present
Restless sleep	Restless sleep
Awakenings with choking	Witnessed apneas/gasping
Weight	
Normal to obese	Commonly obese
Polysomnographic findings	
No airflow resulting in apnea	No airflow resulting in apnea
No ventilatory effort	Obvious ventilatory effort present

apnea is characterized by no respiratory effort throughout the period of apnea. Evaluation of respiratory effort has been performed in two ways, using esophageal pressure measurements and using respiratory-induced wall motion strain. Esophageal balloons have been used in research to measure esophageal pressure but are rarely used in clinical practice.

Other research using respiratory inductive plethysmography (RIP) to measure wall motion consists of a magnetized gauge belt placed on the abdomen and the chest to measure effort during breathing. Most laboratories effectively use a strain belt on the chest and abdomen to measure motion.

Polysomnographic Features of Central Apnea

Central apnea is characterized by an absence of airflow[1] and respiratory effort[2] (see Fig. 2-5). In this case, the patient exhibits absence of airflow. Absence of motion is also noted on the abdominal or thoracic belts, indicating that the patient was not demonstrating effort to breathe. These findings are characteristic of central apnea.

Differential Diagnosis

Differential diagnosis should be considered in patients presenting with persistent daytime symptoms, especially those diagnosed with comorbidities such as cor pulmonale or respiratory failure. Central and obstructive apneas usually occur together. A thorough evaluation for central apnea should include an assessment for obstructive apnea. Central apnea rarely occurs in isolation. Rebound central apneas have been noted in patients with OSAHS immediately after effective treatment with CPAP. Fortunately, this usually resolves without intervention in the patient compliant with this therapy.

Management

Management of patients with nonobstructive central apnea with documented hypoxemia and hypercarbia may include the use of a mask and pressure-cycled ventilation. In the past, tracheostomy was the treatment of choice, because patients requiring this form of treatment usually had hypoventilation resulting from respiratory disease or failure. SDB resolves with adequate treatment for nocturnal ventilatory failure.

Patients who have central apnea frequently also have obstructive apnea. If significant, treatment of the airway obstruction associated with OSAHS should be instituted immediately, with consideration given to the management of central apnea, if unresolved. Supplemental oxygen administration with and without nasal CPAP has been useful in the treatment of nonhypercarbic central apnea.[23] Tracheostomy is a useful intervention for the treatment of respiratory failure but is usually considered as a last resort.

Follow-up

Successful treatment of central apnea is dependent on treatment of OSAHS, CHF, respiratory disease, and other chronic conditions. These conditions, if present, must be managed therapeutically. If the patient is hypoxemic, then home oxygen is necessary and should be instituted immediately. If the patient is not hypoxemic or hypercarbic but continues to complain about disrupted sleep, then sleep-promoting agents may be used—very cautiously, because these agents may also interfere with ventilation and worsen the problem. In this case, patient education and follow-up are essential to the management of SDB.

ASTHMA

Episodic bronchoconstriction is the most common feature of asthma. Asthmatic attacks occur more frequently at night or early in the morning, making nocturnal bronchoconstriction a common cause of SDB.[24] Although management of asthma has become significantly easier with the advances in pulmonary medicine, research indicates that up to 85% of patients with asthma still complain about their symptoms waking them up.

Clinical Presentation

The patient with asthma describes sleep disturbances related to nocturnal wheezing. Wheezing is associated with bronchoconstriction and airway obstruction. Asthma symptoms also include shortness of breath, chest tightness, and cough. The forced expiratory volume in 1 second (FEV_1) and peak expiratory flow (PEF) rates fall in patients with asthma.[25]

Classification

Asthma is characterized by episodic bronchoconstriction, inflammation, and hyperresponsiveness of the airway. Bronchoconstriction is reversible and may vary from mild to severe and unrelenting. Inflammation of the airway involves a complex immune response that is cellular and biochemical.[24] Mast cells, neutrophils, eosinophils, and lymphocytes, as well as leukotriene, histamine,

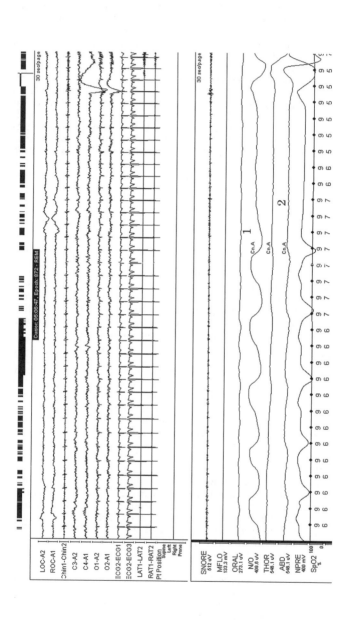

and other mediators, are responsible for the pathophysiologic response that occurs in an asthma attack. Although asthma is noted as a form of SDB, the use of sleep studies such as PSG do not confer additional clinical advantage in the diagnosis and treatment unless it is performed in the settings of suspected sleep apnea.

Epidemiology

Asthma affects 7% to 10% of the population. Research indicates that most in-hospital deaths from asthma occur at night.

Diagnostic Evaluation

Wheezing is a sign of uncontrolled asthma. Sleep disturbance experienced by patients with asthma has been confirmed by EEG studies. Nocturnal wheezing accompanied by frequent arousals result in little or no sleep during the attacks in the night. The frequency of nocturnal asthma is an indicator of asthma severity.[25] Pulmonary function tests are used to establish the diagnosis and severity and to monitor the response to therapy.

The diagnosis of asthma is confirmed by demonstrating airflow limitations on spirometry; these are usually reversible after inhalation of a bronchodilator. Measurement of forced vital capacity (FVC), FEV_1, and PEF yields the essential information. Improvement of FEV_1 after inhalation of a bronchodilator confirms the diagnosis of asthma. However, this finding is not exclusive to asthma because reversible bronchoconstriction can also be elicited in patients with bronchitis and emphysema.

The absence of wheezing does not necessarily mean the absence of bronchoconstriction. In this case, wheezing is misleading. Other clinical findings that occur in asthma are tachypnea, tachycardia, pulsus paradoxus due to exaggerated respiratory effort, hyperinflation, diaphoresis, prolonged expiration, and musical wheezing upon auscultation. Severe attacks may present with exhaustion, difficulty with speech, cyanosis, and use of accessory muscles. Impending respiratory arrest is possible at this stage.

Differential Diagnosis

Nocturnal asthma has been associated with enhanced airway inflammation and hyperresponsiveness. Other factors that might be related to asthma exacerbation during sleep include increased vagal tone, mucus retention, airway cooling and drying, gastroesophageal reflux, CHF, and sleep apnea. The relationship between asthma and OSAHS remains unexplored, although asthma symptoms do decrease after successful treatment of OSAHS with CPAP. Other nonasthmatic causes of wheezing

←

Figure 2-5.   Central sleep apnea. Illustrated in this figure is a 1-minute epoch from a split night polysomnogram of a 43-year-old man. Central sleep apnea characterized by nasal–oral (N/O) breathing cessation (1) in the absence of respiratory effort (2). Channels are as follows: Electrooculogram (left: LOC-A2, right: ROC-A1), chin electromyogram (EMG), electroencephalogram (left central, right central, left occipital, and right occipital), electrocardiogram, limb EMG (left leg and right leg), snoring, MFLO (mask flow before the application of CPAP),—N/O airflow, respiratory effort (thoracic and abdominal), nasal pressure, and oxygen desaturation.

include foreign body airway obstruction, anaphylactic laryngeal edema, COPD, cardiac asthma, pulmonary embolism, and pulmonary carcinoma.

Management

Management of asthma should be approached systematically. Medications play a primary role in the treatment of asthma symptoms. Medications are used in the long-term maintenance of asthma and the immediate treatment of acute attacks. Inhaled corticosteroids are the preferred long-term treatment. Improvement in the control of nocturnal wheezing and episodic dyspnea results in improvement in sleep. Patients who do not improve with initial therapies will require oral steroid therapy.

Follow-up

Factors known to exacerbate asthma include respiratory infections, rhinosinusitis, COPD, obesity, poor physical condition, cardiovascular disease, gastroesophageal reflux disease (GERD), pregnancy, OSAHS, β-blockers, cholinesterase inhibitors, angiotensin-converting enzyme (ACE) inhibitors, and failure to adhere to a prescribed regimen.

CHRONIC OBSTRUCTIVE PULMONARY DISEASE

COPD is a group of diseases associated with increased cough and dyspnea on exertion. Bronchitis and emphysema are two types of COPD. An exacerbation of COPD may result in worsened dyspnea, sleep hypoxemia, nocturnal wheezing, and disturbed sleep. Hypoxemia during sleep results from hypoventilation, a decrease in functional residual capacity, and ventilation–perfusion mismatch. Minute ventilation decreases in all sleep stages in healthy subjects.[26] Patients with COPD become more hypoxemic during sleep, especially during REM sleep. Functional residual capacity is reduced during sleep in healthy patients, although this has not been demonstrated in subjects with COPD. These factors contribute to a ventilation–perfusion mismatch, with resultant nocturnal hypoxemia. Nocturnal hypoxemia presents as worsened dyspnea at night and causes the patients to seek medical attention.

Clinical Presentation

Dyspnea is the most common presenting symptom in a patient with COPD. Other findings include hemoptysis or purulent sputum, hypoxemia, wheezing, coarse crackles or rhonchi, and a prolonged expiratory time. As the severity of the disease increases, more physical signs including decreased caloric intake, barrel-shaped chest, pursed-lip breathing, and emaciation are noted. The patient attempts to compensate for dyspnea by using the body position known as "tripoding." Radiologic examinations demonstrate lung hyperinflation. Displaced apical heart sounds to the midline may occur as a result of severe lung hyperinflation. A loud pulmonic component of S_2 may indicate pulmonary HTN.

Classification

Exacerbation of COPD may result in SDB especially related to worsened dyspnea and hypoxemia. Despite these complaints, there seems to be no clinical advantage in performing PSG for patients presenting with exacerbation of COPD unless a positive history of OSAHS or symptoms of OSAHS exist.

Epidemiology

The prevalence of COPD in the United States has been noted to be as high as 10% of individuals aged 55 to 85 years. COPD and OSAHS can occur concomitantly, although the prevalence of sleep apnea in patients with COPD is no more than that in normal populations. Mortality data indicate that COPD is the fourth leading cause of death.[27]

Diagnostic Evaluation

Previous research has demonstrated that the patients with COPD who were most hypoxic at night were also the most hypoxic during wakefulness.[26] Oxygenation during sleep can be predicted from the arterial tension obtained from the awake patient. Performance of nocturnal PSG provides no clinical advantage in patients with COPD unless it coexists with OSAHS.

Differential Diagnosis

Consequences of sleep hypoxemia include cardiac arrhythmias, pulmonary HTN, and polycythemia. Patients with COPD have poor sleep compared to healthy subjects, although most patients do not demonstrate evidence of increased daytime sleepiness using the Multiple Sleep Latency Test.

Management

Treatment of nocturnal hypoxemia in COPD includes oxygen therapy, β agonists and anticholinergics, CPAP, intermittent positive pressure ventilation through mask, and inspiratory muscle training. Oxygen therapy improves oxygenation during sleep, and most studies indicate that sleep quality is improved with this therapy. Patients reporting morning symptoms after initiation of oxygen therapy should be evaluated by PSG. This may be a sign of CO_2 retention and may be a particular problem if OSAHS coexists.

Avoidance of hypnotic agents and alcohol is recommended. Unfortunately, hypnotics are prescribed for sleep disturbances or alcohol is used as self-treatment in many cases.

Follow-up

Treatment of COPD is considered palliative, not curative. COPD causes many physical activities to be modified because of the dyspnea, so patients need education and encouragement to remain active.

REFERENCES

1. Hoffstein V. Snoring. In: Kryger M, Roth T, Dement WC, eds. *Principles and practice of sleep medicine*. Philadelphia, PA: WB Saunders; 2000:813–826.
2. *The international classification of sleep disorders*. Westchester, IL: American Academy of Sleep Medicine; 2005.
3. Young T, Peppard PE, Gottlieb DJ. Epidemiology of obstructive sleep apnea: A population health perspective. *Am J Respir Crit Care Med*. 2002;165(9):1217–1239.

4. Lugaresi E, Cirignotta F, Montagna P, et al. Snoring: Pathogenic, clinical, and therapeutic aspects. In: Kryger M, Dement WC, Roth T, eds. *Principles and practices of sleep medicine*. Philadelphia, PA: WB Saunders; 1994:621–628.

5. Lugaresi E, Cirignotta F, Piana G. Some epidemiological data on snoring and cardiocirculatory disturbances. *Sleep*. 1980;3:221–224.

6. Honsberg A, Dodge R, Cline M. Incidence and remission of habitual snoring over a 5- to 6-year period. *Chest*. 1995;108:604–609.

7. Johns M. Reliability and factor analysis of the Epworth Sleepiness Scale. *Sleep*. 1992;15:376–381.

8. Mallampati SR, Gatt SP, Gugino LD, et al. A clinical sign to predict difficult tracheal intubation: A prospective study. *Can Anaesth Soc J*. 1985;32(4):429–434.

9. Liistro G, Rombaux P, Belge C, et al. High Mallampati score and nasal obstruction are associated risk factors for obstructive sleep apnoea. *Eur Respir J*. 2003;21(2):248–252.

10. Guilleminault C, Stoohs R, Clerk A. A cause of excessive daytime sleepiness. The upper airway resistance syndrome. *Chest*. 1993;104:781–787.

11. Strobel R, Rosen R. Obesity and weight loss in obstructive sleep apnea: A critical review. *Sleep*. 1996;19:104–115.

12. Sher A. Upper airway surgery for obstructive sleep apnea. *Sleep Med Rev*. 2002;6:195–212.

13. Guilleminault C, Obstructive sleep apnea syndromes. *Med Clin North Am*. 2004;88(3):611–630, viii.

14. American Academy of Sleep Medicine. Sleep related breathing disorders in adults: Recommendations for syndrome definition and measurement techniques in clinical research. *Sleep*. 1999;22:667–689.

15. Bassiri A, Guilleminault C. Clinical features and evaluation of obstructive sleep Apnea-Hypopnea Syndrome. In: Kryger M, Roth T, Dement WC, eds. *Principles and practice of sleep medicine*. Philadelphia, PA: WB Saunders; 2000:869–877.

16. Kripke D, Ancoli-Israel S, Klauber M. Prevalence of sleep-disordered breathing in ages 40–64 years: A population based survey. *Sleep*. 1997;20:65–76.

17. Kryger M. Management of obstructive apnea-hypopnea syndrome: Overview. In: Kryger M, Roth T, Dement WC, eds. *Principles and practice of sleep medicine*, Philadelphia, PA: WB Saunders; 2000:940–954.

18. Ip M, Tsang WT, Lam WK, et al. Obstructive sleep apnea syndrome: An experience in Chinese adults in Hong Kong. *Chin Med J*. 1998;111:257–260.

19. Rechtschaffen A, Kales A, eds. *A manual of standardized terminology, techniques, and scoring system for sleep stages of human subjects*. Los Angeles, CA: Brain Information Service/Brain Research Institute, University of California; 1968.

20. Ayas N, Patel S, Malhotra A. Auto-titrating versus standard continuous positive airway pressure for the treatment of obstructive sleep apnea : Results of a meta-analysis. *Sleep*. 2004;27:249–253.

21. Masa J, Jiménez A, Durán J, et al. Alternative methods of titrating continuous positive airway pressure. A large multicenter study. *Am J Respir Crit Care Med*. 2004;170:1218–1224.

22. Loube DI, Gay PC, Strohl KP, et al. Indications for positive airway pressure treatment of adult obstructive sleep apnea patients: A consensus statement. *Chest.* 1999;115(3):863–866.
23. White D. Central sleep apnea. In: Kryger M, Roth T, Dement WC, eds. *Principles and practice of sleep medicine.* Philadelphia, PA: WB Saunders; 2000.
24. Douglas N. Asthma. In: Kryger M, Roth T, Dement WC, eds. *Principles and practice of sleep medicine.* Philadelphia, PA: WB Saunders; 2000:955–964.
25. Jarjour N. Asthma in adults: Evaluation and management. In: *Adkinson: Middleton's allergy: Principles and practice.* Mosby, Inc.; 2003.
26. Douglas N. Chronic obstructive pulmonary disease. In: Kryger M, Roth T, Dement WC, eds. *Principles and practice of sleep medicine.* Philadelphia, PA: WB Saunders; 2000:965–973.
27. Gay P. Chronic obstructive pulmonary disease and sleep. *Respir Care.* 2004;49(1):39–51.

ADDITIONAL READINGS

1. Bohadana A. Nocturnal worsening of asthma and sleep-disordered breathing. *J Asthma.* 2002;39(2):85–100.
2. Gay P. Chronic obstructive pulmonary disease and sleep. *Respir Care.* 2004;49(1):39–51.
3. Gold A. The symptoms and signs of upper airway resistance syndrome: A link to the functional somatic syndromes. *Chest.* 2003;123(1):87–95.
4. Goldberg A. Noninvasive mechanical ventilation at home: Building upon the tradition. *Chest.* 2002;121(2):321–324.
5. Guilleminault C. Obstructive sleep apnea syndromes. *Med Clin North Am.* 2004;88(3):611–630, viii.
6. Jordan A. Gender differences in sleep apnea: Epidemiology, clinical presentation and pathogenic mechanisms. *Sleep Med Rev.* 2003;7(5):377–389.
7. Wolk R. Cardiovascular consequences of obstructive sleep apnea. *Clin Chest Med.* 2003;24(2):195–205.

INTERNET RESOURCES FOR HEALTH CARE PROFESSIONALS AND PATIENTS

1. American Academy of Allergy Asthma and Immunology. (www.aaaai.org).
2. American Academy of Family Physicians. (http://www.aafp.org/afp/991115ap/2279.html).
3. American Academy of Pediatrics. (http://www.aap.org/policy/re0118.html).
4. American Sleep APNEA Association. (http://www.sleepapnea.org/).
5. Center for Medicare and Medicaid Services. (http://www.cms.hhs.gov/manuals/pub06pdf/pub06pdf.asp).
6. Medline Plus-a service of the National Library of Medicine and the National Institute of Health. (http://www.nlm.nih.gov/medlineplus/ency/article/000811.htm).
7. National Heart, Lung, and Blood Institute of the National Institute of Health and US Department of Health and Human Services. (http://www.nhlbi.nih.gov/health/dci/Diseases/SleepApnea/SleepApnea_WhoIsAtRisk.html).
8. National Sleep Foundation. (www.sleepfoundation.org).

Insomnia

Ruth M. Benca

CLINICAL PRESENTATION

Insomnia is marked by subjective complaints about quantity and/or quality of sleep that result in daytime impairment. Sleep-related symptoms include difficulty in initiating sleep at the beginning of the night, difficulty in staying asleep (i.e., having frequent and/or prolonged periods of wakefulness during the sleep period), waking earlier than the desired time in the morning and being unable to go back to sleep, and the perception of nonrestorative or poor-quality sleep. Patients with insomnia typically report that their sleep is "nonrefreshing" or "nonrestorative" and that they wake up in the morning feeling tired.

It is important to keep in mind that insomnia is a clinical definition, based on subjective patient reports. Although sleep laboratory studies of patients with insomnia generally support the subjective complaints, objective sleep abnormalities do not necessarily correlate with the patient's experience or treatment response. Polysomnographic studies have generally shown that patients with insomnia have prolonged latency to sleep onset, increased time awake during the sleep period, decreased total sleep time, and reduced amounts of slow-wave sleep.[1] All U.S. Food and Drug Administration (FDA)-approved hypnotics significantly improve both subjective and objective sleep parameters.

Classification

A variety of approaches have been used to classify insomnia on the basis of features such as symptoms, frequency, duration, severity, and presumed etiology. Symptom-based classifications, such as sleep-onset insomnia, are generally not useful because symptoms in patients tend to change over time and do not necessarily have clinical utility.[2,3]

More recent clinical definitions, such as the Research Diagnostic Criteria (RDC) for insomnia established by the American Academy of Sleep Medicine, include the requirement of daytime impairment resulting from sleep disturbance. Common daytime sequelae include fatigue, cognitive impairment causing difficulty in functioning in school or at work, and worries about sleep. The RDC are consistent with the diagnostic categories for insomnia in both the *International Classification of Sleep Disorders, second edition* (*ICSD-2*) and the clinical modification of the *International Classification of Diseases, 10th edition* (*ICD-10-CM*) (see Table 3-1).

Frequency, duration, and severity criteria vary considerably across different nosologies and also have limited diagnostic utility, although they may aid in identifying patients in need of treatment and/or in following up treatment response. Duration

Table 3-1. Research diagnostic criteria for insomnia disorder

1. The individual reports one or more of the following sleep-related complaints:
   a. Difficulty in initiating sleep
   b. Difficulty in maintaining sleep
   c. Waking up too early
   d. Sleep that is chronically nonrestorative or poor in quality
2. The sleep difficulty mentioned in the preceding text occurs despite adequate opportunity and circumstances for sleep
3. At least one of the following forms of daytime impairment related to the nighttime sleep difficulty is reported by the individual:
   a. Fatigue/malaise
   b. Attention, concentration, or memory impairment
   c. Social/vocational dysfunction or poor school performance
   d. Mood disturbance/irritability
   e. Daytime sleepiness
   f. Motivation/energy/initiative reduction
   g. Proneness to errors/accidents at work or while driving
   h. Tension headaches and/or GI symptoms in response to sleep loss
   i. Concerns or worries about sleep

GI, gastrointestinal.

of insomnia is probably the best indicator for diagnosis. Insomnias are generally classified as short-term (acute or transient), lasting days to weeks, and chronic, lasting weeks to months. Short-term insomnias are usually due to psychosocial stressors (e.g., stressful life events, pain, and travel), whereas chronic insomnia is frequently associated with a variety of comorbid conditions, as well as behavioral factors that may perpetuate the insomnia. The definition of chronic insomnia ranges from durations of 2 weeks to several months, depending on the nosology used. Lichstein et al. recently proposed a set of criteria for diagnosing chronic insomnia on the basis of experience in clinical trials, which include reported latency to sleep onset or the time spent awake after sleep onset being at least 31 minutes per night, occurring at least three times per week for at least 6 months.[4]

From an etiologic perspective, insomnia is classified as either primary or secondary, the latter on the presumption that the insomnia is caused by another disorder. Many medications, as well as a large number of psychiatric, medical, and sleep disorders, can cause or exacerbate insomnia. It is increasingly recognized that insomnia may be comorbid with many other disorders, meaning that there may not be a simple cause-and-effect relationship between the primary disorder and insomnia. For example, insomnia may not resolve completely when the primary disorder is in clinical remission, such as with depression. Furthermore, insomnia may exacerbate other disorders; for example, patients

Table 3-2.   Medical, psychiatric, and sleep disorders associated with insomnia

Medical Conditions and Disorders

Cancer
Cardiovascular disease (e.g., congestive heart failure)
Chronic pain syndromes
Dermatologic disorders (e.g., eczema, psoriasis and urticaria)
Endocrinal disorders (e.g., thyroid disease)
Gastrointestinal disorders (e.g., gastroesophageal reflux,
    inflammatory bowel disease and irritable bowel disorder)
Infectious disease (e.g., HIV and Lyme disease)
Neurologic disorders (e.g., dementia and Parkinson disease)
Perimenopause
Pulmonary disorders (e.g., asthma and COPD)
Rheumatologic disorders (e.g., arthritis and fibromyalgia)
Urologic disorders (e.g., nocturia and prostatic hypertrophy)

Psychiatric Disorders

Adjustment disorders
Anxiety disorders (e.g., generalized anxiety, panic disorder, and
    post-traumatic stress disorder)
Eating disorders (e.g., anorexia nervosa and bulimia nervosa)
Mood disorders (e.g., major depressive disorder and bipolar disorder)
Schizophrenia
Substance abuse disorders

Primary Sleep Disorders

Circadian rhythm disorders (e.g., advanced or delayed sleep phase,
    shift work, and jet lag)
Parasomnias (e.g., sleepwalking or confusional arousals)
Periodic movement disorder
Restless legs syndrome
Sleep apnea

HIV, human immunodeficiency virus; COPD, chronic obstructive pulmonary disease.

with fibromyalgia report increased pain following a night of poor sleep[5] (see Tables 3-2 and 3-3).

Epidemiology

The prevalence of significant insomnia (as defined by persistent sleep disturbance for a period of at least 2 weeks in the previous year) in the general population is about 10% to 15%.[6,7] Using less-stringent criteria, estimates for insomnia range up to 50% to 60% of the US population in a given year. Women are 1.4 times more likely than men to report insomnia.[3] The prevalence of insomnia is also greater in elderly individuals, with approximately 25% of those older than 65 years in a community survey complaining of insomnia.[8] The age-associated increase in insomnia, however, is likely due at least in part to the greater

Table 3-3. Medications associated with insomnia

Antidepressants
  SSRIs (e.g., fluoxetine, sertraline, citalopram, and paroxetine)
  SNRIs (e.g., venlafaxine and duloxetine)
  Bupropion
Antihypertensives
  α-Blockers, β-blockers
Chemotherapy
Diuretics
Decongestants
  Phenylephrine, pseudoephedrine
Hormones
  Steroids, thyroid hormones
Respiratory agents
  Albuterol, theophylline
Stimulants
  Amphetamine, caffeine, methylphenidate, modafinil

SSRIs, selective serotonin reuptake inhibitors; SNRIs, serotonin–noradrenaline reuptake inhibitors

prevalence of other medical and psychiatric disorders in the elderly population.[9,10]

Although chronic insomnia is usually defined as lasting for at least 2 weeks, in fact most individuals with insomnia tend to have long-standing sleep problems. In a European survey of almost 15,000 individuals, 19.1% complained of insomnia and of those, more than 80% reported having insomnia for at least 1 year.[11]

Rates of insomnia are increased in medical and psychiatric populations. Individuals with insomnia have higher rates of medical disorders and use medical services more frequently than those without sleep complaints.[6,8] In primary care settings, more than half the patients may have insomnia, although two thirds of these patients will not spontaneously report sleep problems to their doctors.[12,13] In patients with medical disorders, those with insomnia have worse outcomes, including higher rates of mortality in patients with cardiovascular disease[14] and institutionalized elderly patients.[15] Among medical disorders, chronic pain is particularly associated with insomnia. In studies of medical populations, the highest odds ratios for insomnia were observed in patients with painful conditions.[16]

Psychiatric illnesses are more highly associated with insomnia than are other medical disorders. Certainly, disturbed sleep is a hallmark of many psychiatric disorders, and most patients with psychiatric disorders complain of insomnia during acute episodes of illness.[17] Epidemiologic studies of the general population have demonstrated that one third to half of the patients with insomnia meet the criteria for primary psychiatric disorders, particularly mood and anxiety disorders. Rates of psychiatric illnesses in patients with insomnia are even higher in primary care settings, with up to 75% of those having diagnosable psychiatric disorders.[6] The specific medical disorder most strongly associated with insomnia in the primary care setting is depression.[18]

The relationship between sleep and psychiatric illness has been studied most extensively in patients with depression. Sleep laboratory studies of these patients show that they have a number of objective changes in their sleep architecture, including prolonged latency to sleep onset, increased time spent awake during the sleep period, and early morning awakening, all of which lead to reduced sleep efficiency and decreased amount of total sleep. In addition, patients with depression, when compared with the age-matched normal controls, tend to have significantly less slow-wave sleep and changes in rapid eye movement (REM) sleep, including reduced time from sleep onset to REM-sleep onset and increased proportion of REM sleep during the night.[1] Subjectively, patients with depression complain of insomnia, nonrestorative or "light" sleep, and disturbing dreams.

Insomnia is a known risk factor for depression. Individuals with insomnia are far more likely to develop depression than those without sleep problems. In a prospective study over a 1-year period, patients with insomnia that had persisted for the period of study were 39.8 times more likely to develop depression than those without insomnia, and those whose insomnia resolved over the course of the year had only a 1.6-fold increased risk for developing depression.[6] In a long-term prospective study of medical students, it was found that insomnia or difficulty in sleeping under stress in young men conferred a significantly elevated risk for developing depression later in life, with the increased rate of depression becoming most robust after several decades of follow-up.[19] Significantly elevated risks for developing depression in patients with insomnia are indicated in these and other studies. Insomnia may also increase the risk for developing other psychiatric disorders, such as anxiety and substance abuse disorders.[6,20]

Not only does insomnia predict an increased risk of developing the new onset of major depression, but it also tends to be the first symptom to appear in recurrent episodes of depression.[21] In a comparison of new-onset and recurrent episodes of depressive illness, Ohayon and Roth demonstrated that insomnia preceded the depressive episode 41% of the time for new onsets of illness and 56.2% of the time in recurrent depressive episodes. In contrast, insomnia was less likely to occur before new or recurrent episodes of anxiety disorders (18% or 23.2%, respectively), but rather tended to occur at the same time or following the onset of the disorder.[11]

Although it is a commonly held belief that insomnia occurring in the context of depression will improve as the mood disorder remits, in fact, patients with histories of depression tend to have chronic sleep problems, even when their psychiatric disorders are in remission. A comparison of patients treated for depression showed that although their insomnia had improved in comparison to when they were acutely depressed, they still had significantly more sleep complaints than normal control subjects.[22] Another study of patients treated for depression demonstrated that sleep disturbance and fatigue were the two most refractory symptoms in depression.[23] Overall, these data suggest that insomnia not only predicts an increased risk for having or developing depression but also is likely to be chronic in those with histories of depression, even when their mood disorder is under control.

In addition to the associations between insomnia and psychiatric and medical disorders, studies have demonstrated decreased quality of life in individuals with insomnia in comparison to those without sleep complaints,[13,24,25] and the decrements in well-being are of comparable magnitude to those seen in patients with medical disorders such as congestive heart failure and major depression.[26] Individuals with insomnia also have significantly more days of limited activity and days in bed and incur greater health care costs than controls do.[27]

Although insomnia has been linked with a broad range of comorbidities, it is not yet known whether the treatment of insomnia improves any of these associated illnesses or outcomes, primarily because studies addressing this question have not been performed. It is certainly likely that untreated insomnia may lead to other health problems, although definitive studies are still lacking. Nevertheless, insomnia is an important risk factor for depression and other psychiatric disorders, as well as poorer medical outcomes; therefore, it should be assessed and treated.

DIAGNOSTIC EVALUATION

The American Academy of Sleep Medicine recommends that all health care practitioners ask all patients about insomnia as part of any general health screening, particularly those patients at increased risk for sleep problems, such as women, elderly patients, and those with multiple medical or psychiatric problems. A complete sleep history should be obtained, including typical routines before bedtime, bedtime and its regularity, sleep pattern across the night, numbers and duration of awakenings, normal wake-up time and its regularity, and quality of sleep. It is equally important to ask about daytime symptoms, including excessive daytime sleepiness and patterns of daytime napping. Typically, individuals with insomnia may complain of daytime fatigue, but they typically do not nap excessively. Patients should also be asked about consequences of insomnia; for example, "How does your sleep problem affect your life?"

Because of the high rates of association between insomnia and medical disorders, especially psychiatric disorders (Table 3-2), a complete medical assessment should be performed for all patients complaining of insomnia. The use of prescription and over-the-counter medications should be assessed because these may interfere with sleep (Table 3-3). Many patients with insomnia tend to self-medicate with alcohol, and although it can initially aid in sleep onset, alcohol tends to disrupt sleep later in the night as blood levels decline. Similarly, other substances such as caffeine, nicotine, and stimulant drugs of abuse can produce insomnia; in some cases, a urine screen for toxic substances may be indicated. Patients may be unaware that their use of over-the-counter drugs are affecting their sleep, but a conversation with their physician can alert them to avoid the possible exacerbation of their condition that these drugs may induce.

Several primary sleep disorders may present with complaints of insomnia. Restless legs syndrome is an uncomfortable or painful sensation leading to an urge to move the legs; it tends to occur in the evening when the patient is lying in bed or sitting quietly. Periodic limb movements are repetitive contractions of the anterior tibialis muscle that may lead to frequent leg movements during sleep and brief arousals; they tend to occur every 20 to 30 seconds, sometimes throughout the night, and can lead to poor-quality or "light" sleep. In severe cases, patients with sleep-related movement disorders tend to have excessive daytime sleepiness, but they may also present with insomnia. Sleep apnea is also a disorder that tends to present with complaints of excessive daytime sleepiness, but in mild cases, and possibly more commonly in women, patients with sleep apnea may complain of sleep disturbance and insomnia, related to frequent arousals at night, caused by their apneic events. Patients with obstructive sleep apnea usually snore loudly and are either overweight or have upper airway problems that contribute to apnea, such as large tonsils or a small airway. Circadian rhythm disorders commonly present as complaints of insomnia. In sleep phase delay, patients are unable to fall asleep until much later than desired but then cannot awaken at the proper time in the morning, sometimes sleeping in and missing work or school. If allowed to sleep according to their desired schedule (e.g., 5 AM until noon), they usually report that they do not have insomnia and would function normally during the day. Because other primary sleep disorders may require specific treatments, their presence should always be assessed in any patient with a sleep problem.

Finally, patients should be asked about environmental and behavioral factors that may contribute to insomnia. Is the bed comfortable, and the bedroom dark and quiet and at the appropriate temperature? Noise and heat, for example, can be highly disruptive of sleep. Behavioral factors are particularly important in chronic insomnia, because behavioral conditioning can become an important perpetuating factor in insomnia. Does the patient worry excessively about sleep and focus efforts on "trying" to sleep? Anxiety about sleep can lead to hyperarousal in the sleep setting, worsening the insomnia. Patients often believe that if they have insomnia, they should spend more time in bed to try to get the "needed" sleep, including extending the nighttime sleep period and napping during the day. Both these practices lead to further sleep fragmentation as sleep becomes less and less consolidated. Does the patient engage in shift work, which may weaken and/or shift the circadian rhythm, making it difficult to sleep at the desired time? Psychosocial stressors can disturb sleep and may be particularly relevant for patients with shorter-term insomnias or for those with frequent bouts of insomnia. For example, is the insomnia correlated with episodes of work-related or interpersonal stress or travel?

During the physical examination, the appearance of patients with insomnia appearance may range from being hyperalert to frankly somnolent, suggesting diagnoses from primary insomnia, hyperthyroidism, abuse of stimulant drugs, or anxiety disorder to sleep deprivation or sleep disorders such as sleep apnea. Hypertension, large neck circumference, enlarged tonsils, and/or narrowed oropharynx may suggest obstructive sleep apnea.

A sleep diary is probably the most helpful diagnostic tool in assessing insomnia, as well as following treatment response. Ideally, a patient should fill out a sleep diary for at least 1 week before the assessment to provide a representative picture of sleep behavior. A representative sleep diary is shown in Figure 3-1. The Epworth Sleepiness Scale (see Appendix A) is helpful in distinguishing patients with hyperaroused insomnia from those with combined effects of insomnia and sleep deprivation. Epworth scores are often quite low in those with insomnia (i.e., <3), but some patients with insomnia may have elevated Epworth scores; those with scores of 12 or more should be screened thoroughly for evidence of sleep deprivation and medical or sleep disorders that cause excessive sleepiness. Polysomnography is rarely performed for complaints of insomnia, but rather is indicated for those with suspected sleep apnea, sleep-related movement disorders, or parasomnias (see Table 3-4).

Table 3-4. Diagnostic assessment of insomnia

Assessment of sleep complaint
    Nature of sleep problem
    Frequency
    Severity
    Duration
    Effect on daytime function
Predisposing factors (e.g., chronic anxiety and reactivity to stress)
Precipitating factors (e.g., illness and stressor)
Behaviors related to sleep
    Sleep schedule, regularity
    Napping
    Maladaptive habits related to sleep
    Exercise pattern
History of prior treatment and response
Medication and substance use
    Over-the-counter medications
    Prescription medications
    Alcohol, caffeine, tobacco
    Recreational drugs
Medical history and examination
Psychiatric history
Screen for sleep disorders
    Sleep apnea (e.g., presence of snoring, obesity, and excessive daytime sleepiness)
    Restless legs/periodic limb movements (uncomfortable sensations or urge to move legs when resting, frequent kicking during sleep)
    Circadian rhythm disorder (sleep period occurring other than at the desired time)
Sleep diary or log
Polysomnography for suspected sleep apnea and periodic movements/restless legs

INSTRUCTIONS:

1. Write the date, day of the week, and type of day: Work, School, Day Off, or Vacation.
2. Put the letter "C" in the box when you have coffee, cola or tea. Put "M" when you take any medicine.
3. Put "A" when you drink alcohol. Put "E" when you exercise.
4. Put a line (I) to show when you go to bed. Shade in the box that shows when you think you fell asleep.
5. Shade in all the boxes that show when you are asleep at night or when you take a nap during the day.
6. Leave boxes unshaded to show when you wake up at night and when you are awake during the day.

SAMPLE ENTRY BELOW: On a Monday when I worked, I jogged on my lunch break at 1 PM, had a glass of wine with dinner at 6 PM, fell asleep watching TV from 7 to 8 PM, went to bed at 10:30 PM, fell asleep around Midnight, woke up and couldn't got back to sleep at about 4 AM, went back to sleep from 5 to 7 AM, and had coffee and medicine at 7:00 in the morning.

Today's Date	Day of the week	Type of Day Work, School, Off, Vacation	Noon	1PM	2	3	4	5	6PM	7	8	9	10	11PM	Mid night	1AM	2	3	4	5	6AM	7	8	9	10	11AM
sample	Mon.	Work		E					A												C M					

week 1

week 2

MANAGEMENT

The management of insomnia includes identifying and treating all medical and psychiatric conditions that may be contributing factors in the case of secondary or comorbid insomnia. Patients with primary insomnia, as well as those with secondary insomnia, need treatment specifically for their sleep complaints. Modalities that have been shown to be effective for insomnia include behavioral and pharmacologic approaches. Although most treatments have been validated in patients with primary insomnia, they are likely also beneficial for patients with secondary or comorbid insomnia.

Nonpharmacologic Treatment

Behavioral treatments for insomnia generally aim at normalizing the two processes that regulate sleep: The circadian rhythm and the homeostatic sleep process.[28] The circadian rhythm of sleep–wakefulness is endogenously generated in the suprachiasmatic nucleus of the hypothalamus, meaning that it is not a passive response to external cues such as day and night. It is, however, entrained to the light–dark cycle through input from the retina to the suprachiasmatic nucleus. Misalignment of the circadian rhythm can result in disorders such as jet lag, in which the internal clock is "set" at a different time than the external environment. Contrary to popular belief, the greatest circadian propensity for sleep is not at the beginning of the night, but rather during the latter portion of the normal nightly sleep period; this is also the time of greatest propensity for REM sleep. Patients with insomnia will sometimes report that if they can get back to sleep in the early morning (around 4 or 5 AM), they can experience some of their best sleep because they take advantage of the circadian drive to sleep at this point in time. Conversely, the strongest circadian propensity of alertness is approximately 12 hours later, in the early evening, which is why many individuals have a period of increased alertness and energy, or a "second wind," at the end of the day.

The homeostatic sleep drive represents the buildup of pressure to sleep produced by sleep deprivation, normally from being awake during the day. Sleep onset at the beginning of the night is largely due to the homeostatic drive, which is why napping or sleeping in late often makes it more difficult to fall asleep at night. Deeper slow-wave sleep is prominent during the first hours of sleep as a response to sleep deprivation. Therefore, the normal progression of sleep across the night consists of sleep onset and the initial period of slow-wave sleep, initiated largely by the homeostatic drive to sleep, followed by the second portion of the sleep period, with greater amounts of REM sleep occurring in response to the circadian drive to sleep. A period of quiet wakefulness in the middle of the night, occurring between these two "pieces" of sleep, is not uncommon or necessarily abnormal

←

Figure 3-1. Two-Week Sleep Diary. (From The American Academy of Sleep Medicine. *Two week sleep diary*. Available from http://www.sleepeducation.com/pdf/sleepdiary.pdf, 2005, [cited 2005 October 31]. With permission.)

Table 3-5.   Sleep hygiene rules

Create a homeostatic need for sleep and reinforce the circadian drive

Wake up at the same time everyday, regardless of when you went to sleep

Maintain a consistent bedtime

Avoid napping; it may interfere with the ability to fall asleep at night

Make the sleep environment conducive to sleep

Use your bed only for sleep and sex; avoid reading in bed and other such activities

Keep your bedroom quiet, cool, and dark (extreme temperatures compromise sleep)

Perform activities that will support good sleep and avoid those that do not:

Exercise regularly, preferably in the late afternoon, but not within 2 h of bedtime

Perform relaxing activities before going to bed

Do not watch the clock at night (clock-watching can create anxiety about lost sleep

Avoid caffeine and nicotine for at least 6 h before bedtime

Drink alcohol only in moderation and avoid consumption for at least 4 h before bedtime

---

as long as it does not result in pathologic arousal, making it difficult to get back to sleep.

The first step in behavioral treatment is the institution of proper sleep hygiene, or good sleep habits (see Table 3-5) (see Appendix E). Sleep hygiene is rarely effective when used alone, particularly in those with severe or chronic insomnia, but it forms the basis for more specific behavioral interventions. Furthermore, failure to follow the rules of good sleep hygiene usually means that the patient is engaged in behaviors that are likely perpetuating or worsening the insomnia problem by interfering with normal homeostatic and/or circadian processes. Sleep hygiene measures are intended to strengthen the physiologic processes that govern sleep. Establishing a regular bedtime and, in particular, a regular wake-up time reinforces the circadian rhythm; in combination with avoiding napping, it allows for a normal buildup of sleep deprivation across the day to create a homeostatic need for sleep at night. Daytime light exposure and physical activity also help entrain the circadian rhythm, whereas bright light or exercise late at night can increase arousal level, as well as lead to a delay in the circadian rhythm. The bedroom environment is important in that light, noise, and heat can all disrupt sleep. Ambient temperature of the room is particularly important; the bedroom should be slightly cool, since temperature set point and, as a result, body temperature drop during the night. Perimenopausal women, for example, may have an exacerbation of nocturnal hot flushes if the bedroom is even slightly warmer than optimal.

Sleep hygiene measures also address issues of substance use and eating behaviors that may interfere with sleep. Substances such as caffeine and nicotine should be avoided before bedtime and eliminated completely if possible. Alcohol can also fragment sleep, particularly later in the sleep cycle. Caffeine, alcohol, and excessive fluid intake later in the day can lead to the need to waken during the night to urinate. Going to bed hungry or overly full can also disturb sleep.

Finally, some sleep hygiene recommendations aim at decreasing arousal levels and negative cognitions related to sleep. Having a relaxing bedtime routine helps decrease the arousal level. Watching the clock during the night is counterproductive because it tends to reinforce patterns of awakening ("I always wake up at 2 AM") or creates anxiety about not being able to fall asleep.

In addition to sleep hygiene rules, there are a number of more specific behavioral therapies that are helpful in treating insomnia. A meta-analysis of 59 behavioral treatment studies involving over 2,000 subjects found that psychological treatments were particularly helpful in reducing latency to sleep onset (effect size 0.88) and decreasing time awake after sleep onset (effect size 0.65) and that these effects were maintained during follow-up periods averaging 6 months.[29] The advantages of behavioral treatments are that they tend to provide long-lasting benefits, thereby making them cost-effective over time, and do not have the side effects associated with pharmacotherapy, such as toxicity, dependence, or abuse liability. The potential disadvantages are that behavioral therapy does not work as quickly as medication.[30] It requires a trained therapist, and the patient must be able to commit to spending the time necessary to learn the techniques and practice them on a nightly basis. Although it is often assumed that in one-on-one sessions significant therapist time is required to perform behavioral treatment, recent studies have suggested that more limited interventions may be helpful; cognitive behavior therapy (CBT), for example, was equally efficacious when provided through group sessions, over the telephone, or in traditional face-to-face sessions.[31]

The American Academy of Sleep Medicine practice guidelines recommend several nonpharmacologic treatments as being efficacious[32]; these treatments have been validated for primary insomnia in controlled clinical trials. In general, nonpharmacologic treatments are aimed at promoting regular sleep schedules, decreasing hyperarousal in bed, correcting negative conditioning to the sleep environment (i.e., associating the bed with anxiety and frustration about difficulty in sleeping), reversing maladaptive habits (e.g., spending a greater than needed amount of time in bed to "try" to get some sleep, which results in further fragmentation of sleep), and removing incorrect beliefs and expectations about sleep.

Stimulus control therapy is a nonpharmacologic treatment for insomnia developed by Bootzin and Epstein[33] and is designed to reestablish the association between the bedroom and rapid sleep onset, as well as strengthen both the circadian rhythm and the homeostatic sleep drive. Because many patients with insomnia have developed a negative association to their beds and bedrooms

Table 3-6.   Stimulus control instructions

1. Go to bed only when sleepy
2. If unable to sleep within 20 min, get out of bed, go to another room, and engage in a relaxing activity such as reading
3. Return to bed when feeling sleepy
4. Repeat steps 2 and 3 until sleep occurs
5. Wake up at the same time every morning, regardless of how much sleep was obtained
6. Do not nap
7. Do not engage in any activities in bed other than sleep or sex

by usually spending many hours in bed in a state of heightened arousal, one of the main principles of stimulus control is to minimize the time spent in bed when not sleeping and to use the bedroom only for sleeping and sex. Patients are instructed only to go to bed when feeling really sleepy, regardless of the time, and not remain in bed for more than approximately 20 minutes if they are not sleeping. If unable to sleep, they are not to be in the bedroom at all, but rather go to another neutral room and engage only in relaxing activities, such as reading. They can only return to the bedroom if they start to feel very sleepy, and, as many times as necessary across the night, they should leave the bedroom if sleep does not occur quickly. Finally, they must arise at the same time every morning, regardless of how little sleep was obtained the previous night, and they are not allowed to nap during the day. As a result, the homeostatic drive for sleep is allowed to build up normally across the day, hopefully increasing the likelihood of more rapid sleep onset the following night. Moreover, a regular waking time is necessary to keep the circadian clock entrained to the normal daily schedule. Although the instructions for stimulus control are fairly simple (see Table 3-6), patient compliance can be problematic, particularly at the beginning.

The primary objective of sleep restriction (see Table 3-7) is to reduce the time spent in bed being awake, and this may be easier for some patients to perform than stimulus control. Bedtimes and waking times are determined by the clinician on the basis of

Table 3-7.   Sleep restriction therapy

1. Determine average hours slept per night from sleep diary
2. Set time in bed equal to average hours slept, not <5 h per night. Bedtime and wake-up time should be consistent day-to-day
3. Calculate average sleep efficiency as time spent sleeping/time in bed. When average sleep efficiency is at least 90% over the preceding 5 d, time in bed may be increased by 15 min for the next 5 d
4. If sleep efficiency falls below 85%, time in bed may be reduced by 15 min for the next 5 d
5. If sleep efficiency is 85%–90%, time in bed need not be altered

the actual amount of time the patient spends sleeping. The total sleep period may not be scheduled for <5 hours per night. The resulting sleep deprivation serves to increase the homeostatic drive for sleep, and by setting the time of the prescribed sleep window, the circadian rhythm is also strengthened. Each week, the allowed time in bed is increased by about 15 to 20 minutes as long as, on average, the patient reports a sleep efficiency of at least 85% (sleep constitutes at least 85% of the time in bed).

Relaxation therapies are aimed at decreasing arousal in the sleep setting. One advantage of relaxation training, which may be combined with other stress management techniques, is that it is often easier to obtain; even therapists not trained in specific approaches for sleep are usually able to teach several types of relaxation techniques. Physical techniques such as progressive muscle relaxation decrease physical tension, whereas techniques such as guided imagery and meditation decrease mental arousal. Many patients with insomnia complain of "racing thoughts" or "inability to turn off thoughts" when they lie in bed at night; this mental hyperarousal leads to problems with sleep onset. Relaxation techniques must be practiced, initially at a time other than bedtime, in order for them to be effective. Not all patients, however, are able to use them productively, and some may even become more aroused rather than relaxed.

An opposite approach to relaxation is paradoxical intention; it is intended to reduce performance anxiety in the sleep setting. Rather than "trying" to relax and sleep, patients are instructed to stay awake (although not engage in arousing activities) and not try to fall asleep. For some patients, interventions intended to promote sleep cause them to become more aroused as they focus on trying to sleep, and by taking away this stress, they can sometimes relax more easily.

Cognitive therapy focuses more directly on dysfunctional beliefs and attitudes about sleep, to help the patient develop more adaptive views. Catastrophizing about the next-day sequelae of a night of insomnia (e.g., "I cannot function without 8 hours of sleep" or "I will get sick if I don't sleep enough tonight") only creates more tension and anxiety about being unable to sleep. Cognitive therapy includes education about sleep to help patients form more realistic views, not only of sleep in general but also about what to expect in terms of improvement in their own sleep patterns.

Cognitive therapy is generally used in combination with other behavioral approaches, in which case it is referred to as *multifaceted CBT* or *multicomponent therapy*. These types of combined approaches, usually incorporating cognitive restructuring and sleep hygiene, sleep restriction, or stimulus control, are becoming the most common approach to treating insomnia. They are effective not only in primary insomnia[34] but also in insomnia secondary to or comorbid with other conditions.[35]

Pharmacologic Treatment

A variety of pharmacologic agents are used in the treatment of insomnia, including those tested and approved for use as hypnotics, as well as a number of prescription and over-the-counter agents that may have sedating properties but have not necessarily been approved for use as hypnotics. The ideal hypnotic should improve sleep through reducing latency to sleep onset, decreasing time awake during the sleep period, increasing total sleep without disturbing normal sleep architecture, producing improved quality of sleep, and leading to better daytime functioning without hangover effects.

All currently available drugs that have an FDA indication for the treatment of insomnia are benzodiazepine receptor agonists (BzRAs) and include both benzodiazepines and newer, nonbenzodiazepine drugs that not only differ in chemical structure but also bind to the benzodiazepine receptor. Other drugs that are frequently used for insomnia include antidepressants, antipsychotics, antihistamines, and anticonvulsants. From the mid-1980s to the mid-1990s, the use of BzRAs declined by more than 50%, whereas the use of sedating antidepressants increased by almost 150%. By 2002, it was estimated that trazodone, a sedating antidepressant, was the most commonly prescribed drug for insomnia, and three out of the top four drugs prescribed for insomnia were antidepressants (see Fig. 3-2).[36]

The declining use of BzRAs over this period is likely due to a combination of factors. First, all BzRAs had short-term indications from the FDA at the time, and chronic use was discouraged. There were concerns that these drugs could cause tolerance, abuse, and dependence, and the longer-acting drugs were associated with hangover effects. Also, concerns originally related to benzodiazepines were transferred onto these newer agents. Clinicians were possibly more comfortable prescribing antidepressants for long-term use because they are nonscheduled drugs. Furthermore, given the high comorbidity between

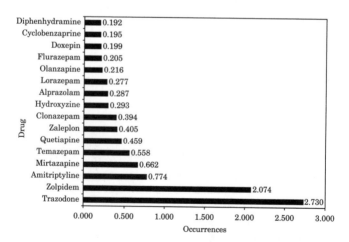

Figure 3-2.   The 16 drugs with the most "drug occurrences," with a desired action of "hypnotic," "promote sleep," or "sedate night" in 2002 from the Verispan Physician Drug and Diagnosis Audit.

insomnia and depression, some clinicians might have felt that they were treating the two disorders simultaneously.

Benzodiazepine Receptor Agonists

BzRAs include the older benzodiazepines and the newer BzRAs; the currently available agents are listed in Table 3-8. All these drugs act as agonists of the benzodiazepine receptor on the γ-aminobutyric acid (GABA) type A receptor complex; their effect is to facilitate the effect of GABA on the receptor, opening chloride channels and inhibiting neural activity. There are several subtypes of GABA A receptors; benzodiazepines bind to all of them with equal affinity, whereas some of the newer agents, including zolpidem, zaleplon, and indiplon, bind preferentially to the α_1 subunit of the receptor, which has been associated with hypnotic and amnestic effects but not with anxiolytic effects. It is possible that receptor subtype selectivity may be associated with differing clinical effects. In general, however, the efficacy of BzRAs is largely related to their half-life and time to onset of action.

Benzodiazepines approved for the treatment of insomnia include the longer-acting agents flurazepam, temazepam, quazepam, and estazolam. Clinical trials have shown that all these agents are effective for sleep induction and sleep maintenance (e.g., decreasing wakefulness after sleep onset) in both subjective reports and objective studies. These benzodiazepines, however, are also associated with next-day sedation and impairments in cognitive and psychomotor functioning.[37] Triazolam, with a shorter half-life, is primarily effective for promoting sleep onset rather than sleep maintenance. It is also less likely to cause next-day impairment but has been associated with rebound insomnia.[38] Benzodiazepines have also been reported to alter normal sleep architecture. They promote sleep, primarily by increasing stage 2 non-REM sleep, whereas they decrease stage 1 sleep and slow-wave sleep and may have a mild suppressive effect on REM sleep as well.

The FDA-approved nonbenzodiazepine BzRAs include zolpidem, zaleplon, and eszopiclone. The first two are more selective for the α_1 subunit of the GABA A receptor, whereas eszopiclone is less specific and also has the longest half-life of these agents, which is why it may be more effective for sleep maintenance; the other agents are primarily effective at sleep onset, although extended-release formulations of zolpidem and indiplon, when available, may also be helpful for sleep maintenance. Zolpidem has been shown to increase total sleep time when dosed at 10 mg, but this may be due to effects earlier in the sleep period because wakefulness after sleep onset or number of awakenings are not significantly reduced.[39] Zaleplon, with a half-life of only approximately 1 hour, is primarily intended for use as a sleep-inducing agent; because of its short half-life, it may even be used later in the night, as long as the patient can spend at least 4 hours in bed after taking it. Doses of <20 mg of zaleplon have not been shown to increase subjectively assessed total sleep time,[40,41] but doses of 20 mg were reported to increase sleep duration and decrease the number of awakenings from sleep.[41] In general, the newer BzRAs seem to preserve sleep architecture at lower therapeutic

Table 3-8.   Benzodiazepine receptor agonists (BzRAs) for insomnia

Drug	Dose Range (mg)	Dose in the Elderly (mg)	Half-life (h)	Effects on Sleep	Side Effects
Benzodiazepine Receptor Agonists: Benzodiazepines					
Estazolam	1–2	0.5 mg	10–24	Total sleep time: ↑ Sleep latency: ↓ WASO: ↓ Stage 1 (%): ↓ Stage 2 (%): ↑ Slow-wave sleep (%): ↓ REM (%): ↓ REM latency: ↑	Dizziness, drowsiness, hypokinesia, abnormal coordination, amnesia, GI symptoms
Flurazepam	15–30	15	47–100	Same as estazolam	Dizziness, drowsiness, lightheadedness, staggering, ataxia, amnesia, increased risk of falling, GI symptoms
Quazepam	7.5–15	7.5	For quazepam and 2-oxoquazepam: 25–41 For N-desakyl-1-oxoquazepam: 70–75	Same as estazolam	Dizziness, drowsiness, dyskinesia, slurred speech, amnesia, GI symptoms

Temazepam	7.5–30	7.5	6–16	Same as estazolam	Drowsiness, dizziness, lightheadedness, difficulty with coordination, amnesia, GI symptoms
Triazolam	0.25–0.5	0.125–0.25	1.5–5.5	Same as estazolam	Drowsiness, dizziness, lightheadedness, coordination disorders/ataxia, amnesia
Benzodiazepine Receptor Agonists: Nonbenzodiazepines					
Eszopiclone	2–3	1–2	5–5.8	Sleep latency: ↓ WASO: ↓	Unpleasant taste, dry mouth, dizziness, drowsiness, amnesia, GI symptoms

(Continued)

Table 3-8. *Continued*

Drug	Dose Range (mg)	Dose in the Elderly (mg)	Half-life (h)	Effects on Sleep	Side Effects
Zaleplon	10–20	5–10	1	Sleep latency: ↓	Dizziness, headache, GI symptoms, myalgia, drowsiness, amnesia
Zolpidem	10	5	1.4–4.5	Sleep latency: ↓	Drowsiness, dizziness, amnesia, GI symptoms
Melatonin Receptor Agonist					
Ramelteon	8	8	1–3	Sleep latency: ↓	Drowsiness, dizziness, interaction with fluvoxamine

WASO, wake after sleep onset; REM, rapid eye movement; GI, gastrointestinal; ↑, increase; ↓, decrease.
From Infante M, Benca RM. Treatment of insomnia. *Primary Psychiatry.* 2005;12(8):47–56. With permission.

doses; decrements in slow-wave sleep, for example, have not been reported.

In contrast to benzodiazepine hypnotics, several of the newer agents have been tested in longer-term controlled studies. In a 12-week study of nonnightly use, zolpidem was shown to have continued efficacy in reducing sleep latency and number of awakenings, increasing total sleep time and improving sleep quality.[42] There was no evidence of rebound insomnia in the nights when medication was not taken. Eszopiclone has been studied in a 6-month placebo-controlled trial and was shown to have continued efficacy in reducing subjective sleep onset and wakefulness during the sleep period, as well as in increasing total sleep time; no evidence of tolerance or rebound insomnia was noted.[43] As a result, eszopiclone is the first BzRA hypnotic that does not have an FDA indication for short-term treatment of insomnia.

Although all the hypnotics described in the preceding text have been shown to improve nocturnal sleep, relatively little data is available about their effects on daytime function. Furthermore, because almost all studies of hypnotics have been performed in patients with primary insomnia, it is unknown whether the treatment of insomnia with hypnotics reduces any of the comorbidities of insomnia. However, in the long-term eszopiclone study, patients reported significant improvement in daytime alertness, sense of well-being, and daytime functioning.[43]

One of the potential side effects of BzRAs is rebound insomnia, which is the transient occurrence of insomnia even worse than the baseline sleep problem on acutely discontinuing the drug; rebound insomnia is more common with shorter-acting drugs, particularly when used at high doses. It is important to distinguish rebound insomnia from recurrence of the baseline sleep problem; many patients believe that they are "dependent" on their medication when they have insomnia on a night that they fail to take medication or that they have rebound insomnia when they are simply experiencing the reemergence of their insomnia. In general, rebound insomnia is not a common occurrence with the newer BzRAs when they are taken at the recommended dosages.

BzRAs have also been associated with amnestic responses. Anterograde amnesia, which is loss of memory for events that occur after ingesting a hypnotic, is a potential side effect of all the BzRAs, including the newer agents, and is more common at higher plasma drug levels. Drugs that attain high plasma levels quickly, such as triazolam and the newer BzRAs, therefore will also have increased liability for producing anterograde amnesia and, therefore, should always be taken only immediately before bedtime.

Although there have been concerns that even the newer, shorter-acting agents such as zolpidem may increase the risk of falls at night in elderly persons,[44] this may be more of a problem with longer-acting benzodiazepines.[45] Furthermore, other classes of drugs used to treat insomnia, including antidepressants and anticonvulsants, also increase the risk of falls in elderly patients.[46] Finally, insomnia itself independently confers a greater risk of falls in this age-group.[47]

Table 3-9.   Antidepressants used for insomnia

Drug	Dose Range (mg)[a]	Dose in the Elderly (mg)[1]	Half-life (h)	Effects on Sleep	Side Effects
Antidepressants					
Amitriptyline	50–100	20	10–28, including the metabolite nortriptyline	Total sleep time: ↑ Sleep latency: ↓ Stage 2 (%): ↑ REM (%): ↓ REM latency: ↑	Drowsiness, dizziness, confusion, blurred vision, dry mouth, constipation, urinary retention, arrhythmias, orthostatic hypotension, weight gain, exacerbation of restless legs, periodic limb movements, or REM-sleep behavior disorder
Doxepin	75–100	25–50	8–24		
Mirtazapine	15–45	7.5–15	20–40	Total sleep time: ↑ Sleep latency: ↓ WASO: ↓	Drowsiness, dizziness, increased appetite, constipation, weight gain

Trazodone	150–400	150	7	Sleep latency: ↓ WASO: ↓ Slow-wave sleep (%): ↑	Drowsiness, dizziness, headache, blurred vision, dry mouth, arrhythmias, orthostatic hypotension, priapism

Anticonvulsants

Clonazepam	0.25–0.5	0.25	18–50	Total sleep time: ↑ Sleep latency: ↓ WASO: ↓ Stage 1 (%): ↓ Stage 2 (%): ↑ Slow-wave sleep (%): ↓ REM (%): ↓ REM latency: ↑	Drowsiness, dizziness, ataxia, depression, nervousness, reduced intellectual ability
Gabapentin	300–600	300	5–7	WASO: ↔ to ↓ Slow-wave sleep (%): ↑	Drowsiness, dizziness, emotional lability, ataxia, tremor, blurred vision, diplopia, nystagmus, myalgia, peripheral edema

(Continued)

Table 3-9. *Continued*

Drug	Dose Range (mg)[a]	Dose in the Elderly (mg)[1]	Half-life (h)	Effects on Sleep	Side Effects
Tiagabine	4–8	4	7–9	WASO: ↓ Slow-wave sleep (%): ↑	Drowsiness, dizziness, ataxia, tremor, new-onset seizures in patients without epilepsy, difficulty in concentration or attention, nervousness, asthenia, abdominal pain, diarrhea, nausea
Antipsychotics					
Olanzapine	5–10	5	21–54	Sleep latency: ↔ to ↓ WASO: ↓ Slow-wave sleep (%): ↑ REM (%): ↔ to ↓	Drowsiness, dizziness, tremor, agitation, asthenia, extrapyramidal symptoms, dry mouth, dyspepsia, constipation, orthostatic hypotension, weight gain, new-onset diabetes mellitus

Quetiapine	25–200	25	6	Insufficient data	Drowsiness, dizziness, asthenia, dry mouth, dyspepsia, constipation, orthostatic hypotension, weight gain, new-onset diabetes mellitus.
Risperidone	1–3	0.5–1.5	20	WASO: ↓ Stage 2 (%): ↑ REM (%): ↓	Drowsiness, dizziness, anxiety, extrapyramidal symptoms, nausea, dyspepsia, constipation, orthostatic hypotension weight gain, new-onset diabetes mellitus

(Continued)

Table 3-9. *Continued*

Drug	Dose Range (mg)[a]	Dose in the Elderly (mg)[1]	Half-life (h)	Effects on Sleep	Side Effects
Over-the-counter agents					
Diphenhydramine	diphenhydramine chloride: 50 Diphenhydramine citrate: 76	25	2.4–9.3	Sleep latency: ↓ WASO: ↔ to ↓ Slow-wave sleep (%): ↔ to ↑ REM %: ↓	Drowsiness, dizziness, dyskinesias, dry mouth, epigastric distress, constipation, tachycardia
Melatonin	Dosages not empirically determined	Dosages not empirically determined	0.5	Sleep latency: ↓	Concentration difficulty, dizziness, fatigue, headache, irritability
Valerian	Dosages not empirically determined	Dosages not empirically determined	Insufficient data	Sleep latency: ↓ Slow-wave sleep %: ↔ to ↑ REM %: ↔ to ↑	Reported adverse effects are rare

[a]Listed are recommended maximum amounts for a single dose.
GABA, γ-aminobutyric acid; WASO, wake after sleep onset; ↔, no change; ↑, increase; ↓, decrease.
From Infante M, Benca RM. Treatment of insomnia. *Primary Psychiatry.* 2005;12(8):47–56. With permission.

Perhaps one of the greatest concerns about BzRAs in the minds of the public is the risk of dependence. In fact, the risk of dependence is quite small because most individuals who use hypnotics do so for only a few weeks.[48] A recent review of case-report literature and a survey of admissions to an addiction treatment center in the United Kingdom suggest that risk for abuse and dependence may be lower for nonbenzodiazepines than for benzodiazepines.[49,50] Abuse and dependence are more common in patients with histories of substance abuse and/or psychiatric illness. Certainly, BzRAs should be used cautiously, if at all, in patients with histories of substance abuse.

Antidepressants

Although no antidepressants are currently indicated for the treatment of insomnia, in recent times they have been prescribed more frequently than BzRAs for insomnia.[51] The most commonly used antidepressants include trazodone, tricyclic antidepressants (particularly amitriptyline and doxepin), and mirtazapine (see Table 3-9). Relatively few studies have been performed to assess their effects on insomnia, and the mechanisms of action for sleep effects are not clear, although tricyclic antidepressants and mirtazapine, and to a lesser extent trazodone, have antihistaminergic effects. When used as sleep agents, sedating antidepressants tend to be used in doses subtherapeutic for depression. They are frequently combined with other, less-sedating or even activating antidepressants (e.g., selective serotonin reuptake inhibitors [SSRIs] such as fluoxetine, sertraline, paroxetine, and citalopram; combined reuptake inhibitors such as venlafaxine and duloxetine; and bupropion) to treat insomnia in patients with depression or are used alone in treating primary insomnia.

Trazodone has been the most widely prescribed antidepressant for insomnia and is probably used clinically almost exclusively for its hypnotic properties rather than as an antidepressant. It is a low-cost medication and has no significant abuse potential. Most studies of its use for insomnia have been performed in patients with underlying depression, and it has been reported to reduce sleep latency, improve sleep efficiency, and increase total sleep time in patients with depression and older patients with primary insomnia.[52–55] It has little effect on sleep architecture and is one of the few antidepressants that do not produce significant REM-sleep suppression. In terms of side effects, it may cause next-day sedation and, possibly, tolerance and rebound insomnia.[15,56] Although trazodone is admittedly safer than the tricyclic antidepressants, it can be associated with orthostatic hypotension and cardiovascular concerns and so should be used with caution in individuals with cardiac disease or elderly patients. Priapism is a rare side effect.

Despite having perhaps one of the most unfavorable side effect profiles of all the medications used for insomnia, tricyclic antidepressants continue to be used frequently, probably because of their low cost. No studies of amitriptyline in primary insomnia have been published, although some evidence suggestive of its sleep-promoting effects has been reported in patients with depression.[57] A recent study of doxepin in patients with primary insomnia showed subjective improvement in sleep quality, total sleep, and sleep efficiency, and objective improvement in sleep laboratory measurement of total sleep and sleep efficiency, although sleep latency was not decreased.[58] Tricyclic antidepressants, however, have a number of drawbacks, including a high toxic-to-therapeutic ratio, significant anticholinergic effects (e.g., arrhythmias, orthostatic hypotension, constipation, urinary retention, and cognitive effects), and daytime sedation. Because they are potent suppressors of REM sleep, they can cause significant REM-sleep rebound, which may produce disturbing dreams and insomnia. They are, therefore, not usually indicated for use on an as-needed basis.

Mirtazapine is a newer antidepressant with lower toxicity than the tricyclics. There are reports that it increased total sleep time and sleep efficiency, as subjectively reported in patients with depression, but no control groups were included in these studies.[59,60] Side effects of mirtazapine include daytime sedation, weight gain, and dizziness.

Antipsychotic Medications

The newer atypical antipsychotic medications, particularly quetiapine and olanzapine, are often used for their sleep-promoting effects. Their primary indication is for the treatment of schizophrenia, and they are also used as mood-stabilizing and antimanic drugs in patients with bipolar disorder. Their primary mechanism of action is to block dopamine type 2 (D_2) receptors, but sleep-inducing effects may be related to antihistamine effects and possibly to effects on antagonism of 5-HT2C receptors. No controlled studies for insomnia have been performed using antipsychotics, although studies of olanzapine on sleep in healthy subjects, in patients with schizophrenia, and in those with depression who were nonresponsive to treatment with SSRIs showed that it increased slow-wave sleep and improved sleep continuity.[61,62]

Although these may be very useful medications for patients with schizophrenia and bipolar disorder, two groups of patients that often have chronic and severe disruption of sleep, particularly when acutely ill,[1] their use in primary insomnia should be discouraged for several reasons. First, their pharmacokinetic profiles include generally long half-lives, leading to daytime sedation. Side effects may be serious and include weight gain, hypotension, extrapyramidal symptoms, and the risk of tardive dyskinesia or neuroleptic malignant syndrome. There are concerns that cerebrovascular accidents may be more common with these agents,[63] and they increase the mortality risk in elderly patients, which has led to a black-box warning about their use in elderly patients.

Over-the-counter Agents

Antihistamines (usually diphenhydramine) are common active ingredients in many over-the-counter sleep aids. They act through antagonism of type 1 histamine (H_1) receptors and therefore enhance sleep by decreasing arousal due to histaminergic neurotransmission. Only a few studies have been performed to assess the effects of diphenhydramine on sleep; these suggest that doses of 25 to 50 mg may reduce latency to sleep onset. There is evidence, however, that tolerance to the sedative effects may develop after only a few days of administration.[64] Antihistamines can also produce daytime sedation and cause psychomotor and cognitive impairment.[65,66]

Melatonin, a hormone produced by the pineal gland, is normally secreted at night. Its secretion is inhibited by light, so that it effectively indicates the length of the night across the changing seasons. Melatonin serves as a modulator of circadian rhythms and of seasonal behaviors (such as reproduction) in some animals. When administered to humans, it seems to promote sleep induction and lower body temperature[67,68] but has not been found to increase total sleep time consistently. Melatonin also has the ability to produce phase shifts in the underlying circadian rhythm,[69] which may make it helpful in treating advanced or delayed sleep phase syndromes, jet lag, or adjustment to shift work. Although little data is available, there are suggestions that low doses (e.g., 0.5 mg) seem to be helpful for circadian applications,[70,71] whereas higher doses (e.g., 5 mg) are usually used for hypnotic effects; however, there are no defined therapeutic doses. In contrast to other sleep-promoting agents, melatonin is typically administered 1 to 2 hours before bedtime. Long-term effects of melatonin are unknown, but its use should be avoided in pregnant or nursing women or in those who wish to become pregnant.

Newer Agents

Indiplon, described in the preceding text in the section on BzRAs, is expected to be available in both an immediate-release formulation with a short half-life, useful primarily for sleep induction, and a sustained-release formulation that will target patients with sleep maintenance problems. The first non-BzRA hypnotic approved by the FDA is ramelteon, an agonist of the melatonin type 1 and type 2 (MT1, MT2) receptors, which are thought to mediate its sleep-inducing and circadian effects. Ramelteon is a nonscheduled medication and may be used for long-term treatment.

Treatment Considerations for Pharmacotherapy

For patients with primary insomnia, BzRAs are generally the pharmacologic treatment of choice. Current guidelines suggest that most BzRAs should be used for short periods, usually not exceeding 1 month, although eszopiclone does not have this restriction. Given that newer agents have generally shown more favorable side effect profiles than older benzodiazepines, possibly because of their shorter half-lives, longer-term use may be considered with caution, although randomized clinical trials are clearly needed.

Choice of drug depends on patient characteristics such as age, sex, concomitant medication use, other medical/psychiatric disorders, and nature of the insomnia complaint. The lowest effective dose should be used for the shortest period, recognizing that some patients with chronic insomnia may need longer-term treatment. Contraindications for BzRA use include the presence of a history of alcoholism or substance abuse, severe sleep apnea (although newer, short-acting agents appear to have minimal effect on mild apnea syndromes), and pregnancy, and the medication is contraindicated in those who need to be alert, if needed, during the night (e.g., a physician on call). Dosages may need to be adjusted in elderly patients or in those with liver disease.

Various dosing schedules may be used, ranging from nightly dosing, particularly in severe, nightly insomnia, to intermittent dosing (e.g., 2 out of 3 nights, or not more than 3–5 nights per week). Intermittent dosing has been shown to be effective with zolpidem[72] in terms of showing no significant rebound insomnia on the nights without medication. Furthermore, particularly with the newer, shorter-acting BzRAs (zolpidem, zaleplon, and indiplon), taking them on an as-needed basis only, after trying to fall asleep first without medication, may minimize use in some patients. Zaleplon and, probably, indiplon can even be used as "rescue" medication in the middle of the night if there are at least 4 hours remaining to sleep.

Relatively little data is available about the use of hypnotics in patients with secondary or comorbid insomnia, although the studies that have been performed suggest that BzRAs are effective in these groups as well. For example, zolpidem was effective in treating insomnia in depressed patients receiving SSRIs.[73]

Sedating antidepressants may be considered for patients who cannot or should not take BzRAs, whereas antipsychotics should preferably be used only in patients who have other indications for their use (e.g., severe psychiatric disorders).

Nonpharmacologic versus Pharmacologic Treatment

Both behavioral and pharmacologic treatments are effective. A comparative meta-analysis of 21 studies for chronic primary insomnia found similar, large-effect sizes for pharmacologic and behavioral treatment for reducing the number of awakenings, time spent awake after sleep onset, total sleep time, and sleep quality. Sleep latency was reduced by both treatments, but the effect size was significantly greater for behavior therapy.[74] A major difference between pharmacotherapy and behavioral treatment is that the effects of behavioral therapy are probably more long-lasting, whereas there is approximately a 50% relapse rate after withdrawal of hypnotics.[75] On the other hand, pharmacotherapy works more quickly.[30] Behavioral treatments may be helpful in tapering patients off medication because relapse rates were lower in patients who received CBT or physician-supervised tapering of medication and were the lowest in patients who received both; subjective sleep was better in patients who had received CBT.[76] All patients with sleep problems should at least receive sleep hygiene training, and the choice of pharmacotherapy, behavioral treatment, or both should be made on the basis of patient characteristics (e.g., preference, motivation, and nature of complaint) and available resources.

Follow-up

Treatment for insomnia should be followed closely, at least initially. If medications are prescribed, the patient should be contacted within a week to determine the efficacy of medication and dosing should be adjusted if needed. Behavior treatment may require several sessions scheduled at regular intervals. Sleep logs or diaries are extremely helpful in monitoring treatment effect because sleep may be variable day-to-day, and treatment effects may be seen more readily over periods of several days or weeks. Patients who end up taking medications more chronically (i.e., longer than 1 month) should be followed up regularly to document continued efficacy of the medication, watch for dosage escalation, and monitor side effects. Setting reasonable treatment goals is important to maximize success; these should include improvements not only in various aspects of nocturnal sleep but also in daytime function. (A summary of the general approach for the evaluation and treatment of insomnia is provided as an algorithm in Appendix F.)

REFERENCES

1. Benca RM, Obermeyer WH, Thisted RA, et al. Sleep and psychiatric disorders: A meta-analysis. *Arch Gen Psychiatry*. 1992;49:651–668.
2. Hohagen F, Kappler C, Schramm E, et al. Sleep onset insomnia, sleep maintaining insomnia and insomnia with early morning awakening—temporal stability of subtypes in a longitudinal study on general practice attenders. *Sleep*. 1994;17(6):551.
3. Ohayon MM. Epidemiology of insomnia: What we know and what we still need to learn. *Sleep Med Rev*. 2002;6(2):97–111.
4. Lichstein KL, Durrence HH, Taylor DJ, et al. Quantitative criteria for insomnia. *Behav Res Ther*. 2003;41(4):427–445.
5. Affleck G, Urrows S, Tennen H, et al. Sequential daily relations of sleep, pain intensity, and attention to pain among women with fibromyalgia. *Pain*. 1996;68(2–3):363–368.
6. Ford DE, Kamerow DB. Epidemiologic study of sleep disturbance and psychiatric disorders: An opportunity for prevention? *J Am Med Assoc*. 1989;262(11):1479–1484.
7. Ohayon MM, Roth T. What are the contributing factors for insomnia in the general population? *J Psychosom Res*. 2001;51(6):745–755.
8. Mellinger GD, Balter MB, Uhlenhuth EH. Insomnia and its treatment. Prevalence and correlates. *Arch Gen Psychiatry*. 1985;42(3):225–232.
9. Foley DJ, Monjan A, Simonsick EM, et al. Incidence and remission of insomnia among elderly adults: An epidemiologic study of 6,800 persons over three years. *Sleep*. 1999;22(suppl 2):S366–S372.
10. Foley D, Ancoli-Israel S, Britz P, et al. Sleep disturbances and chronic disease in older adults: Results of the 2003 National Sleep Foundation Sleep in America Survey. *J Psychosom Res*. 2004;56(5):497–502.
11. Ohayon MM, Roth T. Place of chronic insomnia in the course of depressive and anxiety disorders. *J Psychiatr Res*. 2003;37(1):9–15.
12. Ancoli-Israel S, Roth T. Characteristics of insomnia in the United States: Results of the 1991 National Sleep Foundation Survey. I. *Sleep*. 1999;22(suppl 2):S347–S353.
13. Shochat T, Umphress J, Israel AG, et al. Insomnia in primary care patients. *Sleep*. 1999;22(suppl 2):S359–S365.

14. Mallon L, Broman JE, Hetta J. Sleep complaints predict coronary artery disease mortality in males: A 12-year follow-up study of a middle-aged Swedish population. *J Intern Med.* 2002;251(3):207–216.

15. Manabe K, Matsui T, Yamaya M, et al. Sleep patterns and mortality among elderly patients in a geriatric hospital. *Gerontology.* 2000;46(6):318–322.

16. Sutton DA, Moldofsky H, Badley EM. Insomnia and health problems in Canadians. *Sleep.* 2001;24(6):665–670.

17. Weyerer S, Dilling H. Prevalence and treatment of insomnia in the community: Results from the Upper Bavarian Field Study. *Sleep.* 1991;14(5):392–398.

18. Katz DA, McHorney CA. Clinical correlates of insomnia in patients with chronic illness. *Arch Intern Med.* 1998;158(10):1099–1107.

19. Chang PP, Ford DE, Mead LA, et al. Insomnia in young men and subsequent depression. The Johns Hopkins Precursors Study. *Am J Epidemiol.* 1997;146(2):105–114.

20. Breslau N, Roth T, Rosenthal L, et al. Sleep disturbance and psychiatric disorders: A longitudinal epidemiological study of young adults. *Biol Psychiatry.* 1996;39(6):411–418.

21. Perlis ML, Giles DE, Buysse DJ, et al. Self-reported sleep disturbance as a prodromal symptom in recurrent depression. *J Affect Disord.* 1997;42(2–3):209–212.

22. Reynolds CF 3rd, Hoch CC, Buysse DJ, et al. Sleep in late-life recurrent depression. Changes during early continuation therapy with nortriptyline. *Neuropsychopharmacology.* 1991;5(2):85–96.

23. Nierenberg AA, Wright EC. Evolution of remission as the new standard in the treatment of depression. *J Clin Psychiatry.* 1999;60(suppl 22):7–11.

24. Chevalier H, Los F, Boichut D, et al. Evaluation of severe insomnia in the general population: Results of a European multinational survey. *J Psychopharmacol.* 1999;13(4):S21–S24.

25. Zammit GK, Weiner J, Damato N, et al. Quality of life in people with insomnia. *Sleep.* 1999;22(suppl 2):S379–S385.

26. Katz DA, McHorney CA. The relationship between insomnia and health-related quality of life in patients with chronic illness. *J Fam Pract.* 2002;51(3):229–235.

27. Simon GE, VonKorff M. Prevalence, burden, and treatment of insomnia in primary care. *Am J Psychiatry.* 1997;154(10):1417–1423.

28. Borbely AA, Achermann P. Sleep homeostasis and models of sleep regulation. *J Biol Rhythms.* 2000;14(6):557–568.

29. Morin C, Culbert J, Schwartz S. Nonpharmacological interventions for insomnia: A meta-analysis of treatment efficacy. *Am J Psychiatry.* 1994;151:1172–1180.

30. McClusky HY, Milby JB, Switzer PK, et al. Efficacy of behavioral versus triazolam treatment in persistent sleep-onset insomnia. *Am J Psychiatry.* 1991;148(1):121–126.

31. Bastien CH, Morin CM, Ouellet MC, et al. Cognitive-behavioral therapy for insomnia: Comparison of individual therapy, group therapy, and telephone consultations. *J Consult Clin Psychol.* 2004;72(4):653–659.

32. Chesson AL Jr, Anderson WM, Littner M, et al. Practice parameters for the nonpharmacologic treatment of chronic insomnia.

An American Academy of Sleep Medicine report. Standards of Practice Committee of the American Academy of Sleep Medicine. *Sleep.* 1999;22(8):1128–1133.

33. Bootzin R, Epstein D, Wood JM. Stimulus control instructions. In: Hauri PJ, ed. *Case studies in insomnia.* New York: Plenum Press; 1991:19–28.

34. Edinger JD, Means MK. Cognitive-behavioral therapy for primary insomnia. *Clin Psychol Rev.* 2005;25(5):539–558.

35. Smith MT, Huang MI, Manber R. Cognitive behavior therapy for chronic insomnia occurring within the context of medical and psychiatric disorders. *Clin Psychol Rev.* 2005;5(5):559–592.

36. Walsh JK. Drugs used to treat insomnia in 2002: Regulatory-based rather than evidence-based medicine. *Sleep.* 2004;27(8):1441–1442.

37. Holbrook AM, Crowther R, Lotter A, et al. Meta-analysis of benzodiazepine use in the treatment of insomnia. *CMAJ.* 2000;162(2):225–233.

38. Mauri MC, Gianetti S, Pugnetti L, et al. Quazepam versus triazolam in patients with sleep disorders: A double-blind study. *Int J Clin Pharmacol Res.* 1993;13(3):173–177.

39. Saletu-Zyhlarz G, Anderer P, Brandstatter N, et al. Placebo-controlled sleep laboratory studies on the acute effects of zolpidem on objective and subjective sleep and awakening quality in nonorganic insomnia related to neurotic and stress-related disorder. *Neuropsychobiology.* 2000;41(3):139–148.

40. Elie R, Ruther E, Farr I, et al. Sleep latency is shortened during 4 weeks of treatment with zaleplon, a novel nonbenzodiazepine hypnotic. Zaleplon Clinical Study Group. *J Clin Psychiatry.* 1999;60(8):536–544.

41. Fry J, Scharf M, Mangano R, et al. Zaleplon improves sleep without producing rebound effects in outpatients with insomnia. Zaleplon Clinical Study Group. *Int Clin Psychopharmacol.* 2000;15(3):141–152.

42. Perlis ML, McCall WV, Krystal AD, et al. Long-term, non-nightly administration of zolpidem in the treatment of patients with primary insomnia. *J Clin Psychiatry.* 2004;65(8):1128–1137.

43. Krystal AD, Walsh JK, Laska E, et al. Sustained efficacy of eszopiclone over 6 months of nightly treatment: Results of a randomized, double-blind, placebo-controlled study in adults with chronic insomnia. *Sleep.* 2003;26(7):793–799.

44. Wang PS, Bohn RL, Glynn RJ, et al. Zolpidem use and hip fractures in older people. *J Am Geriatr Soc.* 2001;49(12):1685–1690.

45. Mendelson WB. Clinical distinctions between long-acting and short-acting benzodiazepines. *J Clin Psychiatry.* 1992;53(suppl):4–7, discussion 8–9.

46. Kelly KD, Pickett W, Yiannakoulias N, et al. Medication use and falls in community-dwelling older persons. *Age Ageing.* 2003;32(5):503–509.

47. Brassington GS, King AC, Bliwise DL. Sleep problems as a risk factor for falls in a sample of community-dwelling adults aged 64–99 years. *J Am Geriatr Soc.* 2000;48(10):1234–1240.

48. Roehrs T, Hollebeek E, Drake C, et al. Substance use for insomnia in Metropolitan Detroit. *J Psychosom Res.* 2002;53(1):571–576.

49. Hajak G, Muller WE, Wittchen HU, et al. Abuse and dependence potential for the non-benzodiazepine hypnotics zolpidem and

zopiclone: A review of case reports and epidemiological data. *Addiction*. 2003;98(10):1371–1378.

50. Jaffe JH, Bloor R, Crome I, et al. A postmarketing study of relative abuse liability of hypnotic sedative drugs. *Addiction*. 2004;99(2):165–173.

51. Compton-McBride S, Schweitzer P, Walsh J. Most commonly used drugs to treat insomnia in 2002. *Sleep*. 2004;27(suppl):A255.

52. Parrino L, Spaggiari MC, Boselli M, et al. Clinical and polysomnographic effects of trazodone CR in chronic insomnia associated with dysthymia. *Psychopharmacology*. 1994;116(4):389–395.

53. Scharf MB, Sachais BA. Sleep laboratory evaluation of the effects and efficacy of trazodone in depressed insomniac patients. *J Clin Psychiatry*. 1990;51(suppl):13–17.

54. Montgomery I, Oswald I, Morgan K, et al. Trazodone enhances sleep in subjective quality but not in objective duration. *Br J Clin Pharmacol*. 1983;16(2):139–144.

55. Saletu-Zyhlarz GM, Abu-Bakr MH, Anderer P, et al. Insomnia in depression: Differences in objective and subjective sleep and awakening quality to normal controls and acute effects of trazodone. *Prog Neuropsychopharmacol Biol Psychiatry*. 2002;26(2):249–260.

56. Scharf MB, Roth T, Vogel GW, et al. A multicenter, placebo-controlled study evaluating zolpidem in the treatment of chronic insomnia. *J Clin Psychiatry*. 1994;55(5):192–199.

57. Shipley JE, Kupfer DJ, Griffin SJ, et al. Comparison of effects of desipramine and amitriptyline on EEG sleep of depressed patients. *Psychopharmacology*. 1985;85:14–22.

58. Hajak G, Rodenbeck A, Voderholzer U, et al. Doxepin in the treatment of primary insomnia: A placebo-controlled, double-blind, polysomnographic study. *J Clin Psychiatry*. 2001;62(6):453–463.

59. Winokur A, DeMartinis NA 3rd, McNally DP, et al. Comparative effects of mirtazapine and fluoxetine on sleep physiology measures in patients with major depression and insomnia. *J Clin Psychiatry*. 2003;64(10):1224–1229.

60. Winokur A, Sateia MJ, Hayes JB, et al. Acute effects of mirtazapine on sleep continuity and sleep architecture in depressed patients: A pilot study. *Biol Psychiatry*. 2000;48(1):75–78.

61. Sharpley AL, Vassallo CM, Cowen PJ. Olanzapine increases slow-wave sleep: Evidence for blockade of central 5-HT(2C) receptors *in vivo*. *Biol Psychiatry*. 2000;47(5):468–470.

62. Salin-Pascual RJ, Herrera-Estrella M, Galicia-Polo L, et al. Olanzapine acute administration in schizophrenic patients increases delta sleep and sleep efficiency. *Biol Psychiatry*. 1999;46(1):141–143.

63. Herrmann N, Lanctot KL. Do atypical antipsychotics cause stroke? *CNS Drugs*. 2005;19(2):91–103.

64. Richardson GS, Roehrs TA, Rosenthal L, et al. Tolerance to daytime sedative effects of H1 antihistamines. *J Clin Psychopharmacol*. 2002;22(5):511–515.

65. Rickels K, Morris RJ, Newman H, et al. Diphenhydramine in insomniac family practice patients: A double-blind study. *J Clin Pharmacol*. 1983;23(5–6):234–242.

66. Witek TJ Jr, Canestrari DA, Miller RD, et al. Characterization of daytime sleepiness and psychomotor performance following H1 receptor antagonists. *Ann Allergy Asthma Immunol.* 1995;74(5):419–426.

67. Haimov I, Lavie P, Laudon M, et al. Melatonin replacement therapy of elderly insomniacs. *Sleep.* 1995;18(7):598–603.

68. Hughes RJ, Sack RL, Lewy AJ. The role of melatonin and circadian phase in age-related sleep- maintenance insomnia: Assessment in a clinical trial of melatonin replacement. *Sleep.* 1998;21(1):52–68.

69. Lewy AJ, Ahmed S, Jackson JM, et al. Melatonin shifts human circadian rhythms according to a phase-response curve. *Chronobiol Int.* 1992;9(5):380–392.

70. Lewy AJ, Bauer VK, Hasler BP, et al. Capturing the circadian rhythms of free-running blind people with 0.5 mg melatonin. *Brain Res.* 2001;918(1–2):96–100.

71. Hack LM, Lockley SW, Arendt J, et al. The effects of low-dose 0.5-mg melatonin on the free-running circadian rhythms of blind subjects. *J Biol Rhythms.* 2003;18(5):420–429.

72. Walsh JK, Roth T, Randazzo A, et al. Eight weeks of non-nightly use of zolpidem for primary insomnia. *Sleep.* 2000;23(8):1087–1096.

73. Asnis GM, Chakraburtty A, DuBoff EA, et al. Zolpidem for persistent insomnia in SSRI-treated depressed patients. *J Clin Psychiatry.* 1999;60(10):668–676.

74. Smith MT, Perlis ML, Park A, et al. Comparative meta-analysis of pharmacotherapy and behavior therapy for persistent insomnia. *Am J Psychiatry.* 2002;159(1):5–11.

75. Morin CM, Belanger L, Bastien C, et al. Long-term outcome after discontinuation of benzodiazepines for insomnia: A survival analysis of relapse. *Behav Res Ther.* 2005;43(1):1–14.

76. Morin CM, Bastien C, Guay B, et al. Randomized clinical trial of supervised tapering and cognitive behavior therapy to facilitate benzodiazepine discontinuation in older adults with chronic insomnia. *Am J Psychiatry.* 2004;161(2):332–342.

Hypersomnia and Narcolepsy

Timothy F. Hoban and Ronald D. Chervin

CLINICAL PRESENTATION

Sleepiness can be defined as a high physiologic drive toward sleep, but the term is also frequently used to denote the conscious perception of the need or readiness for sleep. Occasional sleepiness is a normal experience in most individuals, for example, at the end of the day or upon unexpected waking from sleep. However, excessive daytime sleepiness, defined as sleepiness that interferes with daytime activities, productivity, or enjoyment, is usually abnormal and may reflect insufficient sleep, disrupted sleep, or a primary sleep disorder such as narcolepsy. This chapter discusses the clinical assessment of the sleepy patient, diagnostic classification of the major sleep disorders characterized by hypersomnolence, diagnostic and laboratory evaluation of sleepiness, and treatment issues.

Symptoms of sleepiness are notoriously variable in severity. Mild sleepiness is sometimes noted only intermittently or during sedentary activities such as reading, watching television, or traveling for extended distances. Mild or moderate sleepiness may or may not be self-evident to the patient because symptoms often subside with stimulating physical or mental activity or may be misattributed to fatigue or boredom. Chronic sleepiness usually evolves insidiously, and many affected individuals do not realize that the sleepy state is not normal.

Patients with moderate or severe sleepiness often have difficulty sustaining full alertness even during active and stimulating situations. These individuals are especially likely to fall asleep inadvertently during sedentary activities or take naps during daytime. Although some degree of subjective sleepiness is usually apparent to the patient or family members, the severity of the sleepiness and the associated impairment of attention and cognition is frequently under-recognized. When sleepiness is both chronic and severe, patients may experience "sleep attacks," characterized by the recurrent, precipitous, unavoidable need to stop an activity and take a nap.

Associated clinical manifestations of sleepiness are likewise variable. Somnolent individuals may complain of fatigue, tiredness, lack of energy, inattention, impaired concentration, or emotional lability. Severely somnolent individuals often appear visibly sleepy and in extreme cases stuporous or encephalopathic. Visible signs of sleepiness on examination may include drooping of the eyelids, pupillary miosis, nodding of the head, or intermittent loss of postural tone.

Determining whether a pathologic degree of sleepiness is present is not always easy. Brief periods of sleepiness near an individual's regular bedtime or transiently upon awakening are usually normal. Even more substantial sleepiness following sleep restriction or extended wakefulness does not always require detailed assessment when the underlying cause is identifiable and self-limited. Sleepiness that interferes with everyday activities or occurs at inappropriate times is almost always abnormal, particularly if the somnolence is chronic, recurrent, or severe. In general, sleepiness that does not improve when nighttime sleep is lengthened is often a sign of an underlying sleep disorder.[1]

A detailed medical and sleep history is arguably the most important element in the diagnostic evaluation of a sleepy patient. The history alone often allows accurate assessment of whether a patient's sleepiness is likely to be the result of insufficient sleep, disrupted sleep (e.g., secondary to obstructive sleep apnea [OSA]), or a central nervous system disorder such as narcolepsy. Patients with excessive sleepiness commonly exhibit identifiable symptoms that help identify specific underlying causes. Such symptoms include snoring or observed apnea during nighttime sleep, restlessness or jerking of the legs, hypnagogic or hypnopompic hallucinations, sleep paralysis, automatic behavior, cataplexy, and other constitutional symptoms. An algorithm for the workup and treatment of sleepiness is provided in Appendix G.

Snoring and Other Obstructive Symptoms during Sleep

Sleep-related breathing disorders (SRBDs) are frequently associated with daytime sleepiness when respiratory disturbances disrupt the quality or continuity of nighttime sleep. Loud snoring is a cardinal symptom of OSA and upper airway resistance syndrome (UARS) and may be accompanied by mouth breathing, unusual body positions, or visible restlessness during sleep. Respiratory pauses are sometimes witnessed by bed partners or family members, sometimes terminating with a snort or gasp when breathing resumes. Such symptoms are most informative when present; conversely, the absence of observed apnea and even snoring does not rule out the possibility of an obstructive SRBD.

Restless Legs and Symptoms of Excessive Periodic Limb Movements

Restless legs syndrome (RLS) and periodic limb movement disorder (PLMD) may also be associated with excessive daytime somnolence, especially when nighttime insomnia is prominent. RLS is characterized by a desire to move the extremities (with or without dysesthesias), motor restlessness, worsening of symptoms at rest, relief by activity, and worsening of symptoms during evening or nighttime.[2] Children may exhibit "growing pains" as a symptom of RLS.[3] The leg movements of PLMD may be reported by bed partners, ranging from gentle dorsiflexion of the toes or feet to fairly vigorous kicking movements with visible arousal from sleep. However, arousals associated with PLMD may not be caused by the movements and do not predict sleepiness.[4,5]

Hypnagogic or Hypnopompic Hallucinations

Hypnagogic (at sleep onset) and hypnopompic (at waking) hallucinations are brief, dreamlike episodes that last seconds to minutes. Hallucinations are often vivid and distressing despite their brevity. Although these hallucinatory episodes are often reported by patients with narcolepsy, they have also been reported in association with other sleep disorders, a variety of psychiatric conditions, and as a medication side effect.[6,7]

Sleep Paralysis

Sleep paralysis is a condition in which muscle atonia, normally restricted to rapid eye movement (REM) sleep, instead occurs at the interface between sleep and wakefulness. Sleep paralysis may be total or partial and may coincide with hypnagogic hallucinations. Although episodes typically last for only a few minutes, they may be extremely frightening to affected patients and accompanied by sensations of suffocation. Episodes can frequently be terminated by extraneous stimuli such as noise or touch. Sleep paralysis is frequently reported by patients with narcolepsy but may also be seen with other sleep disorders, as a familial condition, or as an occasional phenomenon in normal individuals.[8–10]

Automatic Behavior

Automatic behavior refers to episodes of purposeful but sometimes inappropriate behavior occurring during periods of sleepiness, usually with partial or absent subsequent recollection of the activity.[11] Some varieties of automatic behavior are common and benign, such as an individual briefly arising during nighttime sleep and using the bathroom but not remembering the event the next day. Other varieties are more serious, as might be the case for a drowsy driver arriving at his destination with no memory of how he got there. Automatic behavior during wakefulness that is prolonged, frequent, or a risk to safety is usually indicative of significant sleepiness.

Cataplexy

Cataplexy is characterized by paroxysmal episodes of bilateral muscle weakness or paralysis, triggered by laughing or emotion. The phenomenon reflects muscle atonia, which is normally restricted to REM sleep but, in this condition, is inappropriately expressed during wakefulness. Unlike sleep paralysis, cataplectic episodes usually occur during sustained wakefulness and are triggered by strong emotions such as laughter, surprise, or anger. The duration of cataplexy is usually short, ranging from seconds to minutes, but successive attacks precipitated by extreme emotional stimuli (status cataplecticus) may rarely last as long as 1 hour.[12] Severity of muscle atonia during episodes is highly variable. Mild attacks may consist only of a brief sensation of weakness without externally visible manifestations. Severe episodes may be characterized by complete paralysis, sparing only respiration, eye movements, and sphincters. Most often, loss of muscle tone in cataplexy is partial and may take the form of knee buckling, head drop, slurred speech, or loss of postural tone. Consciousness is maintained during attacks, distinguishing them from syncope and atonic seizure, although in some cases, patients may fall asleep during the immobility of a severe cataplectic attack.

Other Constitutional Symptoms and Signs Associated with Specific Causes of Sleepiness

- Episodes of hyperphagia, hypersexuality, and other behavioral disturbances accompany sleepiness in individuals with Kleine-Levin syndrome (recurrent hypersomnia) or hypothalamic lesions.[13,14]
- Lethargy, weight gain, and unsteady gait may accompany somnolence in patients with hypothyroidism, who are at increased risk for OSA.[15]
- Morning headache or other neurologic complaints are nonspecific symptoms sometimes associated with sleepiness secondary to structural pathology within the central nervous system.[16]
- Hypersomnia can occur in individuals with unipolar or bipolar depression, in whom associated symptoms of anhedonia, fatigue, or intermittent mania may be apparent.[17,18]

CLASSIFICATION AND CLINICAL CHARACTERISTICS

The *International Classification of Sleep Disorders (ICSD)*, introduced in 1990, established a standard nosology for sleep disorders. The second edition in 2005 *(ICSD-2)* groups conditions characterized by primary hypersomnolence into a single category titled *Hypersomnias of central origin not due to a circadian rhythm disorder, sleep related breathing disorder, or other case of disturbed nocturnal sleep*, as summarized in Table 4-1 and outlined in the subsequent text.[12]

Table 4-1. The *International Classification of Sleep Disorders, Second Edition*, (ICSD-2) classification for hypersomnias of central origin

1. Narcolepsy with cataplexy
2. Narcolepsy without cataplexy
3. Narcolepsy due to medical condition
4. Narcolepsy, unspecified
5. Recurrent hypersomnia
   a. Kleine-Levin syndrome
   b. Menstrual-related hypersomnia
6. Idiopathic hypersomnia with long sleep time
7. Idiopathic hypersomnia without long sleep time
8. Behaviorally induced insufficient sleep syndrome
9. Hypersomnia due to medical condition
10. Hypersomnia due to drug or substance
11. Hypersomnia not due to substance or known physiologic condition (nonorganic hypersomnia, not otherwise specified)
12. Physiologic (organic) hypersomnia, unspecified (organic hypersomnia, not otherwise specified)

Adapted from International Classification of Sleep Disorders. *Diagnostic and Coding Manual,* 2nd ed. Westchester: American Academy of Sleep Medicine; 2005. With permission.

Narcolepsy with Cataplexy

Narcolepsy with cataplexy is characterized primarily by excessive daytime somnolence and cataplexy. Sleepiness is usually most evident during sedentary or monotonous activities but may also take the form of irresistible *sleep attacks* that may occur during more active pursuits. Daytime sleep periods in patients having narcolepsy with cataplexy are usually short and refreshing, but followed by recurrent somnolence within hours. The severity of somnolence in affected patients ranges from mild to disabling.

Cataplexy is unique to narcolepsy but often develops years after onset of excessive daytime sleepiness. Episodes are most commonly precipitated by "positive" emotions such as elation or surprise. Attacks may be localized to specific body areas (e.g., face) or involve all skeletal muscle groups in a generalized manner. Respiration is never affected, but subjective sensations of choking or dyspnea are sometimes reported. The frequency of cataplexy in affected patients may range from rare and isolated attacks to innumerable daily episodes.

The nonobligate clinical manifestations frequently exhibited by patients having narcolepsy with cataplexy may include *sleep paralysis, hypnagogic hallucinations*, and *automatic behavior* (described in the section "Clinical Presentation"). These phenomena affect a small proportion of normal sleepers as well. The REM-sleep behavior disorder (RBD)—episodes of complex motor behavior arising during REM sleep—is seen with increased frequency in adults with narcolepsy. Nocturnal sleep disruption is frequently seen in individuals having narcolepsy with cataplexy, often taking the form of excessive night waking. Disrupted nighttime sleep in these patients is often sufficient to cause further exacerbation of daytime sleepiness.

Onset of narcolepsy with cataplexy can appear during early childhood but most commonly occurs during adolescence or young adulthood. Cataplexy usually develops during the first few years after disease onset but may occasionally develop before or long after the hypersomnolence does. Recent evidence suggests that loss of hypocretin-1–secreting cells in the hypothalamus, possibly on an autoimmune basis, plays a pathogenetic role in most cases.[19,20]

Narcolepsy without Cataplexy

Narcolepsy without cataplexy is similar in most clinical respects to narcolepsy with cataplexy except for the lack of definite cataplectic episodes. Because some patients in this category eventually develop cataplexy later in the course of their disease, it is recognized that the diagnostic classification may change for some patients if new symptoms become apparent.[12]

Despite the substantial clinical similarities between narcolepsy without cataplexy and narcolepsy with cataplexy, some evidence suggests that the underlying pathophysiology of the two conditions is not identical. Cerebrospinal fluid (CSF) hypocretin-1 levels are most often normal in narcolepsy without cataplexy, whereas they are substantially decreased or undetectable when cataplexy is present.[20] This suggests that the underlying cause or causes of narcolepsy without cataplexy may not involve loss of hypocretin-1–secreting hypothalamic neurons.

Narcolepsy due to Medical Condition

Narcolepsy with and without cataplexy has been reported in association with a variety of medical and neurologic conditions. Genetic disorders associated with narcolepsy include type C Niemann-Pick disease,[21] Prader-Willi syndrome,[22] and possibly Coffin-Lowry syndrome.[23] Structural lesions in the hypothalamic region, including tumors, sarcoidosis, and multiple sclerosis, may also cause secondary narcolepsy.[24,25] Symptomatic narcolepsy may also be seen in several neurologic disorders not having demonstrable hypothalamic involvement, including acute disseminated encephalomyelitis, multiple system atrophy, and possibly head injury.[26–28]

Narcolepsy, Unspecified

Narcolepsy, unspecified, is defined by the ICSD-2 as a temporary classification for patients who meet clinical and laboratory criteria for narcolepsy but require additional evaluation for more precise classification.

Recurrent Hypersomnia

Recurrent hypersomnias are rare conditions in which prolonged episodes of excessive sleepiness are separated by periods of normal alertness and function. In *Kleine-Levin syndrome*, which typically affects adolescent boys, patients may sleep for all but a few hours daily for periods lasting days to weeks.[29] Somnolence is often accompanied by variable disturbances of mood, cognition, and temperament, often including increased appetite and significantly aggressive or hypersexual behavior. Episodes may occur up to ten times yearly, often with gradual improvement over time.[12] No specific etiology has been established for this syndrome, but intermittent hypothalamic dysfunction or autoimmune etiologies have been postulated.[30]

Menstrual-associated hypersomnia represents a poorly characterized condition in which episodic sleepiness coincides with the menstrual cycle and is postulated to be secondary to hormonal influences.

Idiopathic Hypersomnia with Long Sleep Time

Idiopathic hypersomnia with long sleep time is characterized by pervasive daytime sleepiness despite longer-than-average nighttime sleep.[31,32] Prolonged nighttime sleep of 10 or more hours with few or no awakenings still leave affected patients unrefreshed or confused (*sleep drunkenness*) on waking in the morning. Daytime sleepiness is pervasive and often severe. Daytime naps of these patients tend to be longer and less refreshing than those of the patients with narcolepsy. The condition most often develops during the early adult years with a chronic but stable course. The pathophysiology of the condition is unknown.

Idiopathic Hypersomnia without Long Sleep Time

Although earlier classifications allowed diagnosis of idiopathic hypersomnia only in the context of a prolonged nighttime sleep period, patients with comparable daytime sleepiness but normal to only slightly prolonged nighttime sleep have been reported.[31,33] As a result, *idiopathic hypersomnia without long sleep time* has been established as a separate diagnostic entity in ICSD-2. Although the severe, pervasive daytime somnolence and unrefreshing naps seen in this condition are identical to those seen in idiopathic hypersomnia with long sleep time, the nighttime sleep period is <10 hours.

Behaviorally Induced Insufficient Sleep Syndrome

Excessive daytime sleepiness often results solely from habitually insufficient nighttime sleep. Review of a sleep diary or sleep history of the affected patients usually reveals a chronically shortened nighttime sleep period that is either less than the patient's premorbid baseline or—for children and adolescents—substantially less than normal for age. Daytime symptoms are those of sleep deprivation and may include sleepiness, irritability, disturbed mood, and impaired school or work performance. Symptoms remit with lengthening of the nighttime sleep period, but transiently longer sleep periods, for example, on weekends, holidays, or vacations, often do not provide complete relief.

Hypersomnia due to Medical Condition

Hypersomnia due to medical condition may be diagnosed when sleepiness is thought to be the direct result of a medical or neurologic condition, but the patient does not meet clinical or laboratory criteria for a diagnosis of narcolepsy. Severity of daytime somnolence and length of nighttime sleep vary considerably among patients. Although cataplexy should not be present, symptoms of sleep paralysis or automatic behavior are sometimes observed.

A variety of causes may lead to this disorder. Associated neurologic conditions may include stroke, brain tumor, encephalitis, head trauma, and Parkinson disease.[34–36] Genetic conditions sometimes associated with sleepiness most notably include Prader-Willi syndrome and myotonic dystrophy.[37,38] Endocrine and toxic–metabolic causes include hypothyroidism, hypoadrenalism, hepatic encephalopathy, and renal failure. Drug-induced and psychiatric causes are discussed in the following sections.

Hypersomnia due to Drug or Substance

Hypersomnia due to drug or substance is characterized by excessive nighttime sleep, daytime somnolence, or excessive napping related either to use of drugs or alcohol or to their discontinuation.[39] Sleepiness is often seen in patients who abuse sedative–hypnotic compounds such as alcohol, benzodiazepines, barbiturates, γ-hydroxybutyric acid (GHB), or nonbenzodiazepine sedatives. Somnolence may also complicate the use of medically indicated prescription medications, including antihistamines, anticonvulsants, and many analgesics. Hypersomnia may also occur following abrupt discontinuation of stimulant use or occasionally following its nonabrupt cessation after prolonged prior use.

Hypersomnia Not due to Substance or Known Physiologic Condition (Nonorganic Hypersomnia, Not Otherwise Specified)

In *hypersomnia not due to substance or known physiologic condition*, excessive nighttime sleep, daytime somnolence, or excessive and nonrefreshing napping is associated with an identifiable psychiatric diagnosis, which sometimes becomes apparent only with time and detailed evaluation. Associated psychiatric conditions may include depression and other mood disorders, somatoform disorders, conversion disorders, or other psychiatric disturbances.[40,41] Affected individuals often demonstrate intense preoccupation with their symptoms and may miss substantial amounts of school or work. Sleep diaries often reveal prolonged bedtime in conjunction with delayed sleep latency and fragmented nighttime sleep with variable daytime napping. The condition most commonly presents during early adulthood. Despite patients' subjective complaints, objective sleepiness may be difficult to document on Multiple Sleep Latency Tests (MSLTs).

Physiologic (Organic) Hypersomnia, Unspecified (Organic Hypersomnia, Not Otherwise Specified)

Chronic sleepiness for at least 3 months with MSLT evidence of excessive sleepiness may be classified as *physiologic (organic) hypersomnia, unspecified*, provided that the symptoms are physiologic and do not meet criteria for other disorders of excessive somnolence.

EPIDEMIOLOGY/DEMOGRAPHICS

Despite its high prevalence, excessive daytime sleepiness is under-recognized by both patients and medical providers. In the National Sleep Foundation's 2002 "Sleep in America" poll of 1,010 randomly sampled adults, over one third of respondents reported problematic sleepiness for at least several days monthly, with 16% experiencing daytime sleepiness several days weekly or more.[42] Overall, 6% of respondents to this survey reported use of medications to maintain wakefulness. Other surveys have reported comparably high prevalence of excessive somnolence for more select populations, including senior citizens in North Carolina (25%), Japanese adolescents (33% for boys and 39% for girls), and Australian commercial vehicle drivers (24%).[43–45]

For many affected individuals, sleepiness is a secondary characteristic of sleep disorders that cause disrupted or insufficient nighttime sleep, and the epidemiology of these conditions is reviewed in other chapters of this book.

Among the conditions for which hypersomnolence is a primary element, *narcolepsy* is the most thoroughly studied. The overall prevalence of narcolepsy with cataplexy is 0.02% to 0.18%, with some variance between specific populations or countries.[12,46–48] The prevalence for narcolepsy without cataplexy is unknown, but this condition is estimated to represent 10% to 50% of the narcoleptic population. The onset of narcolepsy is highest in the second decade of life, followed in descending order by the third, fourth, and first.[49] Some series have reported slightly more frequent incidence in men compared to women.[49] Histocompatibility human leukocyte antigen (HLA) associations and hypocretin-1 data for human narcolepsy are reviewed in the section "Diagnostic Evaluation" in this chapter.

The prevalence of *recurrent hypersomnia* is unknown, but the condition is thought to be rare. Most reports of the Kleine-Levin syndrome suggest onset in early adolescence, more commonly in men.[50,51]

Few prevalence or demographic data exist for the *idiopathic hypersomnias*. Although they were once felt to be fairly common, this diagnosis now seems to be made less frequently. The ICSD-2 estimates the prevalence of idiopathic hypersomnia with long sleep time to be one tenth that of narcolepsy, with no prevalence data available for the other classified varieties of idiopathic hypersomnia.[12] The onset of symptoms for the idiopathic hypersomnias usually occurs during adolescence or young adulthood.[32] Familial cases of idiopathic hypersomnia have been reported.[52]

Prevalence and demographic data do not yet exist for *behaviorally induced insufficient sleep syndrome, hypersomnia due to medical condition, hypersomnia due to drug or substance*, or *physiologic (organic) hypersomnia. Hypersomnia not due to substance or known physiologic condition* is thought to present during young adulthood in both sexes and be potentially influenced by the familial patterns sometimes manifested by the associated psychiatric conditions.[12]

DIAGNOSTIC EVALUATION

A careful history is the single most important tool in the diagnosis of a patient with excessive daytime sleepiness. Questions should focus on the degree to which sedentary or more active situations are affected (indicating more severe pathology) and also on the extent to which the sleepiness is considered a problem. Whenever possible, family members or close friends should also be interviewed because their perception of excessive daytime sleepiness can sometimes differ considerably from that of the patient. Effects of sleepiness on quality of life, relationships, leisure activities, work productivity, and safety, particularly motor vehicle crashes or near-misses, should be explored. Lifestyle, sleep habits, medications, caffeine intake, and use of other stimulant substances should be reviewed. Critical clues to the presence of specific causes of hypersomnolence, as noted in the preceding text, can usually be identified in an office-based history.

A sleep diary from recent weeks, which some sleep clinics ask patients to complete before their evaluations, can be particularly helpful in some cases. A detailed office-based history and physical examination, sometimes in combination with a sleep diary that some sleep clinics ask patients to bring to their evaluations, is often sufficient to provide a diagnosis or at least a provisional diagnosis even without additional diagnostic testing. For example, a clear history of cataplexy in a sleepy patient narrows the differential diagnosis to narcolepsy, a history of chronic sleepiness in a teenager who sleeps only 5 hours nightly is most likely to represent behaviorally induced insufficient sleep syndrome, and RLS is often diagnosed by history alone.

A variety of questionnaire assessment tools can be used to help assess patients for sleepiness and its underlying causes. The most commonly used questionnaire for sleepiness during preceding weeks is the *Epworth Sleepiness Scale (Appendix A).*[53] This instrument asks respondents to rate sleep propensity in eight briefly described, variously sedentary situations. Results can help discriminate between patients with and without disorders of hypersomnolence or monitor treatment effects in a standardized manner. The results do not necessarily reflect the severity of an underlying sleep disorder and may show little or no correlation with objective tests of daytime sleepiness.[54]

The *Stanford Sleepiness Scale* generates a standardized patient rating of instantaneous subjective sleepiness (see Appendix H).[55] Other specific instruments may be useful in identifying specific types of sleep disorders. Validated examples include the *Sleep Disorders Questionnaire* (for sleep apnea, narcolepsy, psychiatric sleep disorders, and PLMD) and the *Berlin Questionnaire* (for sleep apnea).[56,57] The *Functional Outcomes of Sleep Questionnaire* discriminates between patients with sleep disorders and healthy controls, correlates with results of generic measures, and also focuses on some more sleep-specific dimensions such as vigilance.[58] Generic quality of life instruments such as the *Medical Outcome Study Short Form-36 (SF-36)* can be sensitive to the presence of disorders that cause hypersomnolence.[59]

In many cases, after a history, examination, and use of any standardized questionnaires, neurophysiologic tests such as *nocturnal polysomnography (PSG)* and *MSLT* are still necessary to confirm a diagnosis, assess its severity, or rule out a primary sleep disorder. *Nocturnal PSG* is valuable in several respects. It provides objective screening for disorders that disrupt nighttime sleep, particularly SRBDs, and also other conditions such as periodic limb movements (PLMs) or nocturnal seizures. In addition, PSG findings may be useful in the diagnosis and classification of the primary hypersomnias.

In patients with narcolepsy, nocturnal PSG often demonstrates REM sleep at sleep onset, generally defined as occurring within the first 15 minutes of sleep. Sleep latency itself is usually short, and subsequent sleep may reflect nonspecific disruption known to afflict patients with narcolepsy, although in practice this can be difficult to distinguish from the "first night effect" of the new sleeping environment and recording equipment. Episodes of complex behavior or electromyographic abnormalities during REM sleep may be recorded on occasion in patients with narcolepsy who have concurrent RBD.

PSG findings in patients with other primary hypersomnias are often less distinctive than those in patients with narcolepsy. Patients with recurrent hypersomnia may show prolonged total sleep time or demonstrate nonspecific findings such as reduced sleep efficiency, increased nighttime waking, or slowing of the electroencephalogram (EEG) background. The PSG in patients with idiopathic hypersomnia may demonstrate normal or prolonged sleep duration, sometimes in conjunction with increased slow-wave sleep or higher-than-expected sleep efficiency. Patients with behaviorally induced insufficient sleep syndrome tend to exhibit short sleep latency, high sleep efficiency, and prolonged sleep time on nocturnal PSG.

The *MSLT* is a series of four to five 20-minute nap opportunities, under conditions conducive to sleep, in which latency to sleep is recorded. The premise is that individuals who are sleepy will tend to fall asleep more quickly, on average throughout the day, than those who are not. Although generally considered the gold standard for objective measurement of sleepiness, the MSLT must be performed under carefully controlled circumstances. In most cases, medications that have the potential to influence sleep should be discontinued at least 15 days (or five times the half-life of the drug or active metabolite) in advance of the MSLT.[12] In addition, the patient's habitual sleep schedule should be maintained for at least 1 week in advance of the MSLT and verified by sleep log or actigraphy. Finally, nocturnal PSG should generally be performed the night before the MSLT to screen for other sleep disorders and to verify that sufficient sleep is obtained ($\geq$6 hours for adults) before the daytime testing.

In adults, a mean sleep latency of >10 to 12 minutes is usually considered abnormal. For diagnostic purposes, an MSLT sleep latency of <8 minutes suggests excessive daytime sleepiness in adults, and a value <5 minutes is often considered severe.[12] Two or more sleep-onset REM periods (SOREMPs) are commonly exhibited by patients with narcolepsy and can be critical to the diagnosis of narcolepsy in the setting of an appropriate history and absence of cataplexy. However, this finding may occasionally be seen in patients with other sleep disorders and can appear in a small proportion (<2%) of healthy adult sleepers.[12,60] Patients with SRBDs are far more numerous at sleep laboratories than those with narcolepsy and may account for many or most of the patients with two or more SOREMPs, although the chance of finding this is greater for a patient with narcolepsy than for a patient with sleep apnea.[61]

Mean sleep latency values for the young—particularly prepubertal children—are significantly higher than those for adults. Detailed norms and diagnostic guidelines for children are available elsewhere.[62]

In patients with *narcolepsy*, the MSLT-derived mean sleep latency is usually <8 minutes, often <5 minutes, but occasionally in the normal or borderline range. In a recent meta-analysis, the mean sleep latency for patients with narcolepsy was 3.1 ± 2.9 minutes.[63] For patients with *idiopathic hypersomnia*, with or without long sleep time, the mean sleep latency is usually <8 minutes but somewhat longer than that exhibited by patients with narcolepsy. In a recent meta-analysis, the mean sleep latency for patients with idiopathic hypersomnia was 6.2 ± 3.0 minutes.[63] Fewer than two SOREMPs are usually seen.

Patients with *behaviorally induced insufficient sleep syndrome* usually demonstrate mean sleep latency of <8 minutes with or without multiple SOREMPs. Consistent MSLT abnormalities have not been identified for patients with *recurrent hypersomnia, hypersomnia due to medical condition, hypersomnia due to drug or substance*, or the other primary hypersomnias.

A variant of the MSLT, called the *maintenance of wakefulness test (MWT)*, is used less commonly but may be useful in specific circumstances or mandated on occasion by certain employers (e.g., by airlines for pilots with sleep disorders). In this test, the patient is asked to try to remain awake for 40 minutes rather than to fall asleep within 20 minutes, lighting is kept dim rather than dark, and the patient is usually semireclined rather than recumbent.[63] These features are designed to test a patient's ability to stay awake rather than the ability to fall asleep. However, aside from the inherent face value of this modified test, data do not yet exist to show that the results of this test better predict functional outcomes than that of the MSLT. In fact, neither test has been well investigated in a prospective manner to show that results predict future motor vehicle crashes or other morbidity associated with sleepiness.

Specific *HLA haplotype* associations have been reported in patients with narcolepsy, but the associations are complex and of limited use in most clinical evaluations. The DQB1*0602 allele has been reported in most patients who have *narcolepsy with cataplexy*, half of patients who have *narcolepsy without cataplexy*, and also approximately 20% of the general population.[64–66] Because of the high prevalence of DQB1*0602 in healthy individuals, its presence in a patient usually cannot be used to support a diagnosis of narcolepsy. On occasion, absence of this allele in a patient with a questionable history of cataplexy may help conclude that narcolepsy is unlikely. In Kleine-Levin syndrome (*recurrent hypersomnia*), the DQB1*0201 has been reported with increased frequency,[30] with additional reports of increased frequency for the occurrence of Cw2 and DR11 alleles in familial cases.[52] Consistent HLA associations have not been identified for the other primary hypersomnias.

Measurement of *hypocretin-1 levels* in CSF represents a promising tool for the assessment of narcolepsy and primary hypersomnias. Deficiencies of hypocretin-1, a neuropeptide produced in the lateral hypothalamus, are strongly associated with *narcolepsy with cataplexy*, with levels <110 pg per mL being highly sensitive and specific for the diagnosis of this condition.[12,67,68] In contrast, low hypocretin-1 levels are identified in only 10% of patients having *narcolepsy without cataplexy* and in an unknown proportion of patients with *narcolepsy due to medical condition*. Although hypocretin-1 levels are normal in patients with *idiopathic hypersomnia*, it remains unknown whether alterations of hypocretin-1 metabolism are associated with other varieties of hypersomnia.

DIAGNOSIS

The ICSD-2 diagnostic criteria for narcolepsy and the hypersomnias are summarized in Table 4-2.

DIFFERENTIAL DIAGNOSIS

While evaluating a patient who presents with excessive sleepiness, the sleep history and, sometimes, a sleep diary are invaluable in formulation of the initial differential diagnosis. Even if a provisional diagnosis cannot be established by history alone, the patient's complaints often can be judged accurately to be secondary to insufficient sleep, extrinsically disrupted sleep, or a primary disorder of hypersomnolence. The PSG provides further screening, mainly for diagnostic patterns of abnormal breathing during sleep and sometimes for clues to other disorders such as narcolepsy, RLS, PLMD, nocturnal seizures, or some causes of insomnia. The MSLT further narrows the differential diagnosis

Table 4-2.   Summary of *International Classification of Sleep Disorders, Second Edition,* (ICSD-2) diagnostic criteria for narcolepsy and hypersomnias of central origin

1. Narcolepsy with cataplexy
    a. Excessive sleepiness is present almost daily for at least 3 mo
    b. Definite history of cataplexy
    c. Where possible, the diagnosis should be confirmed by nocturnal PSG documenting sufficient sleep ($\geq$6 h) followed by MSLT documenting mean sleep latency $\leq$8 min with two or more SOREMPs; alternative confirmation with CSF hypocretin-1 levels $\leq$110 pg/mL or one third of mean normal control values
    d. Hypersomnia is not better explained by other sleep, medical, neurologic, or psychiatric disorders
2. Narcolepsy without cataplexy
    a. Excessive sleepiness is present almost daily for at least 3 mo
    b. Typical cataplexy *not* present, but atypical or doubtful cataplexylike events may be reported
    c. Diagnosis *must* be confirmed by nocturnal PSG documenting sufficient sleep ($\geq$6 h) followed by MSLT documenting mean sleep latency $\leq$8 min with two or more SOREMPs
    d. Hypersomnia is not better explained by other sleep, medical, neurologic, or psychiatric disorders
3. Narcolepsy due to medical condition
    a. Excessive sleepiness is present almost daily for at least 3 mo
    b. One of the following is observed:
        i.   Definite history of cataplexy
        ii. If cataplexy is not present or is very atypical, nocturnal PSG documenting sufficient sleep ($\geq$6 h) followed by MSLT documenting mean sleep latency $\leq$8 min with two or more SOREMPs
        iii. CSF hypocretin-1 levels <110 pg/mL (or 30% of normal control values), provided the patient is not comatose
    c. A significant underlying neurologic or medical disorder accounts for the excessive sleepiness
    d. Hypersomnia is not better explained by other sleep, medical, neurologic, or psychiatric disorders
4. Narcolepsy, unspecified
    a. Patient meets clinical and MSLT criteria for diagnosis of narcolepsy but requires further evaluation to determine the most precise diagnostic classification
5. Recurrent hypersomnia (including Kleine-Levin syndrome and menstrual-related hypersomnia)
    a. Recurrent episodes of sleepiness with duration of 2 d to 4 wk
    b. Episodes recur at least once yearly

Table 4-2. *Continued*

---

    c. Alertness, cognition, and behavior are normal between episodes

    d. Hypersomnia is not better explained by other sleep, medical, neurologic, or psychiatric disorders

6. Idiopathic hypersomnia with long sleep time

    a. Excessive sleepiness is present almost daily for at least 3 mo

    b. Nocturnal sleep time is prolonged ($\geq$10 h), as documented by history, sleep log, or actigraphy; waking up is usually laborious

    c. Nocturnal PSG excludes other causes of sleepiness

    d. Nocturnal PSG shows short sleep latency and major sleep period $\geq$10 h in duration

    e. If MSLT is performed following overnight PSG, mean sleep latency is <8 min with less than two SOREMPs; mean sleep latency in idiopathic hypersomnia with long sleep time averages 6.2 ± 3.0 min

    f. Hypersomnia is not better explained by other sleep, medical, neurologic, or psychiatric disorders

7. Idiopathic hypersomnia without long sleep time

    a. Excessive sleepiness is present almost daily for at least 3 mo

    b. Nocturnal sleep is normal (>6 h and <10 h), as documented by history, sleep log, or actigraphy

    c. Nocturnal PSG excludes other causes of sleepiness

    d. MSLT performed following overnight PSG documents mean sleep latency <8 min with less than two SOREMPs. Mean sleep latency in idiopathic hypersomnia averages 6.2 ± 3.0 min

    e. Hypersomnia is not better explained by other sleep, medical, neurologic, or psychiatric disorders

8. Behaviorally induced insufficient sleep syndrome

    a. Excessive sleepiness is present almost daily for at least 3 mo; in prepubertal children, symptoms may consist of behavioral abnormalities suggesting sleepiness

    b. Sleep duration is less than expected for age, as documented by history, sleep log, or actigraphy

    c. Sleep duration lengthens considerably when habitual sleep schedule is not maintained (e.g., vacations or weekends)

    d. PSG and MSLT are not required for diagnosis; if performed, nocturnal PSG shows sleep latency <10 min and sleep efficiency >90% and MSLT shows mean sleep latency <8 min with or without SOREMPs

    e. Hypersomnia is not better explained by other sleep, medical, neurologic, or psychiatric disorders

9. Hypersomnia due to medical condition

    a. Excessive sleepiness is present almost daily for at least 3 mo

    b. A significant underlying neurologic or medical disorder accounts for the excessive sleepiness

---

(Continued)

Table 4-2.   *Continued*

    c. If MSLT is performed, mean sleep latency is <8 min with less than two SOREMPs following nocturnal PSG documenting sufficient sleep ≥ 6 h

    d. Hypersomnia is not better explained by other sleep, medical, neurologic, or psychiatric disorders

10. Hypersomnia due to drug or substance

    a. Complaint of sleepiness or excessive sleep is present

    b. Sleep-related complaint is believed to be secondary to current use, recent cessation, or prior prolonged use of drugs or prescribed medication

    c. Hypersomnia is not better explained by other sleep, medical, neurologic, or psychiatric disorders

11. Hypersomnia not due to substance or known physiologic condition (nonorganic hypersomnia, not otherwise specified)

    a. Complaint of sleepiness or excessive sleep is present

    b. The sleep complaint is temporally related to a psychiatric diagnosis

    c. Polysomnographic monitoring documents both:

        i. Diminished sleep efficiency with increased frequency and duration of awakenings on PSG

        ii. Variable but often normal mean sleep latency on MSLT

12. Physiologic (organic) hypersomnia, unspecified (organic hypersomnia, not otherwise specified)

    a. Excessive sleepiness is present almost daily for at least 3 mo

    b. MSLT documents mean sleep latency <8 min with less than two SOREMPs

    c. Sleep complaints are believed to be secondary to a physiologic condition

    d. Symptoms and testing do not meet criteria for other hypersomnolence syndromes

PSG, polysomnography; MSLT, multiple sleep latency test; SOREMPs, sleep-onset REM periods; CSF, cerebrospinal fluid.
Adapted from International Classification of Sleep Disorders. *Diagnostic and Coding Manual,* 2nd ed. Westchester: American Academy of Sleep Medicine; 2005. With permission.

with some objective quantification of the degree of sleepiness and demonstration of the presence or absence of SOREMPs—features necessary for appropriate classification of narcolepsy and many of the hypersomnias. Nevertheless, clinicians do encounter a minority of situations in which a precise diagnosis remains uncertain despite extensive clinical and diagnostic evaluation.

For patients with *narcolepsy*, the presence of definite cataplexy in some cases reliably distinguishes the condition from the other primary hypersomnias. Nondefinite cataplexy must be differentiated from other paroxysmal episodes such as near-syncope, atonic seizures, and behaviorally mediated spells. Likewise, hypnagogic or hypnopompic hallucinations must be distinguished from other hallucinatory conditions. Although the early stages of narcolepsy may resemble those of idiopathic hypersomnia, the presence of SOREMPs on the MSLT and the temporarily refreshing nature of naps in patients with narcolepsy help distinguish this condition from idiopathic hypersomnia.

The unusual presentation of *recurrent hypersomnia* may delay the diagnosis of the condition, particularly early in the course of the disorder when its cyclic nature may not yet be evident. Patients presenting with their first episode, or with particularly severe sleepiness and cognitive changes, must sometimes be evaluated for other organic causes of encephalopathy, including encephalitis, hypothalamic or third ventricular lesions, nonconvulsive status epilepticus, or migraine variant. Recurrent sleepiness resembling recurrent hypersomnia may also occur secondary to psychiatric disorders—particularly bipolar disorder and seasonal affective disorder—or due to intermittent sleep restriction.

The *idiopathic hypersomnias* also pose difficulties with respect to classification and differential diagnosis because the conditions may occur in the context of either normal or prolonged sleep times. The pervasive nature of the sleepiness for these conditions and the lack of refreshment from napping help distinguish them from narcolepsy. The sleepiness associated with the idiopathic hypersomnias may resemble that associated with OSA, PLMD, insufficient sleep, or hypersomnia due to medical condition, so care must be exercised in diagnosis. *Long sleepers*—patients who require much more than average amounts of sleep but function normally when they attain it—may resemble patients having *idiopathic hypersomnia without long sleep time* if they do not meet their lengthy sleep requirements.

The diagnosis of *behaviorally induced insufficient sleep syndrome* can usually be established clinically provided accurate estimation of nocturnal sleep time is available. Short sleep times and daytime somnolence also may occur in patients with primary or secondary insomnias, circadian rhythm disorder, or depression. Resolution of daytime sleepiness after lengthening of the nighttime sleep period helps distinguish insufficient sleep syndrome from these other conditions.

In *hypersomnia due to medical condition* and *hypersomnia due to drug or substance*, the cause of sleepiness is sometimes self-evident, but in other cases, a meticulous search for the underlying problem is required. A thorough medical history, medication review, inquiry about alcohol and drug use, and examination may be sufficient. Use of toxicology screens, thyroid levels, full EEG, brain imaging, or other ancillary testing may be helpful in specific circumstances but generally are not obtained on a routine basis.

Hypersomnia not due to substance or known physiologic condition often resembles idiopathic hypersomnia with long sleep time because lengthy nighttime sleep and excessive but unrefreshing daytime sleep is reported by patients in both conditions. Nocturnal PSG helps differentiate between the conditions, generally documenting shorter and less-efficient nighttime sleep than that exhibited by patients with hypersomnia. Likewise, the MSLT tends to show normal sleep latency that contrasts with the

Table 4-3. Medications commonly prescribed for sleepiness and cataplexy

Drug	Available Dosage Forms	Adult Starting Dose	Dosing Regimen	Adult Maintenance Dose	Potential Side Effects
Modafinil (Provigil)	100, 200 mg	100–200 mg q.d.	q.d.–b.i.d.	100–400 mg/d	Headache Nausea Syncope Arrhythmia
Methylphenidate (Ritalin)	5, 10, 20 mg	5–10 mg q.d.–b.i.d.	q.d.–t.i.d.	20–60 mg/d	Anorexia Weight loss Headache Tachycardia Arrhythmia Behavioral changes Seizures Dependence Abuse

| Methylphenidate extended release (Metadate CD) (Metadate ER) (Ritalin LA) (Ritalin SR) | 10, 20, 30 mg SR 10, 20 mg SR 20, 30, 40 mg SR 20 mg SR | 10–20 mg q.d. | q.d.–b.i.d. | 20–60 mg/d | Anorexia Weight loss Headache Tachycardia Arrhythmia Behavioral changes Seizures Dependence Abuse |
| Methylphenidate (Concerta) | 18, 27, 36, 54 mg SR | 18 mg q.d. | q.d. | 18–54 mg/d | Anorexia Weight loss Headache Tachycardia Arrhythmia Behavioral changes Seizures Dependence Abuse |

(Continued)

Table 4-3. *Continued*

Drug	Available Dosage Forms	Adult Starting Dose	Dosing Regimen	Adult Maintenance Dose	Potential Side Effects
Amphetamine/ dextroamphetamine (Adderall)	5, 7.5, 10, 12.5, 15, 20, 30 mg	10 mg q.d.	q.d.–b.i.d.	10–60 mg/d	Anorexia Weight loss Headache Tachycardia Arrhythmia Behavioral changes Hypertension Seizures Dependence Abuse
Amphetamine/ dextroamphetamine extended release (Adderall XR)	5, 10, 15, 20, 30 mg SR	10–20 mg q.d.	q.d.	1060 mg/d	Anorexia Weight loss Headache Tachycardia Arrhythmia Behavioral changes Hypertension Seizures Dependence Abuse

Dextroamphetamine (Dexedrine)	5 mg 5, 10, 15 mg SR	10 mg q.d.	10–60 mg/d	q.d.–b.i.d.	Anorexia Weight loss Headache Tachycardia Arrhythmia Behavioral changes Hypertension Seizures Dependence Abuse
Sodium oxybate (Xyrem)	2.25–4.5 g in 4.5–9.0 mL of fluid	2.25 g	2.25–4.5 g	Taken at bedtime and again 2–3 h later	Confusion Impaired waking Exacerbation of sleepwalking Hallucinations Psychosis Respiratory depression Abuse

severity of the subjective complaints. Symptoms of hypersomnia not due to substance or known physiologic condition may also resemble those of chronic fatigue syndrome or hypersomnia due to medical condition, but the presence of an associated psychiatric diagnosis helps distinguish between these conditions.

MANAGEMENT

Optimal management of sleepiness for patients with narcolepsy or other hypersomnia often requires multimodal treatment strategies that include behavioral interventions, lifestyle modification, and judicious use of wake-promoting medication.

Optimizing nighttime sleep is an important component of treatment for the sleepy patient. Treatable disruptors of nocturnal sleep such as insomnia, OSA, PLMD, or circadian rhythm disorders should be identified and treated. In patients without nocturnal sleep disorders, efforts to ensure adequate sleep length and good sleep hygiene may result in substantial improvements in daytime alertness.

Nonpharmacologic treatment is an appropriate next step in the treatment of several specific types of hypersomnia. *Behaviorally induced insufficient sleep syndrome* is treated by lengthening nighttime sleep rather than by administering wake-promoting medications. Sleepiness in *hypersomnia due to medical condition* and *hypersomnia due to drug or substance* often responds to treatment of the underlying condition. Similarly, *hypersomnia not due to substance or known physiologic condition* often improves when the underlying psychiatric disorder is controlled.

Planned daytime naps benefit some patients with hypersomnia. Patients with *narcolepsy* in particular often report that brief, regularly scheduled naps are refreshing and improve alertness for up to several hours. Naps for patients with *idiopathic hypersomnia* tend to be long, unrefreshing, and sometimes followed by great difficulty waking up. The effect of napping in the other primary hypersomnias is less predictable but occasionally may reduce the need for other interventions.

Wake-promoting medications usually play a central role in the treatment of patients with *narcolepsy* and *idiopathic hypersomnia*, especially when sleepiness is severe enough to impact the patient's job performance, education, quality of life, or safety. Commonly used agents are summarized in Table 4-3. In general, wake-promoting medications should be started at low dosage, with gradual upward titration over time to clinical effect, maximal safe dosage, or limiting side effects. Modafinil and long-acting stimulant preparations can sometimes be administered as a single daily dose, usually at the time of waking in the morning. Medications with short durations of action, or long-acting medications that nonetheless lose effectiveness in the afternoon, may require a second dosing at midday, or just before the period of worsening sleepiness. Care must be taken to ensure that use of late-day medication does not cause insomnia.

Psychostimulants such as methylphenidate and dextroamphetamine have been used to treat narcolepsy for more than 70 years.[69] Stimulants promote wakefulness because they facilitate the action of monoaminergic neurotransmitters, by enhanced release or inhibited reuptake, at the level of the synaptic cleft.

These compounds also facilitate peripheral release of norepinephrine, which increases sympathetic activity and accounts for many of the side effects seen with this class of medication.[70]

The relatively short half-lives of methylphenidate (3 to 6 hours) and dextroamphetamine (12 hours) often necessitate multiple daily doses, usually in the morning, at midday, and occasionally in the mid-afternoon as well. For the sustained-release forms of the psychostimulants (Table 4-3), a single morning dose may sometimes suffice.

Dextroamphetamine and methylphenidate are both thought to be effective in alleviating subjective and objective measures of daytime sleepiness, although large placebo-controlled trials have not been performed. Mean sleep latency on the MSLT may lengthen during treatment.[71] The extent to which treatment effects change or lose effectiveness with time remains uncertain, although it is the authors' experience that tachyphylaxis is occasionally observed in patients receiving long-term therapy.

Side effects of sympathomimetic agents include signs and symptoms of autonomic overactivity, including tachycardia, hypertension, palpitations, and insomnia. Other side effects may include headache, anorexia, or tremor. Psychiatric complications are observed in a minority of patients and may range from minimally altered mood to delusional or psychotic behavior.[69,70] Although psychostimulants in standard doses are usually well tolerated when used for an appropriate medical indication, dependence and addiction risks exists with these agents, so treatment must be carefully and appropriately monitored.

Modafinil is a nonstimulant, wake-promoting medication for which the mechanism of action is unknown. It may promote wakefulness with less risk of causing the sympathetic and autonomic side effects commonly exhibited by the psychostimulants. As a long-acting medication with a half-life of 15 hours, a single morningtime dose is sufficient for many patients.

Modafinil has been the subject of several large randomized, placebo-controlled trials among patients with *narcolepsy*. These studies showed significant improvement of subjective and objective measures of sleepiness during short-term use.[72,73] Modafinil was also reported to improve sleepiness in a small series of patients with *idiopathic hypersomnia*, although few data are available on its use in other varieties of hypersomnia.[74]

Side effects of modafinil are generally mild but may include headache, nausea, and nervousness. Cardiovascular side effects such as hypertension, tachycardia, and palpitations are occasionally encountered but considered uncommon.[75] Birth control pills may not retain adequate effectiveness when modafinil is used concurrently. Modafinil is thought to have less potential for abuse than the psychostimulants.[76]

Medication for cataplexy until recently consisted primarily of antidepressant agents of several classes, particularly the tricyclic agents and selective serotonin reuptake inhibitors. Its precise mechanism of action on cataplexy is unknown, although most agents augment monoaminergic neurotransmission and are potent suppressors of REM sleep. *Clomipramine, imipramine*, and *fluoxetine* represent the antidepressants most frequently reported in the treatment of cataplexy, and a detailed clinical review of their use is available.[77]

Sodium oxybate (GHB) is the first and only U.S. Food and Drug Administration (FDA)-approved medication for the treatment of cataplexy. Sustained improvement of cataplexy was demonstrated during long-term treatment.[78] In addition, a large double blind, placebo-controlled trial found significant improvements in self-reported sleepiness, nighttime waking, and sleep attacks in a dose-related manner.[79] The mechanism of action is not well understood, although the nocturnally administered compound binds strongly to GHB-specific receptors in the brain, increases slow-wave sleep, and improves sleep continuity.[80] Sodium oxybate has a short half-life of approximately 1 hour and is typically administered at bedtime, with a second dose later during the night to avoid rebound insomnia.

The strong and rapid sedative effect of sodium oxybate necessitates that it be administered only at bedtime and the second scheduled nighttime dose. The medication can potentially impair ability to awaken unexpectedly from sleep or cause residual sleepiness following premature waking. Common side effects include nausea, headache, dizziness, enuresis, and exacerbation of any preexisting sleepwalking.[79] More serious adverse events—including delirium, coma, respiratory depression, and death—at higher doses or in combination with alcoholare common when this drug is abused but is markedly rare or unobserved in patients who have been prescribed sodium oxybate for narcolepsy. Nonetheless, because of its notoriety as a drug of abuse, sodium oxybate is classified as a schedule III drug, requires close patient supervision and appropriate safety precautions to be taken, and is administered in the United States through a special centralized national pharmacy.

FOLLOW-UP

Clinical follow-up for patients with excessive sleepiness is strongly influenced by the nature of the specific diagnosis and the severity of symptoms. Patients with *hypersomnia due to drug or substance* or *hypersomnia not due to substance or known physiologic condition* do not always require long-term follow-up because treatment of the associated condition usually results in improvement of associated sleepiness. Intermittent follow-up is required for patients with *recurrent hypersomnia* and *hypersomnia due to medical condition* who exhibit chronic symptoms. Long-term clinical follow-up is usually required for patients with *narcolepsy* and *idiopathic hypersomnia*, chronic conditions that usually require ongoing management.

Regular clinical follow-up ensures that any new symptoms—for example, development of cataplexy in a patient previously exhibiting only excessive sleepiness—or worsening symptoms are reliably identified and treated. Follow-up assessments also allow assessment of medication compliance, provide monitoring for treatment-related side effects, and ensure optimal titration of treatment measures on the basis of the patient's present clinical status.

REFERENCES

1. Aldrich MS. Cardinal manifestations of sleep disorders. In: Kryger MH, Roth T, Dement WC, eds. *Principles and practice of sleep medicine*. Philadelphia, PA: WB Saunders; 1994:418–425.
2. Walters AS, Group TIRLSS. Toward a better definition of the restless legs syndrome. *Mov Disord*. 1996;10:634–642.
3. Rajaram SS, Walters AS, England SJ, et al. Some children with growing pains may actually have restless legs syndrome. *Sleep*. 2004;27(4):767–773.
4. Chervin RD. Periodic leg movements and sleepiness in patients evaluated for sleep-disordered breathing. *Am J Respir Crit Care Med*. 2001;164(8 Pt 1):1454–1458.
5. Karadeniz D, Ondze B, Besset A, et al. EEG arousals and awakenings in relation with periodic leg movements during sleep. *J Sleep Res*. 2000;9(3):273–277.
6. Takata K, Inoue Y, Hazama H, et al. Night-time hypnopompic visual hallucinations related to REM sleep disorder. *Psychiatry Clin Neurosci*. 1998;52(2):207–209.
7. Yorston GA, Gray R. Hypnopompic hallucinations with donepezil. *J Psychopharmacol*. 2000;14(3):303–304.
8. Buzzi G, Cirignotta F. Isolated sleep paralysis: A web survey. *Sleep Res Online*. 2000;3(2):61–66.
9. Overeem S, Mignot E, van Dijk JG, et al. Narcolepsy: Clinical features, new pathophysiologic insights, and future perspectives. *J Clin Neurophysiol*. 2001;18(2):78–105.
10. Dahlitz M, Parkes JD. Sleep paralysis. *Lancet*. 1993;341(8842):406–407.
11. Mahowald MW, Schenck CH. Dissociated states of wakefulness and sleep. *Neurology*. 1992;42(7 Suppl 6):44–51, discussion 52.
12. ICSD—International Classification of Sleep Disorders. *Diagnostic and coding manual*, 2nd ed. Westchester: American Academy of Sleep Medicine; 2005.
13. Oka Y, Kanbayashi T, Mezaki T, et al. Low CSF hypocretin-1/orexin-A associated with hypersomnia secondary to hypothalamic lesion in a case of multiple sclerosis. *J Neurol*. 2004;251(7):885–886.
14. Fenzi F, Simonati A, Crosato F, et al. Clinical features of Kleine-Levin syndrome with localized encephalitis. *Neuropediatrics*. 1993;24(5):292–295.
15. Skjodt NM, Atkar R, Easton PA. Screening for hypothyroidism in sleep apnea. *Am J Respir Crit Care Med*. 1999;160(2):732–735.
16. Happe S. Excessive daytime sleepiness and sleep disturbances in patients with neurological diseases: Epidemiology and management. *Drugs*. 2003;63(24):2725–2737.
17. Douglass AB. Narcolepsy: Differential diagnosis or etiology in some cases of bipolar disorder and schizophrenia? *CNS Spectr*. 2003;8(2):120–126.
18. Fernandes PP, Petty F. Modafinil for remitted bipolar depression with hypersomnia. *Ann Pharmacother*. 2003;37(12):1807–1809.
19. Mignot E. Sleep, sleep disorders and hypocretin (orexin). *Sleep Med*. 2004;5(Suppl 1):S2–S8.
20. Kanbayashi T, Inoue Y, Chiba S, et al. CSF hypocretin-1 (orexin-A) concentrations in narcolepsy with and without cataplexy and idiopathic hypersomnia. [see comment]. *J Sleep Res*. 2002;11(1):91–93.

21. Kanbayashi T, Abe M, Fujimoto S, et al. Hypocretin deficiency in Niemann-Pick type C with cataplexy. *Neuropediatrics*. 2003;34(1):52–53.

22. Tobias ES, Tolmie JL, Stephenson JB. Cataplexy in the Prader-Willi syndrome. *Arch Dis Child*. 2002;87(2):170.

23. Nelson GB, Hahn JS. Stimulus-induced drop episodes in Coffin-Lowry syndrome. *Pediatrics*. 2003;111(3):e197–e202.

24. Marcus CL, Trescher WH, Halbower AC, et al. Secondary narcolepsy in children with brain tumors. [see comment]. *Sleep*. 2002;25(4):435–439.

25. Aldrich MS, Naylor MW. Narcolepsy associated with lesions of the diencephalon. *Neurology*. 1989;39(11):1505–1508.

26. Gledhill RF, Bartel PR, Yoshida Y, et al. Narcolepsy caused by acute disseminated encephalomyelitis. *Arch Neurol*. 2004;61(5):758–760.

27. Melberg A, Hetta J, Dahl N, et al. Autosomal dominant cerebellar ataxia deafness and narcolepsy. *J Neurol Sci*. 1995;134(1–2):119–129.

28. Bruck D, Broughton RJ. Diagnostic ambiguities in a case of post-traumatic narcolepsy with cataplexy. *Brain Inj*. 2004;18(3):321–326.

29. Gadoth N, Kesler A, Vainstein G, et al. Clinical and polysomnographic characteristics of 34 patients with Kleine-Levin syndrome. *J Sleep Res*. 2001;10(4):337–341.

30. Dauvilliers Y, Mayer G, Lecendreux M, et al. Kleine-Levin syndrome: An autoimmune hypothesis based on clinical and genetic analyses. *Neurology*. 2002;59(11):1739–1745.

31. Bassetti C, Aldrich MS. Idiopathic hypersomnia. A series of 42 patients. *Brain*. 1997;120(Pt 8):1423–1435.

32. Black JE, Brooks SN, Nishino S. Narcolepsy and syndromes of primary excessive daytime somnolence. *Semin Neurol*. 2004;24(3):271–282.

33. Bruck D, Parkes JD. A comparison of idiopathic hypersomnia and narcolepsy-cataplexy using self report measures and sleep diary data. *J Neurol Neurosurg Psychiatry*. 1996;60(5):576–578.

34. Scammell TE, Nishino S, Mignot E, et al. Narcolepsy and low CSF orexin (hypocretin) concentration after a diencephalic stroke. [see comment]. *Neurology*. 2001;56(12):1751–1753.

35. Korner Y, Meindorfner C, Moller JC, et al. Predictors of sudden onset of sleep in Parkinson's disease. *Mov Disord*. 2004;19(11):1298–1305.

36. Overeem S, Van Hilten J, Ripley B, et al. Normal hypocretin-1 levels in Parkinson's disease patients with excessive daytime sleepiness. *Neurology*. 2002;58:489–499.

37. Laberge L, Begin P, Montplaisir J, et al. Sleep complaints in patients with myotonic dystrophy. *J Sleep Res*. 2004;13(1):95–100.

38. Helbing-Zwanenburg B, Kamphuisen HA, Mourtazaev MS. The origin of excessive daytime sleepiness in the Prader-Willi syndrome. *J Intellect Disabil Res*. 1993;37(Pt 6):533–541.

39. Schweitzer P. Drugs that disturb sleep and wakefulness. In: Kryger M, Roth T, Dement W, eds. *Principles and practice of sleep medicine*, 3rd ed. Philadelphia, PA: WB Saunders; 2000:1176–1196.

40. Vgontzas AN, Bixler EO, Kales A, et al. Differences in nocturnal and daytime sleep between primary and psychiatric hypersomnia: Diagnostic and treatment implications. *Psychosom Med.* 2000;62(2):220–226.

41. Billiard M, Dolenc L, Aldaz C, et al. Hypersomnia associated with mood disorders: A new perspective. *J Psychosom Res.* 1994;38(Suppl 1):41–47.

42. National Sleep Foundation. *2002 "Sleep in America" Poll.* Washington, DC: National Sleep Foundation; 2002.

43. Hays JC, Blazer DG, Foley DJ. Risk of napping: Excessive daytime sleepiness and mortality in an older community population. [see comment]. *J Am Geriatr Soc.* 1996;44(6):693–698.

44. Ohida T, Osaki Y, Doi Y, et al. An epidemiologic study of self-reported sleep problems among Japanese adolescents. *Sleep.* 2004;27(5):978–985.

45. Howard ME, Desai AV, Grunstein RR, et al. Sleepiness, sleep-disordered breathing, and accident risk factors in commercial vehicle drivers. [see comment]. *Am J Respir Crit Care Med.* 2004;170(9):1014–1021.

46. Wilner A, Steinman L, Lavie P, et al. Narcolepsy-cataplexy in Israeli Jews is associated exclusively with the HLA DR2 haplotype. A study at the serological and genomic level. *Hum Immunol.* 1988;21(1):15–22.

47. Wing YK, Li RH, Lam CW, et al. The prevalence of narcolepsy among Chinese in Hong Kong. *Ann Neurol.* 2002;51(5):578–584.

48. Lavie P, Peled R. Narcolepsy is a rare disease in Israel. *Sleep.* 1987;10(6):608–609.

49. Silber MH, Krahn LE, Olson EJ, et al. The epidemiology of narcolepsy in Olmsted County, Minnesota: A population-based study. *Sleep.* 2002;25(2):197–202.

50. Poppe M, Friebel D, Reuner U, et al. The Kleine-Levin syndrome—effects of treatment with lithium. *Neuropediatrics.* 2003;34(3):113–119.

51. Papacostas SS, Hadjivasilis V. The Kleine-Levin syndrome. Report of a case and review of the literature. *Eur Psychiatry: J Assoc Eur Psychiatr.* 2000;15(4):231–235.

52. Montplaisir J, Poirier G. HLA in disorders of excessive sleepiness without cataplexy in Canada. In: Honda Y, Juji T, eds. *HLA in narcolepsy.* Berlin, Germany: Springer-Verlag; 1988:186.

53. Johns MW. A new method for measuring daytime sleepiness: The Epworth sleepiness scale. *Sleep.* 1991;14(6):540–545.

54. Chervin RD, Aldrich MS. The Epworth sleepiness scale may not reflect objective measures of sleepiness or sleep apnea. *Neurology.* 1999;52(1):125–131.

55. Hoddes E, Dement W, Zarcone V. The development and use of the Stanford Sleepiness Scale (SSS). *Psychophysiology.* 1972;9:150.

56. Douglass AB, Bornstein R, Nino-Murcia G, et al. The sleep disorders questionnaire. I: Creation and multivariate structure of SDQ. *Sleep.* 1994;17(2):160–167.

57. Netzer NC, Stoohs RA, Netzer CM, et al. Using the Berlin questionnaire to identify patients at risk for the sleep apnea syndrome. [see comment]. *Ann Intern Med.* 1999;131(7):485–491.

58. Weaver TE, Laizner AM, Evans LK, et al. An instrument to measure functional status outcomes for disorders of excessive sleepiness. *Sleep.* 1997;20(10):835–843.

59. Moyer C, Sonad S, Garetz S, et al. Quality of life in obstructive sleep apnea: A systematic review of the literature. *Sleep Med.* 2001;3:477–491.

60. Aldrich MS, Chervin RD, Malow BA. Value of the Multiple Sleep Latency Test (MSLT) for the diagnosis of narcolepsy. *Sleep.* 1997;20(8):620–629.

61. Chervin RD, Aldrich MS. Sleep onset REM periods during multiple sleep latency tests in patients evaluated for sleep apnea. *Am J Respir Crit Care Med.* 2000;161(2 Pt 1):426–431.

62. Hoban TF, Chervin RD. Assessment of sleepiness in children. *Semin Pediatr Neurol.* 2001;8(4):216–228.

63. Littner MR, Kushida C, Wise M, et al. Practice parameters for clinical use of the multiple sleep latency test and the maintenance of wakefulness test. [see comment]. *Sleep.* 2005;28(1):113–121.

64. Rogers AE, Meehan J, Guilleminault C, et al. HLA DR15 (DR2) and DQB1*0602 typing studies in 188 narcoleptic patients with cataplexy. *Neurology.* 1997;48(6):1550–1556.

65. Mignot E, Hayduk R, Black J, et al. HLA DQB1*0602 is associated with cataplexy in 509 narcoleptic patients. *Sleep.* 1997;20(11):1012–1020.

66. Mignot E, Young T, Lin L, et al. Nocturnal sleep and daytime sleepiness in normal subjects with HLA-DQB1*0602. *Sleep.* 1999;22(3):347–352.

67. Krahn LE, Pankratz VS, Oliver L, et al. Hypocretin (orexin) levels in cerebrospinal fluid of patients with narcolepsy: Relationship to cataplexy and HLA DQB1*0602 status. *Sleep.* 2002;25(7):733–736.

68. Mignot E, Lammers GJ, Ripley B, et al. The role of cerebrospinal fluid hypocretin measurement in the diagnosis of narcolepsy and other hypersomnias. *Arch Neurol.* 2002;59(10):1553–1562.

69. Nishino S, Mignot E. Pharmacological aspects of human and canine narcolepsy. *Prog Neurobiol.* 1997;52(1):27–78.

70. Banerjee D, Vitiello MV, Grunstein RR. Pharmacotherapy for excessive daytime sleepiness. *Sleep Med Rev.* 2004;8(5):339–354.

71. Mitler MM, Hajdukovic R, Erman MK. Treatment of narcolepsy with methamphetamine. *Sleep.* 1993;16(4):306–317.

72. US Modafinil in Narcolepsy Multicenter Study Group. Randomized trial of modafinil for the treatment of pathological somnolence in narcolepsy. US Modafinil in Narcolepsy Multicenter Study Group. *Ann Neurol.* 1998;43(1):88–97.

73. US Modafinil in Narcolepsy Multicenter Study Group. Randomized trial of modafinil as a treatment for the excessive daytime somnolence of narcolepsy: US Modafinil in Narcolepsy Multicenter Study Group. *Neurology.* 2000;54(5):1166–1175.

74. Bastuji H, Jouvet M. Successful treatment of idiopathic hypersomnia and narcolepsy with modafinil. *Prog Neuropsychopharmacol Biol Psychiatry.* 1988;12(5):695–700.

75. Schwartz JR, Feldman NT, Fry JM, et al. Efficacy and safety of modafinil for improving daytime wakefulness in patients treated previously with psychostimulants. *Sleep Med.* 2003;4(1):43–49.

76. Jasinski DR, Kovacevic-Ristanovic R. Evaluation of the abuse liability of modafinil and other drugs for excessive daytime sleepiness associated with narcolepsy. *Clin Neuropharmacol.* 2000;23(3):149–156.

77. Houghton WC, Scammell TE, Thorpy M. Pharmacotherapy for cataplexy. *Sleep Med Rev*. 2004;8(5):355–366.
78. Group USXMS. Sodium oxybate demonstrates long-term efficacy for the treatment of cataplexy in patients with narcolepsy. *Sleep Med*. 2004;5(2):119–123.
79. A randomized, double blind, placebo-controlled multicenter trial comparing the effects of three doses of orally administered sodium oxybate with placebo for the treatment of narcolepsy. *Sleep*. 2002;25(1):42–49.
80. Scammell TE. The neurobiology, diagnosis, and treatment of narcolepsy. *Ann Neurol*. 2003;53(2):154–166.

5

Motor Disorders of Sleep and Parasomnias

Alon Y. Avidan

Motor disorders of sleep encompass a variety of conditions disrupting sleep and contributing to insomnia and hypersomnia. This chapter addresses the parasomnias (e.g., sleepwalking and rapid eye movement–sleep behavior disorder [RBD]), sleep-related movement disorders (e.g., restless legs syndrome [RLS] and periodic limb movement disorder [PLMD]), and a variety of other conditions that manifest as motor disorders during sleep (e.g., hypnic jerks and nocturnal paroxysmal dystonia [NPD]). Discussion of each disorder begins with epidemiology, clinical manifestations, and diagnostic evaluations and concludes with specific management.

An algorithm for the workup of motor disorders of sleep is provided in Appendix I.

PARASOMNIAS

Parasomnias are undesirable nondeliberate motor or subjective phenomena that take place during transition from wakefulness to sleep or during arousals from sleep.[1–4] Although initially thought to represent a unitary phenomenon, often attributed to behavioral or psychiatric disorders, it is now evident that parasomnias are not a unitary phenomenon but rather the manifestation of a wide variety of completely different conditions, most of which are readily explainable, diagnosable, and treatable.[4–9] Parasomnias may include abnormal movements, behaviors, emotions, and autonomic activity[2] and may be manifestations of central nervous system (CNS) activation. Parasomnias are subdivided into arousal disorders, parasomnias usually associated with rapid eye movement (REM) sleep, and other parasomnias. The most common explanation for parasomnias is that sleep and wakefulness are not mutually exclusive states and the overlap or intrusion of these states into one another causes these abnormalities.[4,5,10] Intrusion of wakefulness into non-REM (NREM) sleep produces arousal disorders, and intrusion of wakefulness into REM sleep produces REM-sleep parasomnias such as RBD.[5,10]

The *International Classification of Sleep Disorders, second edition (ICSD-2)* lists 15 types of parasomnias[11] categorized as disorders of arousal from NREM sleep (confusional arousals, sleepwalking, sleep terrors), parasomnias associated with REM sleep (RBD, recurrent isolated sleep paralysis, and nightmare disorder) and other parasomnias (sleep enuresis, sleep-related eating disorder, and several others that are not addressed here).

Table 5-1 summarizes the key features of these parasomnias with regard to treatment, semiology, and sleep-stage propensity.

Disorders of Arousal

The arousal disorders are classified together because they have a common underlying pathophysiology postulated to involve impaired arousal from sleep. The onset of these disorders in slow-wave sleep (SWS) is the most typical feature. Given that SWS predominates the first third of the sleep cycle, these disorders are more prevalent in the beginning of the night and are common in childhood—usually decreasing in frequency with increasing age.[12,13] Arousal disorders may be triggered by a variety of conditions including fever, alcohol, sleep deprivation, emotional stress, or medications. These precipitators should be viewed as triggering events rather than causal agents in susceptible individuals. A variety of primary sleep disorders such as PLMD, nocturnal epilepsy, or obstructive sleep apneas (OSAs) may also provoke disorders of arousal.[14]

Confusional Arousals

EPIDEMIOLOGY.   Confusional arousal is almost universal in children <5 years of age and is less common in older children. A strong familial pattern exists in the cases of idiopathic confusional arousal. The prevalence of confusional arousal in adults is approximately 4%.[15]

CLINICAL MANIFESTATIONS.   Confusional arousal is associated with confusion and disorientation during and following arousals from sleep, typically during SWS in the first part of the night.[16–18] Patients may exhibit inappropriate behaviors (talking nonsense), have decreased mentation, and respond poorly and slowly to commands or questioning. In children, confusional arousals are characterized by movements in bed, and sometimes thrashing about, or inconsolable crying.[19] Retrograde and anterograde amnesia is present. The confusional behavior generally lasts a few minutes but can be as long as several hours. Confusional arousal can be precipitated by forced awakenings, mainly in the first third of the night. The course of the childhood form is usually benign. The underlying etiology may be related to recovery from sleep deprivation, the presence of circadian rhythm sleep disorders (shift work, jet lag, etc.), the use of CNS depressants (i.e., hypnotics, sedatives, tranquilizers, alcohol, and antihistamines), and the presence of underlying metabolic, hepatic, renal, and toxic encephalopathies. Confusional arousals are often seen in hypersomnias characterized by deep sleep, such as idiopathic hypersomnia, as well as in narcolepsy or OSA. Episodes of confusional arousal are frequent in patients with sleep terror and sleepwalking. Organic causes of confusional arousal are rare but may include lesions in arousal generators, such as the periventricular gray, the midbrain reticular area, and the posterior hypothalamus.

DIAGNOSTIC EVALUATION.   Polysomnographic (PSG) recordings during the episodes demonstrate arousals from SWS, most commonly during the first third of the night. Electroencephalogram (EEG) monitoring during the spell may show brief episodes of delta activity, stage-1 theta patterns, repeated microsleep, or a diffuse and poorly reactive alpha rhythm.

Table 5-1. Differential diagnosis of nocturnal spells

	Confusional Arousals	Sleepwalking (Somnambulism)	Nightmares	REM-Sleep Behavior Disorder
Stage of sleep	First third of night and during SWS	First third of night and SWS	Second half of night, during REM sleep, and also during NREM	REM sleep
Spell symptoms	Sudden arousal, confusion, disorientation, inappropriate behavior	Automatisms, getting out of bed, walking	Sudden awakening with anxiety and dream recall	Talking, arm movements, kicking, punching
Duration	s–10 min	1–5 min, 30–60 min (rare)	5–15 min	s to 20–30 min
Postspell symptoms	No recall of event	Confusion, amnesia about the event, recall is rare	Vivid recall of a frightening dream	Detailed recall of an active dream with theme of violence
EEG pattern during spell	Slow-wave activity, microsleep, poorly reactive alpha rhythm	Transition from SWS to stage 1, diffuse and slow alpha high-amplitude delta bursts	Increased eye movements during REM	REM sleep

Pathophysiology	Incomplete awakening from SWS	Predisposing psychopathology, sleep deprivation, alcohol, strong sleep pressure	Precipitated by daytime stress, drugs (β-blockers), psychopathology	Loss of muscle atonia, pontine/CNS lesions, stress, Parkinson disease
Potential treatments	Relaxation techniques, avoidance of stress	Avoid injury, protect patient, avoid precipitating factors, hypnosis psychotherapy, benzodiazepines, tricyclic antidepressants	Address underlying psychiatric illness, avoid stress, psychotherapy, improve sleep hygiene, rarely REM suppressants	Clonazepam, levodopa–carbidopa, diazepam

SWS, slow-wave sleep; CNS, central nervous system; REM, rapid eye movement; NREM, non-rapid eye movement; EEG, electroencephalogram. From Avidan AY. Sleep in the older person. In: Sirven JI, Malamut BL, eds. *Clinical neurology of the older adult.* Philadelphia, PA: Lippincott Williams & Wilkins; 2002:158–175. With permission.

DIFFERENTIAL DIAGNOSIS.   It is essential to differentiate confusional arousal from other parasomnias in which mental confusion occurs during the sleep period

1. *Sleep terrors*: are differentiated by symptoms of acute autonomic hyperarousal and fear.
2. *Sleepwalking*: includes ambulation and complex motor automatisms.
3. *RBD*: consists of dream enactment and complex movements such as fighting and punching while asleep.
4. *Sleep-related epileptic seizures of the partial complex type with confusional automatisms*: are rare, diurnal, and associated with an epileptic EEG pattern.

MANAGEMENT.   Nonpharmacotherapy includes avoidance of irregular sleep–wake schedule patterns, limiting exposure to CNS depressants, and managing coexisting sleep disorders. Efforts to control the patient's behavior during an episode of confusional arousal should be avoided because these may lead to aggression and prolongation of the spell. The episode of confusional arousal should simply be allowed to run its course, unless there is a potential for injury such as an attempt to walk. Pharmacologic treatment is rarely necessary because most episodes remit with age. Some patients respond to tricyclic antidepressants (TCAs) such as clomipramine.

Sleepwalking (Somnambulism)

EPIDEMIOLOGY.   The prevalence of sleepwalking in the general population is between 1% and 17%. It is common in children aged between 4 and 8 years and is far more common in adults (approximately 4%) than is generally acknowledged.[15,20] Sleepwalking can occur as soon as the child is able to walk.

CLINICAL MANIFESTATIONS.   Sleepwalking consists of complex behaviors during SWS that result in walking during sleep. Sleepwalking can range from simple sitting up in bed to walking and, rarely, to "escape" when severe. On waking up, the patient is sometimes confused and amnestic about the events during the episode. Sleepwalking can occur several times a week or only when precipitating factors are present.[4,10] Sleepwalking may include inappropriate behavior and may result in falls and injuries during attempts to "escape" or when walking into dangerous situations (i.e., walking out through a window). Other parasomnia, such as sleep terrors, can coexist as a "hybrid" in sleepwalking.

Precipitating factors include the use of medications, such as thioridazine hydrochloride, chloral hydrate, and desipramine. Sleep deprivation and fever can induce sleepwalking episodes. Underlying disorders such as OSA may produce severe SWS disruption and can yield sleepwalking spells. Internal stimuli, such as a full bladder, or external stimuli, such as outside noises, can also precipitate episodes.

DIAGNOSTIC EVALUATION.   Sleepwalking originates from SWS and is common during the first third of the night or during times of SWS rebound, such as after sleep deprivation. The PSG shows that sleepwalking begins during SWS, most commonly toward the end of the first or second episode of SWS. The EEG is normal.

DIFFERENTIAL DIAGNOSIS.

1. *Sleep terrors*: are differentiated in that they are often associated with an attempt to "escape" from the terrifying stimulus, and the patients have an associated autonomic hyperarousal such as fear and panic coupled with a scream.
2. *RBD*: is characterized on the basis of the PSG, demonstrating episodes of complex dream enactment during REM sleep.
3. *Sleep-related epilepsy with ambulatory automatism*: can be distinguished by an epileptiform EEG.
4. *Nocturnal eating syndrome*: is characterized by ambulatory behavior of eating.

   MANAGEMENT. Sleepwalking is treated by avoiding the precipitating factors and establishing a safe living quadrant (i.e., removing sharp objects from the bedroom, locking doors, and arranging for a sleeping space on the ground floor). Anticipatory awakening has been studied for treating this disorder in children.[21] When spells are severe and refractory or dangerous to the patients and others, medications such as TCAs or benzodiazepines may be administered.[2,22,23]

Sleep Terrors

   EPIDEMIOLOGY. The prevalence of sleep terror is approximately 3% in children aged between 4 and 12 years. Sleep terror can occur at any age but are most common in prepubertal children. In adults, they are much more prevalent than is generally acknowledged (4% to 5%)[24] and is most common in individuals aged between 20 and 30 years, with a predisposition in men compared to women. They can occur in several members of a family.

   CLINICAL PRESENTATION. Sleep terror is the most dramatic disorder of arousal. It is characterized by a sudden arousal from SWS with a piercing scream or cry and extreme panic, accompanied by severe autonomic discharge (i.e., tachycardia, tachypnea, diaphoresis, mydriasis, and increased muscle tone) and behavioral manifestations of intense fear. During a typical spell, the patient sits in bed, is unresponsive to external stimuli, and, if awakened, is disoriented and confused. The episodes are sometimes followed by prominent motor activity such as hitting the wall and running around or out of the bedroom, even out of the house—resulting in bodily injury or property damage.[4,25,26] Sleep terrors are characterized by amnesia about the episode, which may be incomplete, accompanied by incoherent vocalizations.[27] Sometimes, attempts to escape from bed or to fight can result in harm to the patient or parents responding to him/her. Mental evaluations of adults indicate that psychopathology may be associated with sleep terror. The episodes of sleep terror may become violent and may result in considerable injury to the patient and bed partners—at times with forensic implications.[28,29] Psychopathology is rare in affected children but may play a role in adult patients. Sleep terror typically resolves spontaneously during adolescence. Precipitating factors include fever, sleep deprivation, or the use of CNS-depressant medications.

   DIAGNOSTIC EVALUATION. The PSG shows sleep terror episodes emanating out of SWS, usually in the first third of the major sleep episode. However, episodes can occur in SWS at any time. The recordings demonstrate episodes of tachycardia and other signs of increased sympathetic activation. Differentiating between sleep terror and sleep-related epilepsy (temporal-lobe epilepsy) is sometimes difficult, and the use of an EEG with nasopharyngeal leads may be helpful.

DIFFERENTIAL DIAGNOSIS.

1. *Nightmares*: differentiation of sleep terror from nightmare is most important. Sleep terror is characterized by amnesia about the event compared to the vivid recollection in case of nightmares. Nightmares also occur during the last third of the night but, unlike sleep terror, are confined to REM sleep. Associated with a vivid recollection and normal cognition, nightmares usually lack the sympathetic activation and confusion that is frequent with sleep terror.
2. *Confusional arousals*: are awakenings from SWS without terror or ambulation.
3. Sleep-related epilepsy
4. OSA
5. Nocturnal cardiac ischemia.

MANAGEMENT. Treatment is often unnecessary when episodes are rare. However, when the episodes are frequent, intense, or disruptive to the patient's sleep, a short-acting benzodiazepine may be used in low doses during the night. Examples include diazepam, which may act by suppressing the autonomic excitability that accompanies sleep terror during SWS and also by reducing the time spent in SWS. Paroxetine and trazodone have been reported to be effective in isolated cases.[30,31] Other treatment options include clonazepam and TCA.[22] Adult patients with a history of a psychiatric disorder may benefit from psychotherapy and stress reduction, as well as reassurance.[5,32]

Parasomnias Usually Associated with Rapid Eye Movement Sleep

As the name implies, parasomnias usually associated with REM sleep typically are associated with the REM-sleep stage. They are grouped together because some common underlying pathophysiologic mechanism related to REM sleep possibly underlies these disorders.

Nightmares

EPIDEMIOLOGY. There is no definite agreement between studies as to the frequency of nightmares in the general population. Apparently, 10% to 50% of children aged 3 to 5 years have clinically significant nightmares that disturb their parents. Up to 75% of these children can remember at least one or a few nightmares in the course of their childhood. About half of the adults admit to having an occasional nightmare. Approximately 1% of the adult population is afflicted with frequent nightmares, with an occurrence of one or more incidence per week.

CLINICAL MANIFESTATIONS. Nightmare typically consists of a long, complicated dream pattern that becomes increasingly frightening toward the end, causing patients to arouse from REM sleep. The vivid dreamlike feature is an essential feature in distinguishing this from sleep terror. Recall is common and may occur during the arousals or at a later time. Some personality characteristics such as schizotypal personality, borderline personality disorder, schizoid personality disorder, or schizophrenia appear to have a unique predisposition to nightmare, and patients with frequent spells can be vulnerable to mental illness. Adult patients have been labeled as having *artistic or other creative inclinations*. Nightmares may increase in frequency during times of stress, particularly following traumatic events. Medications such as levodopa (and related drugs) and β-adrenergic blockers and abrupt withdrawal of REM-suppressant medications precipitate nightmares. The episodes usually start at 3 to 6 years of age but can occur at any age. Whereas in children, the sex ratio is equal, in adults there is a ratio of 2:1 to 4:1 favoring women.

DIAGNOSTIC EVALUATION. The PSG shows an abrupt awakening from REM sleep, typically lasting 10 minutes, with an associated increased REM-sleep density associated with variability in heart and respiratory rates. The spells may also be encountered in NREM sleep, especially stage 2, following traumatic events.

DIFFERENTIAL DIAGNOSIS.

1. *Sleep terrors*: unlike nightmares rarely have dream content, occur later during the night, and do not have autonomic hyperarousal. The utility of PSG is somewhat low in the laboratory confirmation of nightmares because their occurrence in the sleep laboratory is lower than that at home.
2. *RBD*: is distinguished by explosive complex-movement activity during REM sleep and is more common in elderly patients.

MANAGEMENT. Treatment of nightmares is often in the form of reassurance because the episodes seem to diminish in frequency and intensity over the course of the patient's lifespan. However, for severe and refractory cases, the use of REM-suppressing agents such as TCA or selective serotonin reuptake inhibitors (SSRIs) for a short period may be helpful.[32–34]

Recurrent Isolated Sleep Paralysis

EPIDEMIOLOGY. Sleep paralysis occurs at least once in a lifetime in 40% to 50% of healthy subjects. It is far less common as a chronic complaint. Surveys of healthy subjects have indicated that sleep paralysis occurred in 3% to 6% of respondents, many of whom had rare episodes. Among patients with narcolepsy, 17% to 40% have reported to have sleep paralysis.

CLINICAL MANIFESTATIONS. Sleep paralysis is associated with the inability to perform voluntary motor function at sleep onset (hypnagogic or predormital form) or on awakening (hypnopompic or postdormital form). Movements of the skeletal muscles of the limbs, trunk, and head are not possible, although ocular and respiratory movements remain intact. Cognition is intact, and patients often report that the episode is very frightening, especially if there is respiratory compromise. Hypnagogic imagery may be present and is often threatening, adding to the individual's discomfort. Sleep paralysis lasts 1 to a few minutes and may be aborted spontaneously or on external stimulation (touch by another person or when the patient performs vigorous eye movements). Sleep paralysis occurs as an isolated episode in healthy subjects (upon awakening), as a genetically transmitted familial disorder (at sleep onset), and as one of the classic tetrad of the narcolepsy syndrome. Precipitating factors include sleep deprivation and disturbances of the sleep–wake cycle. Isolated sleep paralysis can occur during periods of jet lag, shift work, and mental stress. Episodes typically begin in adolescence and show no sexual predominance. The underlying pathology is probably related to dysfunction in the mechanism controlling the normal motor paralysis of the REM state.

DIAGNOSTIC EVALUATION.   PSG performed during episodes of sleep paralysis demonstrate suppression of the electromyogram (EMG) tone associated with an EEG pattern of wakefulness and the presence of eye movement and blink patterns in the electrooculogram that is typical of the wake state. Formal polysomnography and a multiple sleep latency test can be important when sleep paralysis has to be differentiated from narcolepsy.

Histocompatibility testing for the DQB1*0602 antigen may be helpful in cases suspicious for narcolepsy without cataplexy.

DIFFERENTIAL DIAGNOSIS.

1. *Narcolepsy*: in which severe excessive daytime sleepiness (EDS), cataplexy, and often vivid hypnagogic hallucinations occur, should be readily distinguishable from sleep paralysis. Cataplexy is differentiated by precipitation by emotional stimuli.

2. *Hysterical paralysis and catatonia*: must be distinguished from sleep paralysis but are usually evident by their associated clinical features.

3. *Atonic generalized epileptic seizures*: can be differentiated by their usual occurrence in the daytime waking state.

4. *Atonic drop attacks*: occur in patients with vertebrobasilar vascular insufficiency, are more common in older patients during wakefulness, lacks a precipitating event (other than orthostatic hypotension), and is unrelated to sleep–wake transitions.

5. *Peripheral-nerve compression*: arises from an unusual sleeping posture ("saturday-night palsy") and may be confused with sleep paralysis but are generally localized to a specific limb paresis.

6. *Hypokalemic periodic paralysis*: is associated with low serum potassium levels during attacks and last hours or even days. The disorder can be provoked by the ingestion of high-carbohydrate meals or alcohol and is reversible by correcting the hypokalemia.

MANAGEMENT.   When the episodes are infrequent, treatment of sleep paralysis is unnecessary. In most cases, reassurance is all that is needed. Avoidance of precipitating factors such as irregular sleep habits and disturbances of the sleep–wake cycle will reduce the frequency of sleep paralysis. When sleep paralysis is severe and anxiety provoking, the use of anxiolytic medications may be indicated. Frequent episodes of sleep paralysis in the presence of narcolepsy can be treated with stimulants.[35]

Rapid Eye Movement Sleep Behavior Disorder

EPIDEMIOLOGY. The overall prevalence of violent behaviors during sleep is estimated at 2% on the basis of a recent phone survey of >4,900 individuals aged between 15 and 100 years. Of these behaviors, one fourth were probably due to RBD, giving an overall prevalence of 0.5% for the disorder.[36] Important demographic features of RBD include the predilection to affect men (approximately 90%) and the highest incidence after the age of 50 years. Subjective reports indicate that one fourth of patients with Parkinson disease have dream enactment behaviors suggestive of RBD, and studies utilizing PSG found RBD in up to 47% of patients with Parkinson disease with sleep complaints.[37,38]

CLINICAL MANIFESTATIONS. RBD is characterized by augmentation of EMG tone during REM sleep and elaborate and complex motor activity associated with dream mentation. Spells consist of punching, kicking, yelling, and running from the bed and usually correlate with the reported dream imagery. The injury associated with the spells often brings the patient or bed partner to medical attention. Spells are likely to occur 90 minutes after sleep onset and more commonly during the second half of the night, when REM sleep is more common. The frequency of the violent spells is about once per week but may occur as frequent as four times per night over several consecutive nights.

An acute (or transient) form of RBD may occur in the setting of toxic or metabolic disorders. These most commonly include withdrawal of alcohol[39] and abrupt withdrawal of sedative–hypnotic agents that accompany REM rebound. Drug-induced cases of loss of REM atonia (due to TCA and biperiden ingestion) have been documented.[40–44] Other agents that have documented association with RBD include monoamine oxidase inhibitor (MAOI),[45] cholinergic agents,[46,47] and, frequently, the SSRI.[48,49] Excessive ingestion of caffeine and chocolate have been implicated.[50,51] A prodromal history of other spells such as sleeptalking, yelling, or limb jerking may be present. With time, the dream content may become more complex, action-filled, violent, or unpleasant, coinciding with the onset of RBD. If sleep becomes fragmented, other symptoms such as EDS may appear. Potential injury (e.g., lacerations, ecchymoses, and fractures) to the patient or bed partner is of major concern.

Advanced age is a predisposing factor for the idiopathic and chronic form of RBD, which is more common and typically begins in late adulthood, progresses over time, and often stabilizes. Approximately 60% of cases are idiopathic; the remaining cases are associated with underlying neurologic disorders such as neurodegenerative disorders (synucleinopathies such as olivopontocerebellar atrophy [OPCA] and diffuse Lewy body disease [DLBD] with a characteristic α-synuclein inclusion in the nerve cell bodies), subarachnoid hemorrhage (SAH), cerebrovascular accident (CVA), multiple sclerosis (MS), and brain stem neoplasm. The presence of RBD may differentiate pure autonomic failure from multiple system atrophy (MSA) with autonomic failure.[52]

RBD usually presents in the sixth or seventh decade; however, it may begin at any age (particularly the symptomatic variety).

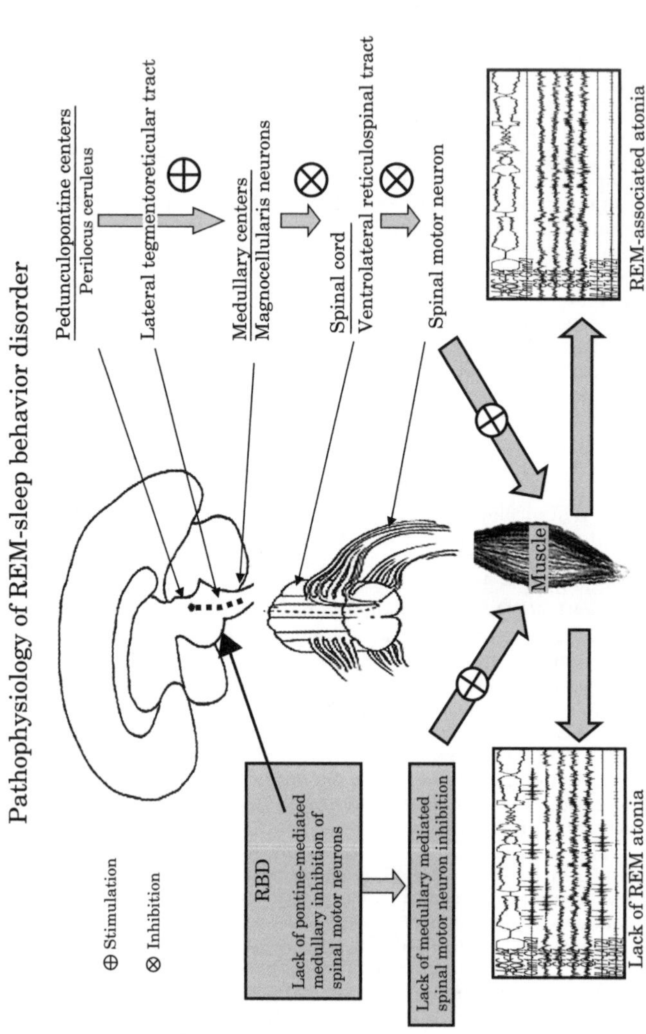

Pathophysiology of REM-sleep behavior disorder

⊕ Stimulation
⊗ Inhibition

Pedunculopontine centers
Perilocus ceruleus
Lateral tegmentoreticular tract

Medullary centers
Magnocellularis neurons

Spinal cord
Ventrolateral reticulospinal tract

Spinal motor neuron

REM-associated atonia

RBD
Lack of pontine-mediated medullary inhibition of spinal motor neurons

Lack of medullary mediated spinal motor neuron inhibition

Muscle

Lack of REM atonia

RBD may be the first manifestation of these disorders and may precede the clinical manifestation of the underlying neuropathologic lesion process by more than a decade.[53–57] There is a higher incidence of RBD in patients with narcolepsy. Medications such as TCA, SSRI, and MAOI, which can be used to treat cataplexy, can sometimes exacerbate or trigger RBD in these patients.[58] RBD is much more predominant in men than in women; however, the reason for this is unclear.

The underlying pathophysiology may be related to the abnormal brain stem control of medullary inhibitory regions (see Fig. 5-1). An identical syndrome was seen in cats with experimentally induced bilateral lesions of the pontine regions adjacent to the locus coeruleus, causing absence of the REM-related atonia associated with REM sleep and abnormal motor behaviors during REM sleep.[59] Dopaminergic abnormalities have recently been implicated in RBD on the basis of neuroimaging studies. Single-photon emission computed tomography (SPECT) studies have demonstrated decreased striatal dopaminergic innervation and reduced striatal dopamine transporters.[60–62] Positron emission tomography (PET) and SPECT studies have shown reduced nigrostriatal dopaminergic projections in patients with MSA and RBD.[63] In patients with idiopathic RBD, impaired cortical activation, as determined by EEG spectral analysis, supports the relationship between RBD and neurodegenerative disorders.[64]

DIAGNOSTIC EVALUATION. PSG reveals augmented muscle tone during REM sleep, exceeding the normal REM-sleep–related EMG twitches (see Fig. 5-2). These motor phenomena may be highly integrated (repeated punching and kicking or more complex limb and trunk movements) and are often associated with emotionally charged utterances. When awoken from an episode, patients may report dream mentation appropriate to the observed behavior. In NREM sleep, periodic movements involving the legs, and occasionally the arms, and periodic movements of all extremities have been reported. There is frequently a pronounced increase in both the REM density and percentage of SWS. The results of the neurologic history and examination may

←

Figure 5-1. **The normally generalized muscle atonia during rapid eye movement (REM) sleep results from pontine-mediated perilocus coeruleus inhibition of motor activity. This pontine activity exerts an excitatory influence on medullary centers (magnocellularis neurons) through the lateral tegmentoreticular tract. These neuronal groups in turn hyperpolarize the spinal motor neuron postsynaptic membranes through the ventrolateral reticulospinal tract. In REM-sleep behavior disorder (RBD), the brain stem mechanisms generating the muscle atonia normally seen in REM sleep may be disrupted. The pathophysiology of RBD in humans is based on the cat model, in which bilateral pontine lesions result in a persistent absence of REM atonia associated with prominent motor activity during REM sleep, similar to that observed in RBD in humans. The pathophysiology of the idiopathic form of RBD in humans is still not well understood but may be related to reduction of striatal presynaptic dopamine transporters. (From Avidan AY. Sleep disorders in the older patient.** *Primary Care: Clin Office Practice.* **2005;32(2):563–586. With permission.)**

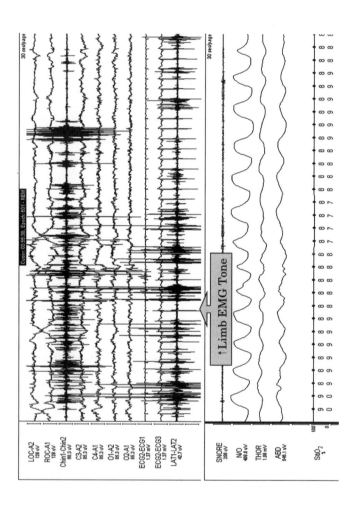

indicate the need for other neurologic testing, including a CT scan or MRI of the brain to identify structural lesions of underlying neurodegenerative processes.

DIFFERENTIAL DIAGNOSIS. The differential diagnosis includes any complex phenomenon during sleep:

1. Sleep-related seizures
2. Confusional arousals
3. Sleepwalking
4. Sleep terrors
5. Post-traumatic stress disorder
6. Nightmares

MANAGEMENT. It is prudent to ensure environmental safety of patients with likely RBD. Pharmacotherapy for RBD may be in the form of clonazepam (0.25 to 1 mg PO q.h.s.), which is effective in 90% of cases with little evidence of tolerance or abuse.[10,65,66] This drug has little or no effect on the characteristic elevated limb EMG tone during the night, but it acts to prevent the arousals associated with the REM-sleep disassociation. Clonazepam's safety for use during pregnancy has not been established. Caution should be exercised when the drug is used in patients with chronic respiratory diseases (e.g., chronic obstructive pulmonary disease) or impaired renal function, and it is contraindicated in patients with documented hypersensitivity, severe liver disease, or acute narrow-angle glaucoma. Abrupt discontinuation of clonazepam can precipitate withdrawal symptoms.[66]

Other agents that may be helpful include imipramine (25 mg PO q.h.s.) and carbamazepine (100 mg PO t.i.d.), as well as pramipexole or levodopa[67,68] in cases where RBD is associated with Parkinson disease. Recent studies have also demonstrated improvement with the use of melatonin, which is believed to exert its therapeutic effect by restoring REM-sleep atonia. One study reported that melatonin was effective in 87% of patients at a dose of 3 to 9 mg at bedtime,[69] whereas a later study reported resolution of symptoms in those taking 6 to 12 mg of melatonin at bedtime.[70] The reader is reminded that melatonin, a food supplement, is not approved by the U.S. Food and Drug Administration (FDA) and is poorly regulated in terms of pharmacologic preparation. It should be used, especially in elderly patients, with great

---

Figure 5-2. A 30-second epoch from the diagnostic polysomnogram of an 80-year-old man who was referred to the sleep disorder clinic for evaluation of recurrent violent nighttime awakenings. Illustrated in this figure is a typical spell that this patient was experiencing. He was noted to yell, jump from bed, and have complex body movements. The *box* and *arrow* demonstrate the normal REM-associated muscle atonia in the left anterior tibialis muscle. The channels are as follows: Electrooculogram (left—LOC-A2, right—ROC-A1), chin electromyogram (EMG), electroencephalogram (left central, right central, left occipital, right occipital), two ECG channels, limb EMG (LAT), snore channel, nasal–oral airflow, respiratory effort (thoracic, abdominal), and oxygen saturation (SaO$_2$). (From Avidan AY. Sleep disorders in the older patient. *Primary Care: Clin Office Practice.* 2005;32(2):563–586. With permission.)

care because it has been found to be vasoactive in laboratory animals and its side effects have not been widely studied.

SLEEP-RELATED MOVEMENT DISORDERS

Sleep-related movement disorders constitute a variety of clinical syndromes. The most common are RLS and PLMD. Sleep-related leg cramps, rhythmic movement disorder (RMD), and bruxism were previously classified as parasomnias, but the new ICSD classifies them as movement disorders.[11] Both PLMD and RLS involve nocturnal involuntary limb movements causing sleep disruption. Unlike PLMDs, which are diagnosed by PSG, the diagnosis of RLS is made by meeting established clinical criteria.[71,72] In addition, PLMD can occur in RLS and with other sleep disorders, as well as in healthy patients, and are therefore nonspecific findings.[71]

Restless Legs Syndrome

Epidemiology

Symptoms of RLS have been identified in 5% to 15% of healthy subjects, 11% of pregnant women, 15% to 20% of patients with uremia, and up to 30% of patients with rheumatoid arthritis. RLS symptom prevalence in the general population varies significantly among countries. The highest prevalence is in Western European countries, with rates as high as 10%, whereas studies from Asia—India, Singapore, and Turkey—have reported lower prevalence rates (0.8%, 0.6% and 3.2%, respectively).[73–76] Among patients with clinically significant RLS in whom the incidence of symptoms are as high, >15 times per month, only a quarter or a third may benefit most from therapy.[77]

Clinical Manifestations

The most recent diagnostic criteria developed at a workshop held by the National Institutes of Health with the members of the International Restless Legs Syndrome Study Group (IRLSSG) requires four essential criteria for the diagnosis of RLS.[78]

RLS is characterized by a tetrad of:

1. Disagreeable leg sensations that usually occur before sleep onset
2. Irresistible urge to move the limbs
3. Partial or complete relief from discomfort on leg movement
4. Return of the symptoms on cessation of leg movements.

The most disabling complaint is the irresistible and profound urge to move the limbs. Patients describe a building of the sensation to a point where they must give in and move their legs. RLS has been described as arising from rest, and the symptoms are present only at rest and just before the patient sleeps. The symptoms sometimes interfere with sleep onset and may cause insomnia and prolonged awakenings, leading to significantly reduced total sleep time (TST); patients often report averaging <4 hours sleep per night[79] The sensory complaints are often very difficult to describe and are left to subjective interpretation by the patients, who may use multiple terms to describe the discomfort (e.g., *creepy crawly, ache, burning, creeping, crawling, pulling, prickling, tingling,* or *itching*). RLS symptoms improve when the patients engage in challenging activities such as playing a mentally consuming game, or sometimes arguing. Getting up and ambulating typically provides immediate relief, which is shortlived and abates soon after the activity ceases.

Typical symptoms involve the ankle and the knee, but when RLS is severe, the thighs or feet, and rarely the arms, can also become involved. The symptoms are typically bilateral and can be asymmetric in both severity and frequency, but are rarely unilateral. RLS can occur at other times of the day but become more pronounced during times of prolonged inactivity, particularly when in an airplane or when driving long distances. The symptoms usually last for a few minutes or several hours. There is evidence that patients with RLS may have symptoms consistent with anxiety and depression and that affected patients may have lower scores on quality-of-life measures,[80,81] suggesting that the sleep disturbances associated with RLS are probably the "tip of the iceberg."

RLS has a clearly established circadian tendency for symptoms to be maximal in the evening, increasing in intensity toward the early sleep period. Most patients with RLS describe that their best sleep quality is generally earlier in the morning, with a relatively "protected" time between 6 and 10 AM that is relatively free of RLS symptoms.

Both PLMD and RLS show a maximal severity in timely coincidence with the falling phase of the core body temperature. There is some evidence that the amplitude of circadian rhythm of dopaminergic function is increased in RLS, with hypofunction occurring at night.[82] This finding, in addition to the fact that RLS responds to dopamine and is exacerbated by dopamine antagonists, fuels the hypothesis that the underlying pathophysiology may be related to dopamine dysfunction. Yet another hypothesis concerns iron storage deficiency in the brain during RLS[83] and the fact that patients with RLS have reduced CSF iron content as compared to healthy controls.[84]

RLS has two forms with separate etiologies and age of onset:

1. *Early onset RLS*: Age of onset is <45 years, tends to cluster in families, has a slower progression, and has a female-to-male ratio of approximately 2:1.
2. *Late-onset RLS*: Age of onset is >45 years, has an equal female-to-male ratio, has a more rapid progression, is more severe with more frequent daily symptoms, has little or no family history, and is more commonly associated with underlying medical conditions such as neuropathy, radiculopathy, or myelopathy.[81]

RLS can be associated with pregnancy (typically after the 20th week of gestation), anemia, and uremia. The prevalence rate of RLS in patients with renal failure requiring hemodialysis ranges from 20% to 50% but may go even higher.[85,86] The prevalence rate seen in pregnancy is approximately 23%.[87–90] The common factor in these conditions is iron deficiency anemia that once treated results in a reversal of the RLS.[88,91] Higher prevalence rates of RLS have also been reported in other neurologic conditions, such as Parkinson disease[76,92] and spinocerebellar ataxia (SCA-3),[93,94] and in low back pain, myelopathy, and arthropathy.[95] Medications that may exacerbate RLS and PLMD include dopamine antagonists (particularly, antiemetics), antihistamines (H_1 antagonists), antidepressants such as the TCA and SSRI that worsen PLMD, and neuroleptics.[96–99]

Most patients with RLS have PLMD, whereas PLMD is less common in patients with RLS. Patients may experience features of intense anxiety and depression in association with RLS. In some patients, the emotional distress may be severe and associated with psychosocial dysfunction. RLS occurs with the waxing and waning cycle of symptoms. The condition is rare in infancy and may be seen for the first time in advanced old age. The peak onset is usually in middle age and is more common in women. RLS is most often seen as an isolated case, but a definitive familial pattern has been reported assuming an autosomal dominant inheritance. RLS may cause severe insomnia, psychologic disturbance, and depression, sometimes producing severe social dysfunction.

Differential Diagnosis

Table 5-2 lists the clinical conditions that should be considered in the differential diagnosis of RLS. Many of these can be ruled out by history and clinical examination.

Diagnostic Evaluation

All patients need to fulfill the diagnostic criteria for RLS and undergo a screening neurologic evaluation for underlying neuropathy. Although sleep studies for RLS are not indicated when the clinical diagnostic criteria have been met,[100,101] PSG can be helpful in excluding other underlying primary sleep disorders such as OSA or when the RLS does not respond to conventional therapy. All patients with RLS should undergo testing for serum ferritin level, and those in whom the serum ferritin level is low (<45 μg per L) are at a higher risk of having RLS.[102,103] Patients should be followed up and observed closely to avoid the development of iron overload.

Management

The treatment of RLS is outlined in Table 5-3. The first approach for patients with symptoms consistent with those of RLS is to determine the serum ferritin level. Patients with levels <45 μg per L should be started on iron replacement therapy[102] with iron sulfate. When iron stores are normal, dopamine (D_3) agonists such as ropinirole and pramipexole may be started. At the time of writing this book, the only medication with clear FDA approval for RLS is ropinirole. Dopamine agonists are preferred because they control RLS symptoms throughout the night.[104] If symptoms persist despite these therapies, other medications including benzodiazepines, such as clonazepam or temazepam,[105] and levodopa/carbidopa[106] may be considered. Both levodopa and dopamine agonists ameliorate RLS symptoms, decrease PLMD, and improve sleep.[107,108] The drawback of levodopa therapy is the potential for augmentation, which is the increase in severity of symptoms earlier in the day.[109] Of the anticonvulsants, both carbamazepine and gabapentin have been proposed, with

Table 5-2. Differential diagnosis of restless legs syndrome

Diagnosis	Clinical Features	Circadian Timing
RLS	Clinical symptoms of uncomfortable sensation experienced during inactivity or rest, with relief once movement commences	Night
PLMD	PSG findings characterized by periodic episodes of repetitive and stereotyped limb movements that occur during sleep; lack sensory symptoms of RLS	Night
Nocturnal leg cramps ("Charley horse cramps")	Painful and palpable muscular contractions relieved by stretching	Night
Painful peripheral neuropathy	Sensory symptoms described as numbness, burning, and pain, typically not relieved while walking or during sustained movement	Diurnal, increased at night
Neuroleptic-induced akathisia	Described as a "whole body sensation" rather than centered only in limbs; do not improve with movement; positive history of specific medication exposure	None
Arthritis of lower limb	Discomfort is centered in the joints	None
Volitional movements, foot tapping, leg rocking	Occurs in fidgety patients, during times of anxiety or boredom; typically lack sensory symptoms, discomfort, or the urge to move	None
Positional discomfort	Associated with prolonged sitting or lying in the same position, relieved on changing position	None
Burning or painful feet and moving toes	Described as continuous slow writhing or repetitive movements of toes; primary involvement of the feet	None

RLS, restless legs syndrome; PLMD, periodic limb movement disorder; PSG, polysomnography.
Adapted from Lesage S, Hening WA. The restless legs syndrome and periodic limb movement disorder: A review of management. *Semin Neurol.* 2004;24(3):249–259.

Table 5-3.   Pharmacotherapy for restless legs syndrome

Drug—class (generic/brand)	Dosage	Risks
Iron: Ferrous sulfate	325 mg b.i.d./t.i.d. Recommended for ferritin levels <50 μg	GI side effects: constipation; role in treatment currently under investigation
Dopaminergic agents: Levodopa and carbidopa (Sinemet)	25/200 mg—half tablet–three tablets 30 min before bedtime	Nausea, sleepiness, augmentation of daytime symptoms, insomnia, GI disturbances
Dopamine agonists: Pramipexole (Mirapex) Pergolide (Permax) Ropinirole (Requip)	0.125–0.5 mg, 1 h before bedtime; start low and increase slowly 0.05–1.0 mg 1 h before bedtime; divided doses; gradually increase as needed 0.25–2 mg 1 h before bedtime[a]	Severe sleepiness, nausea reported in some cases
Anticonvulsants: Gabapentin (Neurontin)	300–2,700 mg/d divided t.i.d.	Daytime sleepiness, nausea
Benzodiazepines: Clonazepam (Klonopin)	0.125–0.5 mg 30 min before bedtime	Nausea, sedation, dizziness
Centrally acting α_2-agonist: Clonidine (Catapres)	0.1 mg b.i.d.; may be helpful in patients with hypertension	Dry mouth, drowsiness, constipation, sedation, weakness, depression (1%), hypotension
Opioids: Darvocet (Darvocet-N) Propoxyphene (Darvon) Codeine	300 mg/d 65–135 mg at bedtime 30 mg	Nausea, vomiting, restlessness, constipation. Addiction, tolerance may be possible

GI, gastrointestinal.
[a] Only FDA-approved drug for RLS as of October, 2005.

gabapentin being effective in controlling the leg movements as well.[110] For refractory cases of RLS, opiates, which are generally reserved as the treatment of last resort, have a proven efficacy[111] with methadone, which can be utilized for the most severe cases of RLS.

Periodic Limb Movement Disorder

Epidemiology

PLMDs are rare in children but become increasingly more common with advancing age. PLMD may be found in up to 34% of patients >60 years; they are very common in a variety of sleep disorders including RLS (80% to 90%), RBD (≈70%), and narcolepsy (45% to 60%),[112] and have been reported to occur in 1% to 15% of patients with insomnia.

Clinical Manifestations

Also known as nocturnal myoclonus, PLMDs are found on PSG, characterized by periodic episodes of repetitive and stereotyped limb movements that occur during sleep. The term *PLMDs* is more appropriate here as opposed to periodic limb movements because the upper limbs may also be involved. The movements usually occur in the legs and consist of extension of the big toe in combination with partial flexion of the ankle, knee, and sometimes the hip. The movements are often associated with a partial arousal or awakening; however, the patient is usually unaware of the limb movements or the frequent sleep disruption. Between the episodes, the legs are still. Patients experience symptoms of frequent nocturnal awakenings and unrefreshing sleep. Patients who are unaware of the sleep interruptions may have symptoms of excessive sleepiness. It is probable that the nature of the patient's complaint is affected by the frequency of the movement, as well as the associated awakenings. The clinical significance of the movements needs to be decided on an individual basis. PLMD may be an incidental finding, and medication that reduces the frequency of limb movements can produce little or no change in sleep duration or sleep efficiency. It is possible that a centrally mediated event can give rise to both the periodic movements and the related sleep disturbance. It is necessary to integrate the clinical history and the PSG findings to assess the role of this phenomenon in a sleep disorder. This disorder can produce anxiety and depression related to the chronicity of the sleep disturbance.

PLMD appears to increase in prevalence with advancing age. In individuals with RLS, PLMD is usually detected during PSG monitoring. PLMD can accompany narcolepsy and OSA. PLMD can be associated with, or evoked by, a variety of medical conditions. Episodes of limb movements can develop in patients with chronic uremia and other metabolic disorders. The use of TCA and MAOI can induce or aggravate this disorder, as does withdrawal from a variety of drugs, such as anticonvulsants, benzodiazepines, barbiturates, and other hypnotic agents. PLMD associated with ingestion or withdrawal from drugs should be distinguished from the disorder in the drug-free patient. Clinically, PLMD can result in fragmented, restless sleep and can eventually contribute to symptoms of insomnia or EDS. The limb

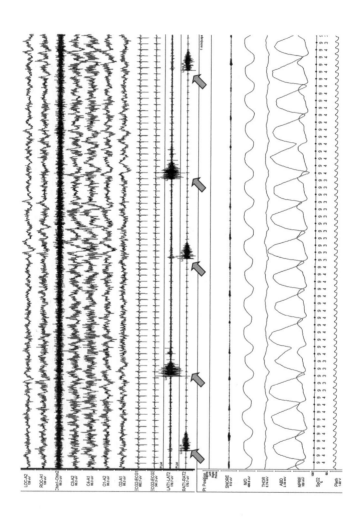

movements can disrupt the sleep of a bed partner. Some patients with severe PLMD can also have the movements during wakefulness.

Diagnostic Evaluation

PSG reveals repetitive EMG contractions of the anterior tibialis lasting 0.5 to 5 seconds (mean duration: 1.5 to 2.5 seconds).[113] PLMDs are diagnosed when more than five leg movements occur per hour of sleep. Four or more consecutive movements are required, and the interval between movements is typically 20 to 40 seconds. Movements that are separated by an interval <5 or >90 seconds are not counted when determining the total number of movements or movement indexes. PLMDs can appear immediately with the onset of light NREM sleep, decrease in frequency in SWS, and are usually absent during REM sleep. Typically, both lower limbs are monitored for the presence of the limb movements; however, movement of the upper limbs may be sampled if clinically indicated. The movement may begin with a leg jerk, followed by a short interval (milliseconds) and a tonic contraction. There may often be repeated myoclonic jerks occurring at the beginning of each movement. The movements may affect one or both the lower limbs, although usually both extremities are involved, but not necessarily in a symmetric or simultaneous pattern. The events may show some alternations from leg to leg. Contractions occurring during drowsiness, before the onset of stage-1 sleep, are not counted as part of the sleep disorder. PLMD can occur in discrete episodes that last a few minutes to several hours or may be present throughout the entire recording. The PLMD index is reported as the number of movements per hour of TST, as determined by the PSG of the major sleep episode; an index of five or more is regarded as abnormal. The PLMD-arousal index is the number of PLMDs associated with an arousal, expressed per hour of TST. Figure 5-3 demonstrates the typical PSG findings in PLMD.

Differential Diagnosis

1. *Hypnic jerks*: occur exclusively during wake-to-sleep transition and not during the major sleep period.

Figure 5-3. This is a 60-second sleep epoch from a diagnostic polysomnogram of a 66-year-old woman with difficulty falling asleep, excessive daytime sleepiness, and uncomfortable sensation in her legs associated with an irresistible urge to move her legs. Her husband reports that she has frequent nighttime kicking and jerking movements, which disrupt his sleep. Illustrated in this figure is a succession of five periodic limb movements occurring in the right and left anterior tibialis muscles. The channels are as follows: Electrooculogram (left—LOC-A2, right—ROC-A1), chin EMG (Chin1-Chin2), EEG (left central [C3-A2], right central [C4-A1], left occipital [O1-A2], right occipital [O2-A1]), electrocardiogram (ECG), limb EMG (left leg [LAT] and right leg [RAT]), patient position (Pt Position), snoring (SNORE), nasal–oral airflow (N/O), respiratory effort (thoracic [THOR] and abdominal [ABD]), nasal pressure (NPRE), oxygen saturation (SpO_2), and plethysmography channel. (From Avidan AY. Sleep disorders in the older patient. *Primary Care: Clin Office Practice.* 2005;32(2):563–586. With permission.)

2.   *OSA*: may produce leg movements and sleep fragmenta-
     tions resembling PLMD but disappear on treatment with
     continuous positive airway pressure (CPAP).
3.   *Nocturnal seizures and myoclonic epilepsy*: may appear as
     abrupt stereotyped focal limb movement resembling PLMD.
     Epileptiform EEG discharge generally accompanies the
     movement.

Management

The treatment of PLMD and RLS are somewhat similar, in that
many patients respond to agents such as low-dose dopamine
agonist and benzodiazepines (e.g., clonazepam). However, compared to RLS, opiates are generally regarded as less beneficial in
PLMD.[72] Another important consideration when treating PLMD
is that many patients may have coexistent OSA[114,115] and agents
that may worsen sleep apnea (e.g., benzodiazepines) should be
used cautiously.[116]

Sleep-Related Leg Cramps

Epidemiology

Sleep-related leg cramps may be present in up to 16% of healthy
individuals, particularly following vigorous exercise, with an
increased incidence among elderly individuals. The peak onset is
usually in adulthood but may be seen for the first time in old age.

Clinical Manifestations

"Charley horse" or nocturnal leg cramps are painful muscular
tightness usually involving the calf, but occasionally the foot, that
occur during sleep. The symptom may last for a few seconds and
remit spontaneously. The cramp often results in arousal or awakening from sleep. Patients with nocturnal leg cramps will often
experience one to two incidence nightly, several times a week. Leg
cramps can occur in some patients primarily during the daytime,
and sleep disturbance is usually not a feature in these patients.
The natural history of leg cramps is not well understood. Many
patients describe a waxing and waning course of many years'
duration. Predisposing factors include pregnancy, diabetes mellitus, and metabolic disorders. The disorder can be associated
with prior vigorous exercise, pregnancy, arthritis, and with fluid
and electrolyte disturbances. Nocturnal leg cramps may be more
prevalent in women because of the frequent occurrence of leg
cramps during pregnancy. The major complications include insomnia and occasional EDS due to interruptions in sleep.

Diagnostic Features

PSG studies of patients with chronic nocturnal leg cramps reveal
nonperiodic bursts of leg EMG activity. Episodes occur during
sleep without any specific preceding physiologic changes.

Differential Diagnosis

The following conditions should be differentiated by clinical history and physical examination:

1.   RLS
2.   Chronic myelopathy

3. Peripheral neuropathy
4. Akathisia

Management

The cramp can usually be relieved by local massage, application of heat, or movement of the affected limb. Quinine sulfate, an antimalarial drug, has been widely used as an effective therapy for idiopathic leg cramps and works by decreasing motor end plate excitability, thereby reducing the muscle contractility. Quinine is not without side effects.[117,118] The drug should be used in a low dose and cautiously, especially in elderly individuals and patients with renal failure, and should be avoided in patients with hepatic disease.[119]

Propriospinal Myoclonus at Sleep Onset

Propriospinal myoclonus (PSM) is a spinal cord–mediated movement disorder, occasionally associated with acquired spinal cord lesions. The patient typically complains of sudden jerks of the abdomen, neck, and trunk occurring during periods of relaxation during times of sleep–wake transition.[11,120] PSM may be confused with hypnic jerks, PLMD, and myoclonic seizures.[121] It can result in severe insomnia, particularly at sleep onset.[122] Clonazepam or antiepileptic drugs may be effective in alleviating these movements.[123]

Sleep-Related Bruxism

Epidemiology

Eighty-five percent to 90% of individuals grind their teeth to some degree during their lifetime. In approximately 5% to 10% of these patients, bruxism will present as a clinical condition resulting in moderate to severe tooth wear and jaw discomfort.[124] Children appear to be affected as frequently as adults, but longitudinal studies are lacking. The condition is prevalent among institutionalized individuals with mental retardation, among whom 58% experience significant tooth wear from bruxism.[125]

Clinical Presentation

Sleep bruxism is a stereotyped movement disorder characterized by grinding or clenching of the teeth during sleep.[11] The sounds made by friction of the teeth are usually perceived by the bed partner as being very unpleasant.[124] The disorder is typically brought to medical attention to eliminate the disturbing sounds, although the first signs of the disorder may be recognized by a dentist. Bruxism can lead to abnormal wear of the teeth, periodontal tissue damage, or jaw pain.[124]

Bruxism has two distinct patterns: Diurnal and nocturnal, which are etiologically different phenomena, although their effects on dentition may be similar. Other symptoms include facial muscle and tooth pain and headache. Psychologic assessment of otherwise healthy adults suggests a close correlation with stress from situational or psychological sources. Predisposing factors include malocclusion and anatomic defects, such as rough cusp ends. Medications such as SSRI, levodopa, amphetamine, and alcohol have been shown to exacerbate bruxism.[124,126,127] This condition induces dental damage with abnormal wear to the teeth and damage to the structures surrounding the teeth. Over time, this leads to recession and inflammation of the gums, alveolar bone resorption, and hypertrophy of the muscles of mastication and temporomandibular joint, and is often associated with facial pain.

Diagnostic Evaluation

The diagnosis of bruxism is based on the presence of tooth wear on dental evaluation. The maxillary canines are the first to show wear. Additional evidence is obtained by observations of bite lesions and ridging of the lateral borders of the tongue and buccal mucosa adjacent to the molars. Tenderness or hypertrophy of the muscles of mastication may also be helpful in confirming the diagnosis.

Polysomnographic Features

PSG monitoring is rarely indicated. The electrographic hallmark of bruxism is an increased rhythmic masseter and temporalis muscle activity during sleep. Bruxism can occur during all stages of sleep but is more prevalent during stage-2 sleep. The sound of bruxism can be very loud and unpleasant. Two nights of PSG monitoring may be needed to either confirm the diagnosis or rule out associated epilepsy. However, because bruxism does not occur every night, PSG has a high false-negative rate, even in patients with significant clinical conditions.[128] An EEG may be indicated if a seizure disorder is suspected.

Differential Diagnosis

The rhythmic jaw movements associated with partial complex or generalized seizure disorders need to be considered in the differential diagnosis. Idiopathic myoclonus and parasomnias, such as sleeptalking, can be mistaken for bruxism.[129]

Management

Patients with severe disease may benefit from a protective mouth splint (or mouth guard), which is worn during the night. This occlusal bite splint may provide protection against tooth damage or fracture. Although the splint does not prevent the bruxism episodes, it does help prevent tooth wear. Stress reduction, hypnosis, or psychologic counseling may help patients with stress- or anxiety-related bruxism. In rare and refractory cases, benzodiazepine therapy may be helpful.

Sleep-Related Rhythmic Movement Disorder

Epidemiology

The reported prevalence of head banging in childhood varies from 5% to 15%. Men are three to four times more likely to be affected compared to women. By 9 months of age, some form of rhythmic activity is found in 67% of all infants; by 18 months, the prevalence declines to less than 50%; and by 4 years, it is only 8%. Body rocking is more common in the first year, but head banging and head rolling are more frequent in older children. Persistence into adulthood is not uncommon.[130,131]

Clinical Manifestations

RMD consists of stereotyped, repetitive movements of the head and neck occurring during drowsiness or sleep. Several types of RMD may exist:

- *Head banging*—the child moves the head back and forth down into the pillow or mattress. This is the most disturbing form of the disorder.
- *Head rolling*—the movements occur in a side-to-side manner.
- *Body rocking*—this may involve the entire body and occurs when the child rocks forward and backward without head banging.

Any of the types of RMD may be accompanied by rhythmic humming or chanting and may be very loud. RMD occurs at a frequency between 0.5 and 2 per second, with a total duration of <15 minutes. Persistence of RMD into childhood or adulthood may be associated with autism, mental retardation, or other significant psychopathology.

Environmental stress and lack of environmental stimulation have also been proposed as causative factors. Traumatic injury is rare but may result in retinal petechiae or subdural hematoma. Severe and chronic head banging can produce callus formation. Violent rhythmic body movements can produce loud noises when the patient hits the bed frame, which can be very disturbing to other family members.

Diagnosis Evaluation

RMD can be diagnosed on the basis of its characteristic clinical features. PSG is rarely indicated but may be helpful when the differential diagnosis includes epilepsy. The PSG shows the RMD activity manifesting during all sleep stages: Light NREM sleep, less frequently during SWS, and only rarely during REM sleep.[132,133] An EEG may be necessary to differentiate this behavior from that due to epilepsy. EEG studies have shown normal activity between episodes of rhythmic behavior.

Differential Diagnosis

RMD of sleep must be distinguished from other repetitive movements as bruxism, rhythmic sucking of the pacifier, thumb sucking, and PLMD. There are usually few diagnostic dilemmas, and rarely does the disorder need to be differentiated from epilepsy.

Management

No systematic studies of pharmacologic or behavioral treatment have been reported. The disorder will generally resolve spontaneously. Behavioral therapy can be helpful, and only in very rare and refractory cases are short-acting benzodiazepines indicated.[134,135]

ISOLATED SYMPTOMS, APPARENTLY NORMAL VARIANTS, AND UNRESOLVED ISSUES

Sleeptalking (Somniloquy)

Epidemiology

Although extensive epidemiologic studies are lacking, sleeptalking is apparently very common. Among children aged between 3 and 10 years, approximately 50% sleeptalk at least once a year, and approximately 10% sleeptalk on a nightly basis.[136] Sleeptalking that significantly disturbs others is rare. In adults, this condition seems to be more common in men than in women, and it has a familial tendency.

Clinical Manifestations

Sleeptalking consists of utterances of speech or sounds that occur during the sleep episode without awareness of the event. The noise may be disturbing to bed partners or other household members. The episodes are generally brief, infrequent, and devoid of signs of emotional stress. However, it can sometimes consist of frequent, nightly, prolonged speeches and may include long speeches and hostile or angry outbursts. Sleeptalking may be spontaneous or induced by conversation with the sleeper. The course is usually self-limited and benign. Precipitating factors include sleep deprivation, emotional stress, febrile illness, or sleep disorders such as sleep terror, confusional arousal, sleep apnea, and RBD.

Diagnostic Features

When sleeptalking is isolated, it does not require any diagnostic workup. However, if other underlying sleep disorders are suspected, such as sleep apnea or RBD, further workup including PSG may be needed. Studies demonstrate sleep talking during all stages of sleep. Dream mentation is associated with episodes occurring during REM sleep in 79% of patients with sleeptalking, stage-2 sleep in 46%, and SWS in 21%.[137,138]

Differential Diagnosis

Sleeptalking, when severe, should be differentiated from talking during nocturnal awakenings, which may be normal phenomena or reflect psychopathology. Sleeptalking can also manifest in other sleep disorders, such as RBD or OSA.

Management

There is no specific therapy for sleeptalking. However, close attention to proper sleep hygiene and treatment of an underlying sleep disorder that may precipitate the sleeptalking is usually helpful.[139]

Hypnic Jerks

Epidemiology

Hypnic jerks can occur at any age and are universal components of the sleep-onset process. The episodes are quite prevalent, occurring in approximately 60% to 70% of the population. Excessive hypnic jerks have been reported in patients with Parkinson disease,[140] in those with postpolio syndrome,[141] and in pediatric patients with migraine.[142]

Clinical Manifestations

The episodes occur at sleep onset and consist of sudden and brief contractions of the limbs. The jerks may occur either spontaneously or secondary to a stimuli. Pure sensory phenomena in the absence of a body jerk, "sensory sleep starts," can also occur, in which case they are associated with a subjective impression of falling, a sensory flash, or a visual hypnagogic dream or hallucination.[143] A sharp cry or utterance may occur. When hypnic jerks are excessive or multiple in the degree of motor activity or frequency, they may cause awakenings, and repetitive episodes can produce sleep-initiation insomnia.

Precipitating factors include prior intense exercise, excessive stimulant or caffeine intake, and emotional stress. Chronic and unremitting episodes may eventually cause chronic anxiety and fear of falling asleep. Injury is uncommon but may occur when the patients suddenly move their foot against a bedstead or kick a bed partner.

Diagnostic Features

The clinical features of hypnic jerks are typically diagnostic. When myoclonic epilepsy is in the differential diagnosis, formal PSG with EEG montage and extra limb EMG channels may be helpful. Hypnic jerks occur in isolation or in succession during transitions from wakefulness to sleep, primarily at the beginning of the first sleep episode. The superficial EMG recordings of the muscles involved demonstrate brief high-amplitude potentials during drowsiness.

Differential Diagnosis

Sleep starts must be differentiated from a number of movement disorders that occur at sleep onset or during sleep.[144]

1. *Periodic limb movement disorder (PLMD)*: in which the muscle contractions are much longer in duration, involve mainly the lower extremities, show stereotypical periodicity, and occur during sleep.
2. *RLS*: consists of unpleasant and unbearable sensations that are temporarily relieved by getting up and exercising.
3. *Brief epileptic myoclonus*: can be differentiated by the presence of other features of epileptic seizures, coexistent EEG discharge, and the presence of the myoclonus during both wakefulness and sleep, unlike hypnic jerks, which occur at sleep onset.
4. *Fragmentary myoclonus*: are small-amplitude jerks or twitches that occur in an asynchronous, symmetrical, and bilateral manner at sleep onset, as well as within all sleep stages.
5. *Benign neonatal sleep myoclonus*: consists of marked twitching of the fingers, toes, and face during sleep in infants. The condition disappears by the age of 3 to 4 months and represents a normal maturational phenomenon of sleep.[145]

Management

Most patients need reassurance, and no further workup or treatment is indicated. Benzodiazepines (i.e., clonazepam) and short-acting hypnotic medications may be suggested when hypnic jerks are refractory and produce sleep-initiation insomnia.

Excessive Fragmentary Myoclonus

Epidemiology

Fragmentary myoclonus occurs in 5% to 10% of patients having EDS. It has a strong male predominance. The phenomenon was found to be associated with sleep-related respiratory problems, PLMD, narcolepsy, intermittent hypersomnia, and sometimes, insomnia.[146] It also occurs in association with EDS as an isolated finding.

Clinical Manifestations

The condition presents with multiple, brief, twitchlike movements occurring asynchronously and asymmetrically in different body areas.[144,147] Muscles of the arms, legs, and face may be involved. The twitches persist irregularly for several minutes, and sometimes up to an hour or more. The patient is usually not aware of the twitchlike movements. Patients with prolonged episodes of twitching may have coexistent EDS. Any cause of chronic sleep fragmentation, such as OSA, CSA, central alveolar hypoventilation syndrome, narcolepsy, and PLMD, may be associated with marked fragmentary myoclonus.[148] In patients with apnea, the twitching intensifies during periods of increased hypoxemia.

Diagnostic Features

The episodes are associated with brief asymmetrical and asynchronous jerks and involve the muscles of the face, arms, and legs and can last from 10 minutes to several hours. They often appear at sleep onset, continue through NREM sleep stages, and may persist during REM sleep, in which they appear superimposed on the normal phasic clusters of physiologic REM myoclonus. The EEG is normal and does not show any cortical potentials related to the twitches.[148]

Differential Diagnosis

1. *PLMDs*: occur at longer duration and have a stereotyped pattern of occurrence.
2. *Sleep-onset hypnic jerks*: occur in isolation or succession during transitions from wakefulness to sleep.
3. *Transient REM-sleep myoclonus*: is limited to the REM sleep and is associated with other REM-sleep phenomena such as autonomic irregularity and REMs.
4. *Myoclonic epilepsy*: myoclonic muscle activity during the seizure is readily distinguishable by epileptiform EEG and the clinical history.

Management

Treatment is in the form of reassurance.

OTHER PARASOMNIAS

This group of parasomnias comprises those parasomnias that cannot be classified in other sections of this chapter. In future editions of the ICSD, some common conditions may be focused on to subdivide what is likely to be a growing list.

Sleep-Related Expiratory Groaning (Catathrenia)

Groaning during sleep has been termed *catathrenia*.[149] The behaviors are characterized by prolonged, often very loud and socially disruptive, groaning sounds during expiration. The disorder has a predilection to occur intermittently during either REM or NREM sleep. It is poorly understood and awaits further definition and therapeutic studies.[150] There is no known effective treatment.

Sleep Enuresis

Enuresis refers to the inability to maintain urinary control during sleep. Primary enuresis refers to the inability to attain urinary control from infancy, whereas secondary enuresis denotes an enuretic relapse after control has been achieved. Sleep enuresis is characterized by recurrent involuntary micturition that occurs during sleep. Please refer to Chapter 7 for additional discussion.

Nocturnal Paroxysmal Dystonia

NPD is characterized by repeated dystonia or dyskinetic (ballistic, choreoathetoid) episodes that are stereotypical and occur during NREM sleep. It was initially thought to represent a syndrome of sleep-related motor attacks that comprises two variants, characterized by short- and long-lasting seizures.[151] Currently, NPD is categorized as a form of sleep-related epilepsy.[11]

It exists in two clinical varieties:

1. *Short episodes* are 15 to 60 seconds in duration, characterized by movements not >1 minute in duration. Episodes can recur up to 15 times per night, usually preceded by a clinical and EEG arousal. They occur nearly every night. Dystonic posturing is associated with ballistic or choreoathetoid movements. The episodes are stereotypic and often associated with vocalizations. At the end of the episode, the patient is coherent and, when left undisturbed, usually resumes sleep. Generalized tonic-clonic epilepsy has been reported in patients with the short-episode type of NPD.
2. *Prolonged episodes* are up to 60 minutes in duration. The prolonged-episode type shows similar clinical features, but episodes can last up to 1 hour. The condition has been known to antedate the onset of Huntington disease by as much as 20 years.

NPD can contribute to severe sleep disruption and produce a complaint of insomnia. The sleep of a bed partner may also be disturbed. The movements may be so severe that injuries due to striking a hard object can occur. There may also be sporadic, unclassifiable episodes, such as a sudden urge to start walking or, on the contrary, a feeling of being unable to move. These particular episodes are suggestive of frontal-lobe epileptic seizures, although evidence of NPD being a manifestation of a seizure disorder has not been established. Onset typically is from infancy to the fifth decade of life. The dystonic episodes usually do not subside spontaneously, and patients have been known to have had episodes for over 20 years.

Diagnostic Features

PSG demonstrates episodes appearing during sleep NREM (stage 2 and SWS). EEG shows desynchronization, indicating arousal, which usually precedes the motor events by a few seconds. The EEG is often obscured by movement artifact, but epileptiform features are not seen preceding, during, or immediately following the dystonic episodes. Routine EEG may demonstrate epileptiform features that are not associated with paroxysmal dystonia episodes.

Differential Diagnosis

NPD must be differentiated from parasomnias such as sleep terror and RBD. The duration of episodes, the dystonic–dyskinetic features, and the recurrence rate are distinguishing features.

Management

Carbamazepine, sometimes at low doses, usually produces therapeutic benefit.

REFERENCES

1. Mahowald MW, Ettinger MG. Things that go bump in the night: The parasomnias revisited. *J Clin Neurophysiol.* 1990;7(1): 119–143.
2. Broughton R. *Behavioral parasomnias.* Boston, MA: Butterworth-Heinemann; 1998:635–660.
3. Brooks S, Kushida CA. Behavioral parasomnias. *Curr Psychiatry Rep.* 2002;4(5):363–368.
4. Mahowald MW, Bornemann MC, Schenck CH. Parasomnias. *Semin Neurol.* 2004;24(3):283–292.
5. Mahowald MW. *Overview of parasomnias.* National Sleep Medicine Course: American Academy of Sleep Medicine, 1999.
6. Kowey PR, Mainchak RA, Rials SJ, et al. Things that go bang in the night. *N Engl J Med.* 1992;327:1884.
7. Thorpy MJ, Glovinsky PB. Parasomnias. *Psychiatr Clin North Am.* 1987;10(4):623–639.
8. Stores G. Dramatic parasomnias. *J R Soc Med.* 2001;94(4): 173–176.
9. Parkes JD. The parasomnias. *Lancet.* 1986;2:1021–1025.
10. Mahowald MW, Ettinger MG. Things that go bump in the night: The parasomnias revisited. *J Clin Neurophysiol.* 1990;7: 119–143.
11. American Academy of Sleep Medicine. *The international classification of sleep disorders.* Westchester, IL: American Academy of Sleep Medicine; 2005.
12. Fisher C, Kahn E, Edwards A, et al. A psychophysiological study of nightmares and night terrors. I. Physiological aspects of the stage 4 night terror. *J Nerv Ment Dis.* 1973;157:75–98.

13. Fisher C, Kahn E, Edwards A, et al. A psychophysiological study of nightmares and night terrors. III. Mental content and recall of stage 4 night terrors. *J Nerv Ment Dis*. 1974;158:174–188.

14. Mahowald MW, Schenck CH. NREM parasomnias. *Neurol Clin*. 1996;14:675–696.

15. Ohayon M, Guilleminault C, Priest RG. Night terrors, sleepwalking, and confusional arousal in the general population: Their frequency and relationship to other sleep and mental disorders. *J Clin Psychiatry*. 1999;60:268–276.

16. Parkes JD. The parasomnias. *Lancet*. 1986;2(8514):1021–1025.

17. Thorpy MJ, Glovinsky PB. Parasomnias. *Psychiatr Clin North Am*. 1987;10(4):623–639.

18. Zaiwalla Z. Parasomnias. *Clin Med*. 2005;5(2):109–112.

19. Rosen G, Mahowald MW, Ferber R. Sleepwalking, confusional arousals, and sleep terrors in the child. In: Ferber R, Kryger M, eds. *Principles and practice of sleep medicine in the child*. Philadelphia, PA: WB Saunders; 1995:99–106.

20. Klackenberg G. Somnambulism in childhood—prevalence, course and behavior correlates. A prospective longitudinal study (6–16 years). *Acta Paediatr Scand*. 1982;71:495–499.

21. Tobin JD Jr. Treatment of somnambulism with anticipatory awakening. *J Pediatr*. 1993;122(3):426–427.

22. Nino-Murcia G, Dement WC. Psychophysiological and pharmacological aspects of somnambulism and night terrors in children. In: Meltzer HY, ed. *Psychopharmacology: The third generation of progress*. New York: Raven Press; 1987:873–879.

23. Reid WH, Ahmed I, Levie CA, et al. Treatment of sleepwalking: A controlled study. *Am J Psychother*. 1981;35:27–37.

24. Crisp AH. The sleepwalking/night terrors syndrome in adults. *Postgrad Med J*. 1996;72:599–604.

25. Mahowald MW, Rosen GM. Parasomnias in children. *Pediatrician*. 1990;17:21–31.

26. Mahowald MW, Ettinger MG. Things that go bump in the night—the parasomnias revisited. *J Clin Neurophysiol*. 1990;7:119–143.

27. Kahn E, Fisher C, Edwards A. Night terrors and anxiety dreams. In: Ellman SD, Antrobus JS, eds. *The mind in sleep. Psychology and psychophysiology*, 2nd ed. New York: John Wiley & Sons; 1991:437–447.

28. Mahowald MW, Bundlie SR, Hurwitz TD, et al. Sleep violence-forensic science implications: Polygraphic and video documentation. *J Forensic Sci*. 1990;35:413–432.

29. Mahowald MW, Schenck CH, Goldner M, et al. Parasomnia pseudo-suicide. *J Forensic Sci*. 2003;48:1158–1162.

30. Lillywhite AR, Wilson SJ, Nutt DJ. Successful treatment of night terrors and somnambulism with paroxetine. *Br J Psychiatry*. 1994;164:551–554.

31. Balon R. Sleep terror disorder and insomnia treated with trazodone: A case report. *Ann Clin Psychiatry*. 1994;6:161–163.

32. Mahowald MW, Schenck CH. NREM sleep parasomnias 1996. *Neurol Clin*. 1996;14(4):675–696.

33. Aldrich MS. *Sleep medicine*, Vol. 53: Oxford University Press; 1999.

34. Wise MS. Parasomnias in children. *Pediatr Ann*. 1997;26(7):427–433.

35. Mitler MM, Hajdukovic R, Erman M, et al. Narcolepsy. *J Clin Neurophysiol.* 1990;7(1):93–118.

36. Ohayon MM, Caulet M, Priest RG. Violent behavior during sleep. *J Clin Psychiatry.* 1997;58(8):369–376, quiz 77.

37. Comella CL, Nardine TM, Diederich NJ, et al. Sleep-related violence, injury, and REM sleep behavior disorder in Parkinson's disease. *Neurology.* 1998;51:526–529.

38. Eisehsehr I, Parrino L, Noachtar S, et al. Sleep in Lennox-Gastaut syndrome: The role of the Cyclic Alternating Pattern (CAP) in the gate control of clinical seizures and generalized polyspikes. *Epilepsy Res.* 2001;46:241–250.

39. Tachibana M, Tanaka K, Hishikawa Y, et al. A sleep study of acute psychotic states due to alcohol and meprobamate addiction. *Adv in Sleep Research.* 1975;2:177–205.

40. Passouant P, Cadilhac J. M. R. Les privations de sommeil avec mouvements oculaires par les anti-depresseurs. *Rev Neurologique.* 1972;127:173–192.

41. Guilleminault C, Raynal D, Takahashi S, et al. Evaluation of short-term and long-term treatment of the narcolepsy syndrome with clomipramine hydrochloride. *Acta Neurol Scand.* 1976;54:71–87.

42. Besset A. Effect of antidepressants on human sleep. *Adv Biosci.* 1978;21:141–148.

43. Shimizu T, Ookawa M, Iijuma S, et al. Effect of clomipramine on nocturnal sleep of normal human subjects. *Ann Rev Pharmacopsychiat Res Found.* 1985;16:138.

44. Bental E, Lavie P, Sharf B. Severe hypermotility during sleep in treatment of cataplexy with clomipramine. *Isr J Med Sci.* 1979;15:607–609.

45. Akindele MO, Evans JI, Oswald I. Mono-amine oxidase inhibitors, sleep and mood. *EEG Clin Neurophysiol.* 1970;29:47–56.

46. Carlander B, Touchon J, Ondze B, et al. REM sleep behavior disorder induced by cholinergic treatment in Alzheimer's disease. *J Sleep Res.* 1996;5(Suppl 1):28.

47. Ross JS, Shua-Haim JR. Aricept-induced nightmares in Alzheimer's disease: 2 case reports. *J Am Geriatr Soc.* 1998;46:119–120.

48. Schenck CH, Mahowald MW, Kim SW, et al. Prominent eye movements during NREM sleep and REM sleep behavior disorder associated with fluoxetine treatment of depression and obsessive-compulsive disorder. *Sleep.* 1992;15:226–235.

49. Schutte S, Doghramji K. REM behavior disorder seen with venlafaxine (Effexor). *Sleep Res Online.* 1996;25:364.

50. Stolz SE, Aldrich MS. REM sleep behavior disorder associated with caffeine abuse. *Sleep Res Online.* 1991;20:341.

51. Vorona RD, Ware JC. Exacerbation of REM sleep behavior disorder by chocolate ingestion: A case report. *Sleep Med.* 2002;3:365–367.

52. Plazzi G, Cortelli P, Montagna P, et al. REM sleep behavior disorder differentiates pure autonomic failure from multiple system atrophy with autonomic failure. *J Neurol Neurosurg Psychiatry.* 1998;64:683–685.

53. Pareja JA, Caminero AB, Masa JF, et al. A first case of progressive supranuclear palsy and pre-clinical REM sleep behavior

disorder presenting as inhibition of speech during wakefulness and somniloquy with phasic muscle twitching during REM sleep. *Neurologia*. 1996;11:304–306.

54. Boeve BF, Silber MH, Ferman JT, et al. Association of REM sleep behavior disorder and neurodegenerative disease may reflect an underlying synucleinopathy. *Mov Disord*. 2001;16:622–630.

55. Boeve BF, Silber MH, Parisi JE, et al. Synuceinopathy pathology often underlies REM sleep behavior disorder and dementia or parkinsonism. *Neurology*. 2003;61:40–45.

56. Schenck CH, Bundlie SR, Mahowald MW. Delayed emergence of a parkinsonian disorder in 38% of 29 older men initially diagnosed with idiopathic rapid eye movement sleep behavior disorder. *Neurology*. 1996;46:388–393.

57. Montplaisir J, Petit D, Decary A, et al. Sleep and quantitative EEG in patients with progressive supranuclear palsy. *Neurology*. 1997;49:999–1003.

58. Schenck CH, Mahowald MW. Motor dyscontrol in narcolepsy: Rapid-Eye-Movement (REM) sleep without atonia and REM sleep behavior disorder. *Ann Neurol*. 1992;32:3–10.

59. Jouvet M, Delorme F. Locus coeruleus et sommeil paradoxal. *CR Soc Biol*. 1965;159:895–899.

60. Eisehsehr I, Linke R, Noachtar S, et al. Reduced striatal dopamine transporters in idiopathic rapid eye movement sleep behavior disorder. Comparison with Parkinson's disease and controls. *Brain*. 2000;123:1155–1160.

61. Eisehsehr I, Linke R, Tatsch K, et al. Increased muscle activity during rapid eye movement sleep correlates with decrease of striatal presynaptic dopamine transporters. IPT and IBZM SPECT imaging in subclinical and clinically manifest idiopathic REM sleep behavior disorder, Parkinson's disease, and controls. *Sleep*. 2003;26:507–512.

62. Albin RL, Koeppe RA, Chervin RD, et al. Decreased striatal dopaminergic innervation in REM sleep behavior disorder. *Neurology*. 2000;55:1410–1412.

63. Gilman S, Koeppe RA, Chervin R, et al. REM sleep behavior disorder is related to striatal monoaminergic deficit in MSA. *Neurology*. 2003;61:29–34.

64. Fantini ML, Gagnon JF, Petit D, et al. Slowing of electroencephalogram in rapid eye movement sleep behavior disorder. *Ann Neurol*. 2003;53(6):774–780.

65. Schenck CH, Mahowald MW. Polysomnographic, neurologic, psychiatric, and clinical outcome report on 70 consecutive cases with REM sleep behavior disorder (RBD): Sustained clonazepam efficacy in 89.5% of 57 treated patients. *Cleve Clin J Med*. 1990;57(Suppl):S9–S23.

66. Mahowald MW, Schenck CH. *REM sleep behavior disorder*. Philadelphia, PA: WB Saunders; 1994:574–588.

67. Fantini ML, Gagnon J-F, Filipini D, et al. The effects of pramipexole in REM sleep behavior disorder. *Neurology*. 2003; 61:1418–1420.

68. Tan A, Salgado M, Fahn S. Rapid eye movement sleep behavior disorder preceding Parkinson's disease with therapeutic response to levodopa. *Mov Disord*. 1996;11:214–216.

69. Takeuchi N, Uchimura N, Hashizume Y, et al. Melatonin therapy for REM sleep behavior disorder. *Psychiatr Clin Neurosci.* 2001;55(3):267–269.
70. Boeve B. Melatonin for treatment of REM sleep behavior disorder: Response in 8 patients. *Sleep.* 2001;24(Suppl):A35.
71. Lesage S, Earley CJ. Restless legs syndrome. *Curr Treat Options Neurol.* 2004;6(3):209–219.
72. Lesage S, Hening WA. The restless legs syndrome and periodic limb movement disorder: A review of management. *Semin Neurol.* 2004;24(3):249–259.
73. Rothdach AJ, Trenkwalder C, Haberstock J, et al. Prevalence and risk factors of RLS in an elderly population: The MEMO study. Memory and morbidity in augsburg elderly. *Neurology.* 2000;54(5):1064–1068.
74. Tan EK, Seah A, See SJ, et al. Restless legs syndrome in an Asian population: A study in Singapore. *Mov Disord.* 2001;16(3):577–579.
75. Sevim S, Dogu O, Camdeviren H, et al. Unexpectedly low prevalence and unusual characteristics of RLS in Mersin, Turkey. *Neurology.* 2003;61(11):1562–1569.
76. Krishnan PR, Bhatia M, Behari M. Restless legs syndrome in Parkinson's disease: A case-controlled study. *Mov Disord.* 2003;18(2):181–185.
77. Hening WA, Walters AS, Allen RP, et al. Impact, diagnosis and treatment of Restless Legs Syndrome (RLS) in a primary care population: The REST (RLS epidemiology, symptoms, and treatment) primary care study. *Sleep Med.* 2004;5(3):237–246.
78. Allen RP, Picchietti D, Hening WA, et al. Restless legs syndrome: Diagnostic criteria, special considerations, and epidemiology: A report from the restless legs syndrome diagnosis and epidemiology workshop at the National Institutes of Health. *Sleep Med.* 2003;4(2):101–119.
79. Allen RP, Earley CJ. Defining the phenotype of the Restless Legs Syndrome (RLS) using age-of-symptom-onset. *Sleep Med.* 2000;1:11–19.
80. Saletu M, Anderer P, Saletu B, et al. EEG mapping in patients with restless legs syndrome as compared with normal controls. *Psychiatr Res.* 2002;115(1–2):49–61.
81. Berger K, Luedemann J, Trenkwalder C, et al. Sex and the risk of restless legs syndrome in the general population. *Arch Intern Med.* 2004;164(2):196–202.
82. Garcia-Borreguero D, Larrosa O, de la Llave Y. Circadian aspects in the pathophysiology of the restless legs syndrome. *Sleep Med.* 2002;3(Suppl):S17–S21.
83. Earley CJ, Allen RP, Beard JL, et al. Insight into the pathophysiology of restless legs syndrome. *J Neurosci Res.* 2000;62(5):623–628.
84. Earley CJ, Connors JR, Allen RP. RLS patients have abnormally reduced CSF ferritin compared to normal controls. *Neurology.* 1999;52(Suppl 2):A111–A1A2.
85. Hui DS, Wong TY, Ko FW, et al. Prevalence of sleep disturbances in Chinese patients with end-stage renal failure on continuous ambulatory peritoneal dialysis. *Am J Kidney Dis.* 2000;36(4):783–788.

86. Hui D, Wong T, Li T, et al. Prevalence of sleep disturbances in Chinese patients with end stage renal failure on maintenance hemodialysis. *Med Sci Monit*. 2002;8(5):CR331–CR336.
87. Collado-Seidel V, Kohnen R, Samtleben W, et al. Clinical and biochemical findings in uremic patients with and without restless legs syndrome. *Am J Kidney Dis*. 1998;31(2):324–328.
88. Lee KA, Zaffke ME, Baratte-Beebe K. Restless legs syndrome and sleep disturbance during pregnancy: The role of folate and iron. *J Womens Health Gend Based Med*. 2001;10(4):335–341.
89. Suzuki K, Ohida T, Sone T, et al. The prevalence of restless legs syndrome among pregnant women in Japan and the relationship between restless legs syndrome and sleep problems. *Sleep*. 2003;26(6):673–677.
90. Winkelman JW, Chertow GM, Lazarus JM. Restless legs syndrome in end-stage renal disease. *Am J Kidney Dis*. 1996;28(3):372–378.
91. Winkelmann J, Stautner A, Samtleben W, et al. Long-term course of restless legs syndrome in dialysis patients after kidney transplantation. *Mov Disord*. 2002;17(5):1072–1076.
92. Ondo WG, Vuong KD, Jankovic J. Exploring the relationship between Parkinson disease and restless legs syndrome. *Arch Neurol*. 2002;59(3):421–424.
93. Abele M, Burk K, Laccone F, et al. Restless legs syndrome in spinocerebellar ataxia types 1, 2, and 3. *J Neurol*. 2001;248(4):311–314.
94. Schols L, Haan J, Riess O, et al. Sleep disturbance in spinocerebellar ataxias: Is the SCA3 mutation a cause of restless legs syndrome? *Neurology*. 1998;51(6):1603–1607.
95. Banno K, Delaive K, Walld R, et al. Restless legs syndrome in 218 patients: Associated disorders. *Sleep Med*. 2000;1(3):221–229.
96. Agargun MY, Kara H, Ozbek H, et al. Restless legs syndrome induced by mirtazapine. *J Clin Psychiatry*. 2002;63(12):1179.
97. Bakshi R. Fluoxetine and restless legs syndrome. *J Neurol Sci*. 1996;142(1–2):151–152.
98. Hargrave R, Beckley DJ. Restless leg syndrome exacerbated by sertraline. *Psychosomatics*. 1998;39(2):177–178.
99. Sanz-Fuentenebro FJ, Huidobro A, Tejadas-Rivas A. Restless legs syndrome and paroxetine. *Acta Psychiatr Scand*. 1996;94(6):482–484.
100. Chesson AL Jr, Ferber RA, Fry JM, et al. The indications for polysomnography and related procedures. *Sleep*. 1997;20(6):423–487.
101. Littner M, Hirshkowitz M, Kramer M, et al. Practice parameters for using polysomnography to evaluate insomnia: An update. *Sleep*. 2003;26(6):754–760.
102. O'Keeffe ST, Gavin K, Lavan JN. Iron status and restless legs syndrome in the elderly. *Age Ageing*. 1994;23(3):200–203.
103. Sun ER, Chen CA, Ho G, et al. Iron and the restless legs syndrome. *Sleep*. 1998;21(4):371–377.
104. Silber MH, Girish M, Izurieta R. Pramipexole in the management of restless legs syndrome: An extended study. *Sleep*. 2003;26(7):819–821.

105. Mitler MM, Browman CP, Menn SJ, et al. Nocturnal my-
     oclonus: Treatment efficacy of clonazepam and temazepam.
     Sleep. 1986;9:385–392.
106. Kaplan P, Allen RP, Buchholz DW, et al. A double-blind,
     placebo-controlled study of the treatment of periodic limb move-
     ments in sleep using carbidopa/levodopa and propoxyphene.
     Sleep. 1993;16(8):717–723.
107. Hening W, Allen R, Earley C, et al. The treatment of restless legs
     syndrome and periodic limb movement disorder. An American
     Academy of Sleep Medicine Review. *Sleep*. 1999;22(7):970–999.
108. Hening WA, Allen RP, Earley CJ, et al. An update on the
     dopaminergic treatment of restless legs syndrome and periodic
     limb movement disorder. *Sleep*. 2004;27(3):560–583.
109. Allen RP, Earley CJ. Augmentation of the restless legs syn-
     drome with carbidopa/levodopa. *Sleep*. 1996;19(3):205–213.
110. Garcia-Borreguero D, Larrosa O, de la Llave Y, et al. Treatment
     of restless legs syndrome with gabapentin: A double-blind,
     cross-over study. *Neurology*. 2002;59(10):1573–1579.
111. Kavey N, Walters AS, Hening W, et al. Opioid treatment of
     periodic movements in sleep in patients without restless legs.
     Neuropeptides. 1988;11(4):181–184.
112. Wetter TC, Pollmacher T. Restless legs and periodic leg
     movements in sleep syndromes. *J Neurol*. 1997;244(4, Suppl
     1):S37–S45.
113. The Atlas Task Force. Recording and scoring leg movements.
     Sleep. 1993;16(8):748–759.
114. Ancoli-Israel S, Kripke DF, Mason W, et al. Sleep apnea and
     periodic movements in an aging sample. *J Gerontol*. 1985;40(4):
     419–425.
115. Carelli G, Krieger J, Calvi-Gries F, et al. Periodic limb move-
     ments and obstructive sleep apneas before and after continuous
     positive airway pressure treatment. *J Sleep Res*. 1999;8(3):
     211–216.
116. Ancoli-Israel S, Bliwise DL, Mant A. *Sleep and breathing in the
     elderly*. New York: Mercel Dekker; 1993:673–693.
117. Brasic JR. Quinine-induced thrombocytopenia in a 64-year-old
     man who consumed tonic water to relieve nocturnal leg cramps.
     Mayo Clin Proc. 2001;76(8):863–864.
118. Crum NF, Gable P. Quinine-induced hemolytic-uremic syn-
     drome. *South Med J*. 2000;93(7):726–728.
119. Mandal AK, Abernathy T, Nelluri SN, et al. Is quinine effective
     and safe in leg cramps? *J Clin Pharmacol*. 1995;35(6):588–593.
120. Vetrugno R, Provini F, Meletti S, et al. Propriospinal myoclonus
     at the sleep-wake transition: A new type of parasomnia. *Sleep*.
     2001;24(7):835–843.
121. Plazzi G, Provini F, Liguori R, et al. Propriospinal myoclonus
     at the transition from wake to sleep. *Sleep Res*. 1996;26:438.
122. Vetrugno R, Provini F, Meletti S, et al. Propriospinal myoclonus
     at the sleep-wake transition: A new type of parasomnia. *Sleep*.
     2001;24:835–843.
123. Montagna P, Provini F, Plazzi G, et al. Propriospinal myoclonus
     upon relaxation and drowsiness: A cause of severe insomnia.
     Mov Disord. 1997;12:66–72.
124. Rugh JD, Harlan J. Nocturnal bruxism and temporomandibular
     disorders. *Adv Neurol*. 1988;49:329–341.

125. Richmond G, Rugh JD, Dolfi R, et al. Survey of bruxism in an institutionalized mentally retarded population. *Am J Ment Defic*. 1984;88(4):418–421.
126. Gerber PE, Lynd LD. Selective serotonin-reuptake inhibitor-induced movement disorders. *Ann Pharmacother*. 1998;32(6):692–698.
127. Ellison JM, Stanziani P. SSRI-associated nocturnal bruxism in four patients. *J Clin Psychiatry*. 1993;54(11):432–434.
128. Lavigne GJ, Rompre PH, Montplaisir JY. Sleep bruxism: Validity of clinical research diagnostic criteria in a controlled polysomnographic study. *J Dent Res*. 1996;75(1):546–552.
129. Kato T, Montplaisir JY, Blanchet PJ, et al. Idiopathic myoclonus in the oromandibular region during sleep: A possible source of confusion in sleep bruxism diagnosis. *Mov Disord*. 1999;14(5):865–871.
130. Happe S, Ludemann P, Ringelstein EB. Persistence of rhythmic movement disorder beyond childhood: A videotape demonstration. *Mov Disord*. 2000;15:1296–1297.
131. Kohyama J, Masukura F, Kimura K, et al. Rhythmic movement disorder: Polysomnographic study and summary of reported cases. *Brain Dev*. 2002;24:33–38.
132. Kempenaers C, Bouillon E, Mendlewicz J. A rhythmic movement disorder in REM sleep: A case report. *Sleep*. 1994;17:274–279.
133. Gagnon P, De Koninck J. Repetitive head movements during REM sleep. *Biol Psychiatry*. 1985;20:176.
134. Kuhn BR, Elliott AJ. Treatment efficacy in behavioral pediatric sleep medicine. *J Psychosom Res*. 2003;54(6):587–597.
135. Hoban TF. Rhythmic movement disorder in children. *CNS Spectr*. 2003;8(2):135–138.
136. Reimao RN, Lefevre AB. Prevalence of sleep-talking in childhood. *Brain Dev*. 1980;2(4):353–357.
137. Arkin AM, Toth MF, Baker J, et al. The degree of concordance between the content of sleep talking and mentation recalled in wakefulness. *J Nerv Ment Dis*. 1970;151(6):375–393.
138. Arkin AM, Toth MF, Baker J, et al. The frequency of sleep talking in the laboratory among chronic sleep talkers and good dream recallers. *J Nerv Ment Dis*. 1970;151(6):369–374.
139. Leo G. Parasomnias. *WMJ*. 2003;102(1):32–35.
140. Clouston PD, Lim CL, Fung V, et al. Brainstem myoclonus in a patient with non-dopa-responsive parkinsonism. *Mov Disord*. 1996;11(4):404–410.
141. Bruno RL. Abnormal movements in sleep as a post-polio sequelae. *Am J Phys Med Rehabil*. 1998;77(4):339–343.
142. Bruni O, Galli F, Guidetti V. Sleep hygiene and migraine in children and adolescents. *Cephalalgia*. 1999;19(Suppl 25):57–59.
143. Sander HW, Geisse H, Quinto C, et al. Sensory sleep starts. *J Neurol Neurosurg Psychiatry*. 1998;64(5):690.
144. Montagna P. Sleep-related non epileptic motor disorders. *J Neurol*. 2004;251(7):781–794.
145. Vaccario ML, Valenti MA, Carullo A, et al. Benign neonatal sleep myoclonus: Case report and follow-up of four members of an affected family. *Clin Electroencephalogr*. 2003;34(1):15–17.

146. Broughton R, Tolentino MA, Krelina M. Excessive fragmentary myoclonus in NREM sleep: A report of 38 cases. *Electroencephalogr Clin Neurophysiol*. 1985;61(2):123–133.

147. Lins O, Castonguay M, Dunham W, et al. Excessive fragmentary myoclonus: Time of night and sleep stage distributions. *Can J Neurol Sci*. 1993;20(2):142–146.

148. Vetrugno R, Plazzi G, Provini F, et al. Excessive fragmentary hypnic myoclonus: Clinical and neurophysiological findings. *Sleep Med*. 2002;3(1):73–76.

149. Vetrugno R, Provini F, Plazzi G, et al. Catathrenia (nocturnal groaning): A new type of parasomnia. *Neurology*. 2001;56:681–683.

150. DeRoeck J, Van Hoof E, Cluydts R. Sleep-related expiratory groaning: A case report. *Sleep Res*. 1983;12:237.

151. Lugaresi E, Cirignotta F, Coccagna G, et al. Nocturnal myoclonus and restless legs syndrome. *Adv Neurol*. 1986;43:295–307.

Circadian Rhythm Sleep Disorders

Brandon S. Lu, Prasanth Manthena, and Phyllis C. Zee

OVERVIEW OF CIRCADIAN BIOLOGY

Human beings have adapted to living in a 24-hour environment by developing an internal timing system that exhibits circadian (Latin for *about a day*) rhythmicity. When humans are isolated from time-indicating external stimuli, such as the light/dark cycle and social cues, this endogenous rhythm cycles with a period that is slightly longer.[1] The master clock of the body is the suprachiasmatic nucleus (SCN) located in the anterior hypothalamus.[2] In addition to governing the 24-hour cycle of sleep and wakefulness, the SCN also maintains the circadian rhythm of other physiologic variables such as temperature and cortisol and melatonin levels.[3]

To entrain the body and its various circadian rhythms to the 24-hour day, the SCN inputs information about time from a variety of sources, ranging from physical exertion to social activity. The strongest *zeitgeber* (German, *for time giver*) is light. The SCN receives input about light levels from the retina, not from the rods and cones responsible for vision but from specialized ganglion cells in the retina, which produce the photopigment melanopsin and are particularly sensitive to light from the blue spectrum.[4] Exposure to light at various times of the day will either advance or delay the circadian rhythm, the direction and magnitude of which is depicted on a phase response curve.

Another important *zeitgeber* is melatonin. This hormone produced by the pineal gland not only is secreted under the direct influence of the SCN but also can shift circadian rhythms and act to promote sleep onset.[5] Melatonin levels are low during the day and begin to rise just before sleep onset in humans. It peaks during the night around the time when the temperature is at its nadir. Light suppresses melatonin secretion, whereas darkness has the opposite effect. Exogenous melatonin taken in the evening will facilitate sleep onset, causing advancement in sleep phase and when taken in the morning will lead to a later bedtime, thereby having opposite phase-shifting effects as light.[6]

CIRCADIAN RHYTHM SLEEP DISORDERS

Circadian rhythm sleep disorders (CRSDs) should be considered in the differential diagnosis of patients who present with symptoms of insomnia or hypersomnia. Affected individuals can present with various sleep complaints, ranging from insomnia to excessive daytime sleepiness (EDS) and early awakenings. The *International Classification of Sleep Disorders, Second Edition,* (*ICSD-2*) recognizes nine types of CRSDs (see Appendix J). The

Table 6-1. Overview of the presentation and treatment of circadian rhythm sleep disorders (CRSD)

Circadian Disorder	Main Complaints	Preferred Sleep/Wake Time	Treatment
Delayed sleep phase type	1. Inability to fall asleep at night 2. Difficulty waking up in the morning	Sleep time: 2–6 AM Wake time: 10 AM–1 PM	Sleep hygiene Bright light therapy: 2,000–2,500 lux for 2–3 h starting from 6 AM Melatonin 1–3 mg—5–7 h before sleep time
Advanced sleep phase type	1. Inability to stay awake at night 2. Inability to stay asleep in the morning	Sleep time: 6–9 PM Wake time: 2–5 AM	Bright light therapy: 2,000 lux for 4 h starting from 8 PM or 4,000 lux for 2–3 h starting from 8 or 9 PM
Free-running type	Changes with time: Varies from insomnia to excess daytime sleepiness	Sleep time: changes Wake time: changes	Melatonin 10 mg 1 h before bedtime (maintenance dose may be reduced to 1 or 0.5 mg)
Irregular sleep/wake type	No consolidated sleep period: Will fall asleep or be awake at inappropriate times	Irregular pattern of sleep and wake times	Increase light exposure and social activity during daylight hours

Shift-work sleep disorder	1. Excessive sleepiness during work associated with work schedule 2. Insomnia when trying to sleep during the day	Varies according to work schedule	Circadian alignment and promotion of sleep Bright light therapy: 5–10,000 lux during the first half of the night shift (intermittent or continuous) Melatonin 2–5 mg—prior to bedtime Stimulants for excessive sleepiness—caffeine and modafinil
Jet lag	Excessive sleepiness and/or insomnia depending on length and direction of travel	Varies according to time zone	Timed bright light Melatonin 2–5 mg—after arrival, taken before bedtime Zolpidem 10 mg—after arrival, taken before bedtime

general criteria for CRSDs are that (i) persistent or recurrent pattern of sleep disturbance is thought to be primarily due to either an alteration in the circadian timing system or a misalignment between endogenous circadian rhythms and external factors that affect the timing of sleep; (ii) sleep disturbance leads to insomnia, excessive sleepiness, or both; or (iii) sleep disturbance is associated with impairment of function (see Table 6-1).

This chapter discusses the most commonly encountered CRSDs: Delayed sleep phase type (DSPT), advanced sleep phase type (ASPT), free-running type, irregular sleep–wake type, shift-work sleep disorder, and jet lag. It is important to note that although CRSDs are important in clinical practice, the practice parameters for the treatment of most of these disorders have not been established. Pharmacologic approaches that are discussed in this chapter represent off-label use, and melatonin is non-U.S. Food and Drug Administration (FDA) approved.

Delayed Sleep Phase Type

DSPT is the most common of the CRSDs.[7] It was first characterized by Weitzman et al. in 1981, and patients with DSPT report a chronic inability to fall asleep at a desired clock time to meet their work schedules but describe undisturbed late sleep on vacations.[8] The exact pathophysiology of DSPT is unknown. However, several mechanisms could potentially explain the persistent delayed sleep phase relative to the 24-hour environment.

One proposed explanation is that patients with DSPT have a longer endogenous circadian period that regulates the sleep-–wake cycle.[9] Evidence also suggests that some patients with DSPT may be hypersensitive to evening light, which can serve as a delaying signal to the circadian clock,[10] or have reduced retinal sensitivity to morning light, which can decrease the phase-advancing effects of light in the morning. Although DSPT is often regarded as resulting from alteration in circadian timing, recent studies indicate that the homeostatic regulation of sleep may also be impaired.[8,11,12] Finally, genetic factors are likely to play a role in the pathogenesis of DSPT. For example, there are familial forms of DSPT, and polymorphisms in circadian *genes* such as *Per3, arylalkylamine N-acetyltransferase, HLA*, and *Clock* have been reported in "evening" types and DSPT.[13–16]

Clinical Presentation

Although DSPT can present at any age, most patients are adolescents or young adults. Individuals with DSPT will present with sleep-onset insomnia and difficulty waking in the morning. Patients usually fall asleep between 2 and 6 AM and wake up between 10 AM and 1 PM[8] (see Fig. 6-1). Early daytime sleepiness may be present, and these patients will score as "evening" types on self-assessment questionnaires such as the Horne and Ostberg.[17] Like "evening" types, patients with DSPT are most alert and active in the late evening hours; however, enforced conventional wake times will lead to chronic sleep deprivation and a persistent inability to fall asleep at an earlier time. In this sense, patients with DSPT are not able to "adapt" themselves to waking up early by going to sleep earlier, unlike unaffected individuals. If a college student who is used to a delayed sleep–wake cycle

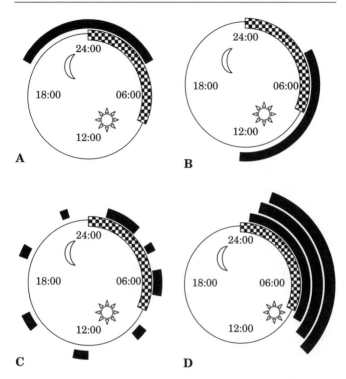

Figure 6-1. Schematic representation of the four major types of circadian rhythm sleep disorders. Advanced sleep phase type (A). Delayed sleep phase type (B). Irregular sleep–wake type (C). Free-running type (D). *Checkered bars* represent conventional sleep time and *black bars* represent sleep times of different disorders.

joins the workforce, he or she will complain of morning fatigue. This individual does not have DSPT if he or she can adjust to the morning work routine within a few days or weeks.

Failure to attend morning classes or be on time for work will often lead to poor grades at school or disciplinary actions at work. On weekends or vacations, patients with DSPT will usually extend their sleep time significantly beyond that during the weekdays.[18] Usually, a variety of methods of phase advancement (e.g., earlier bedtime and multiple alarm clocks) have been tried without success. Pharmacologic means of inducing sleep are also frequently tried (e.g., sedatives and alcohol) but may result in drowsiness next morning or may lead to substance abuse.[19]

Epidemiology

DSPT is estimated to be present in approximately 0.17% of the general population,[20] and most reports show a male:female ratio of 10:1.[11] A survey of adolescents, however, indicated a prevalence of $>7\%$.[21] DSPT also accounts for approximately 7% of patients with chronic insomnia presenting to sleep clinics.[8]

Classification

The American Academy of Sleep Medicine revised the classification of sleep disturbances in the *ICSD-2*.[22] "Circadian rhythm sleep disorder, delayed sleep phase type" has the same classification and name in *Diagnostic and Statistical Manual, Text Revision (DSM-IV-TR, 2000)*.[23] The ICD-9 code is 327.31.

Diagnostic Evaluation

The diagnosis of DSPT is usually evident from a detailed history and a sleep diary or actigraphy for at least 7 days, which should include weekends with less strict social and work restrictions to ensure that the patient exhibits a delayed sleep–wake pattern Actigraphy uses a wrist-worn motion detector (usually designed to look like a wristwatch) to monitor sleep and wake activity for prolonged periods (up to several weeks). Provided that a normal neurologic examination is performed, overnight polysomnography may be indicated when complaints of sleep maintenance and daytime somnolence are present to rule out other sleep disorders such as sleep apnea and periodic limb movement disorders.[8] If performed at the patient's desired sleep–wake times, the sleep architecture should be normal with the exception of sleep latency that may be prolonged.[19]

Diagnosis

The diagnostic criteria for DSPT set forth by the *ICSD-2*[22] are:

1. A delay in the phase of the major sleep period in relation to the desired sleep time and wake-up time is present.
2. When allowed to set their schedule, patients will exhibit normal sleep quality and duration for age and maintain a delayed, but stable, phase of entrainment to the 24-hour sleep–wake pattern.
3. Sleep log or actigraphy monitoring for at least 7 days demonstrates a stable delay in the timing of the habitual sleep period.
4. The sleep disturbance is not better explained by another disorder.

Differential Diagnosis

DSPT must be distinguished from "normal" sleep patterns in which an individual has a late schedule (delayed bedtime and rise time) that does not cause personal, social, or occupational distress. This is most commonly seen in adolescents and young adults. Other causes of sleep-initiation insomnia, such as primary and secondary insomnias, should be included in the differential. Insomnia will not be present in patients with DSPT if they are allowed to sleep and rise on their own accord. EDS may also be caused by other sleep disturbances (e.g., sleep-related breathing disorders, insomnias, and sleep-related movement disorders), as well as medical, neurologic, and psychiatric disorders. The circadian nature of DSPT, however, should differentiate it from other disorders with similar complaints. There is a strong association of DSPT with many psychiatric disorders including depression, personality disorder, and hypochondriasis.[9,24–26] It is prudent, therefore, to screen for psychiatric disorders in patients with DSPT.

Management

Several modalities of treatment of DSPT have been reported in the literature, including chronotherapy, bright light therapy, and pharmacologic intervention. Just as there are many possible causes of DSPT, patients will respond differently to the various treatment options. Successful treatment of a patient may require alteration of therapy on the basis of response.

CHRONOTHERAPY. Chronotherapy, first described by Czeisler et al. in 1981, refers to progressive phase delay by 3 hours every 2 days until the desired sleep time is achieved.[27] This principle is based on the analogy of Weitzman in which he likened DSPT to driving in a one-way street and being unable to back up even one or two houses. The best treatment in this case would be to "drive around the block" or progressively delay bedtime and wake time until the desired timing has been reached.[9] Although success with chronotherapy has been reported, the process is disruptive to the daily routine and requires full patient compliance.[8,27] Originally implemented on an in-patient basis, chronotherapy is now performed at home following a well-structured protocol that is patient-dependent. Its rigid design and lengthy process, however, are the downfall of the procedure, limiting its clinical use. Maintenance of an early schedule after successful phase advancement is also difficult.[28] Cases of free-running syndrome (see section on "Free-Running [nonentrained] Type") have also been described after chronotherapy for DSPT, in which patients develop a persistent 25-hour sleep–wake cycle that lies outside the range of entrainment.[29]

BRIGHT LIGHT THERAPY. Bright light therapy is based on a phase response curve, which predicts that light pulse given before the time of body temperature minimum will delay the circadian system, whereas light given after the minimum will advance it.[30,31] Lewy et al. first proposed the use of bright light therapy for the treatment of DSPT, and Rosenthal et al. demonstrated that a combination of 2-hour bright light treatment of 2,500 lux in the morning and use of dark goggles in the evening significantly phase advanced patients with DSPT by 1 hour and 25 minutes compared to controls.[32,33] On the basis of level II and III evidence, the American Academy of Sleep Medicine maintains that light therapy appears to have a potential utility in the treatment of DSPT, although the minimum or optimal duration of therapy is unknown.[34] As with other therapies, patient compliance may be problematic, especially when bright light therapy has to be given early in the morning (see Fig. 6-2). With recent studies illustrating an increased effectiveness of low-wavelength and less intense light in phase-shifting the circadian rhythm, a potentially less noxious therapy may improve patient compliance in the future.

PHARMACOTHERAPY. Of the pharmacologic options for DSPT, melatonin has been studied most extensively. When administered in the evening, melatonin can advance the phase of

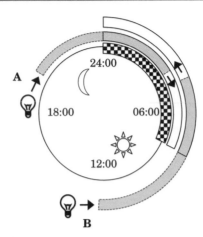

Figure 6-2. Schematic representation of light therapy for circadian rhythm sleep disorders. Evening light therapy will phase delay advanced sleep phase types (A). Morning light therapy will phase advance delayed sleep phase types (B). *Checkered bar* represents conventional sleep time and *gray bars* represent disordered sleep times being phase shifted.

circadian rhythm and sleep.[6] Melatonin 5 mg taken at 10 PM significantly advanced sleep-onset time and wake time without hangover effects next morning[35] and improved quality of life in patients with DSPT.[36] Other small trials have yielded similar results, although the dose and administration time of melatonin have varied in these studies.[37–39] A recent study showed that melatonin doses lower than 3 mg when given approximately 7 hours before sleep time can also be effective.[40] However, because of the lack of large randomized placebo-controlled studies and the variability in the dose and timing of melatonin administration in the available studies, clinical guidelines for the use of melatonin has not been established. Potential adverse effects of melatonin include its vasoconstrictive properties and endocrine effects; therefore, caution should be used when prescribing this drug to patients with cardiovascular disease and to children.[41]

Other pharmacologic measures used for DSPT include hypnotics and vitamin B_{12}. Three studies have documented successful treatment of long-standing DSPT after vitamin B_{12} administration, with two studies being case reports.[28,42,43] A multicenter, double-blind study of patients with DSPT, however, showed no difference in night sleep, daytime mood, or drowsiness between the vitamin B_{12} and the control groups.[44] Ozaki et al. successfully treated a patient with DSPT using a combination of triazolam and chronotherapy, but another patient became more depressed on triazolam.[45] Clearly well-designed studies are needed to better define the role of pharmacologic therapies for the treatment of DSPT.

Because the etiology of DSPT is likely multifactorial, a single treatment strategy will not be effective for every patient. Several investigators have attempted to treat patients with DSPT using one or more of the options mentioned in the preceding text. Okawa et al. treated 20 adolescent patients with DSPT with chronotherapy, bright light therapy, vitamin B_{12}, and/or melatonin. Thirteen of the 20 patients were successfully treated in this study.[46] Yamadera et al. reported a marked or moderate improvement in 42% of patients with DSPT treated with vitamin B_{12}, bright light therapy, and/or hypnotic medication.[43]

Follow-up

Patients with DSPT should be carefully monitored once therapy begins. For patients on chronotherapy, compliance must be strictly enforced and progress followed. Bright light therapy should be administered daily, with or without dark goggles in the evening, and patients given pharmacologic therapy should be assessed for toxicities.

General Approach to Evaluation and Treatment of Delayed Sleep Phase Type

EVALUATION.

- DSPT should be considered in patients with sleep-onset insomnia, difficulty waking up, and excessive sleepiness (particularly in the morning).
- When allowed to go to bed and wake up at the preferred later times of the patients, sleep quality is essentially normal.
- Careful attention should be paid to rule out other sleep disorders, as well as medical and psychiatric disorders.
- Behavioral factors (e.g., irregular sleep schedules, voluntarily delaying bedtime, light exposure, exercise, and caffeine) should be considered in the evening, particularly in adolescents and young adults.
- To confirm the diagnosis, sleep logs or actigraphy monitoring for 7 days is recommended (patients will usually show further delay in sleep and wake times on weekends or vacation).

MANAGEMENT.

- Good sleep habits to promote sleep and advance circadian rhythms.
    - Maintain regular sleep and wake time
    - Avoid naps
    - Avoid exposure to bright light after 9 PM
    - Encourage exposure to bright light in the morning
    - Exercise regularly
- Bright light exposure
    - Bright light therapy should be provided as soon as possible after awakening (usually 6 to 8 AM; but time needs to be adjusted if sleep and wake times are extreme)
    - This is usually done with a light intensity starting around 2,000 to 2,500 lux (intensity of most commercial light sources)
    - Patient should be encouraged to maintain daily treatment as much as possible for approximately 1 hour per morning (Note: There are no guidelines for the duration of therapy)

- Melatonin (no established clinical practice parameters for use and not FDA approved)
  - Melatonin 1 to 3 mg (available over the counter) can be given 5 to 7 hours before habitual sleep time (8 to 10 PM) for patients who typically fall asleep between 2 to 4 AM. This early administration time is recommended to promote the largest possible advancement of the circadian rhythm.[40]
  - Melatonin has also been shown in small studies to be effective when taken within 1 hour of bedtime.
- If no significant improvement is observed any time after evaluation and initial behavioral therapies, referral to a sleep specialist is appropriate.

Advanced Sleep Phase Type

ASPT is characterized by sleep/wake times that are several hours earlier than the desired or conventional time. Patients have a habitual sleep time of 6 to 9 PM and staying up past 9 PM is extremely difficult. The usual wake time is between 2 and 5 AM, and these patients will score as "morning-types" on the Horne and Ostberg questionnaire.

Similar to DSPT, the pathogenesis of ASPT is not clearly defined and could be multifactorial. Shortening of the endogenous circadian period could offer a potential explanation, and this is corroborated by the finding of a short circadian period in a patient with familial ASPT.[47] Another factor that could contribute to the development of ASPT is exposure to early morning light, which can serve to advance circadian rhythms. Furthermore, "morning-type" individuals may have increased retinal sensitivity to light in the morning compared to "evening-type" individuals.[48] Similarly, by going to bed early, these patients are not exposed to light in the phase delay region of the curve, resulting in a perpetual advanced phase.[49]

Recently, a human *Per2* gene mutation that caused hypophosphorylation of the *Per2* protein was associated with ASPT in only one member of a family with ASPT.[50] This fact speaks for the heterogeneity of the disease. Another study showed an autosomal dominant mode of inheritance of ASPT in a large family.[51] Further genetic analysis and genomics research should better elucidate the pathogenesis of ASPT.

Clinical Presentation

Individuals affected with ASPT will complain of sleepiness in the late afternoon or early evening, early morning–awakening insomnia, or sleep-maintenance insomnia. When required to keep a conventional schedule by delaying bedtime, these patients will still have early rising time, leading to chronic sleep deprivation. The use of hypnotics, stimulants, or alcohol to combat sleep-maintenance insomnia and daytime sleepiness may lead to substance abuse in these individuals.

Epidemiology

The estimated prevalence of ASPT is substantially lower than that of DSPT. Ando et al.[52] estimated a prevalence of 1% in middle-aged adults, and in a survey of 10,000 adult Norwegians, no case of ASPT was identified.[20] Non–age-related ASPT is uncommon, with only a few reported cases.[53,54] A potential reason for the low prevalence of ASPT in the general population is underreporting. It may be that an "early person" is less likely to seek medical attention because having an early schedule does not interfere with school or work, unlike a "night owl" who is constantly late for morning events. Older individuals may not complain of an advanced sleep/wake cycle because it does not interfere with their lives or it may be perceived as a normal aging process.

Classification

The *ICSD-2* classifies ASPT as "circadian rhythm sleep disorder, advanced sleep phase type," whereas in the *DSM-IV-TR* this disorder is known as "circadian rhythm sleep disorder, unspecified type."[22,23] It carries an ICD-9 code of 327.32.

Diagnostic Evaluation

A history of chronic early evening sleepiness and early morning awakening/insomnia is always present. As stated, patients will complain of daytime sleepiness when required to conform to a conventional schedule because of chronic sleep deprivation. A sleep log or actigraphy over 7 days can be used to confirm ASPT. Again, 7 days is recommended to allow for data collection from days when the patient is relatively free of social and work demands and can sleep at desired bedtimes. Polysomnography performed at the patient's desired sleep times will show normal sleep architecture and total sleep time for age with a long period of wakefulness at the end of the night.[19] Polysomnography may be useful to exclude other causes of hypersomnia.

Diagnosis

The criteria given by the *ICSD-2*[22] for the diagnosis of ASPT are:

1. An advance in the phase of the major sleep period in relation to the desired sleep time and wake-up time is present.
2. When allowed to set their schedule, patients have normal sleep quality and duration for age in an advanced, but stable, phase of entrainment to the 24-hour sleep–wake pattern.
3. Sleep log or actigraphy monitoring for at least 7 days demonstrates a stable advance in the timing of the habitual sleep period.
4. The sleep disturbance is not better explained by another disorder.

Differential Diagnosis

The diagnosis of ASPT should only be made in a patient with advanced sleep schedules if it is associated with functional impairment. Other causes of early morning awakening/insomnia, such as primary and secondary insomnias, should also be excluded. Because early morning awakening is a prominent feature of major depression, mood disorders must also be considered.

Management

Similar to DSPT, bright light therapy and chronotherapy have been used to normalize the timing of the sleep–wake cycle. Lack and Wright reported their success with treating patients with ASPT using bright light therapy from 8 PM to 12 AM for two consecutive nights. Although sleep-onset time did not change, final wake time was delayed by >1 hour and resulted in increased total sleep time. Other measures of circadian rhythm were also delayed (temperature and melatonin rhythms).[55] Another study of older individuals with sleep-maintenance insomnia treated for 12 days with evening bright light therapy demonstrated a significant reduction in waking time during sleep and increased sleep efficiency.[56]

Chronotherapy, with phase advancement of bedtime by 3 hours every 2 days, was shown to be effective in one patient with ASPT.[57] Behavioral therapies such as bright light therapy and chronotherapy are notorious for poor compliance if the task is difficult or inconvenient. Melatonin therapy could potentially cause phase delay if administered in the morning. The sedating effect of melatonin, however, may limit its use during the morning. To date, there has been no data proving the efficacy of using melatonin for ASPT.

Follow-up

The two available therapies for treating ASPT require close monitoring and follow-up. Before treatment is completed, it is imperative to monitor the patient to ensure adherence to the proposed protocol. After successful treatment, behavioral strategies should be set to prevent phase advancement (i.e., avoid early bedtime, keep active in the evening).

General Approach to Evaluation and Treatment of Advanced Sleep Phase Type

EVALUATION.

- ASPT should be considered in patients with early morning awakening and excessive sleepiness (particularly in the early evening).
- When allowed to go to bed and wake up at the preferred earlier times of the patients, sleep quality is essentially normal.
- Careful attention should be paid to rule out other sleep disorders, as well as medical and psychiatric disorders.
- Behavioral factors such as irregular sleep schedules, voluntarily waking up early, and light exposure in the early morning should be considered, particularly in older adults.
- To confirm the diagnosis, sleep logs or actigraphy monitoring for 7 days is recommended (patients will usually show a stable advanced sleep–wake cycle, which persists on weekends and vacation).

MANAGEMENT.

- Good sleep habits to promote sleep and normalize phase of circadian rhythms
    - Avoid bright light exposure too early in the morning (5 to 7 AM)
    - Increase exposure to light in the late afternoon and early evening (7 to 9 PM)

- Maintain a regular sleep–wake schedule
- Exercise regularly
- Avoid naps
- Bright light
  - Bright light of 2,000 lux for 4 hours starting from 8 PM or 4,000 lux for 2 to 3 hours starting from 8 or 9 PM
  - Referral to a sleep specialist should be considered if symptoms do not improve.

Free-Running (Nonentrained) Type

The sleep and wake times of patients with free-running type vary because their circadian rhythm is not stably entrained to the 24-hour day. The free-running endogenous circadian period is usually slightly longer than 24 hours; therefore, the sleep period will usually drift later each day. As the rhythm drifts, at different times, sleep and wake times will be in phase with the external 24-hour physical environment for a short period (days to weeks). Because light is the strongest external synchronizer, most patients with free-running type are blind or have impaired light perception.

The precise etiology of free-running type in sighted individuals is unknown. In blind individuals it is thought to be due to lack of photic entrainment.[58] However, some blind individuals are able to respond to bright light.[59] In sighted individuals, decreased exposure or sensitivity to light and social and physical activity cues may contribute to a nonentrained circadian rhythm.[60]

Similar to patients with DSPT, a long circadian period outside the range of entrainment has been proposed as part of the pathophysiology in those with free-running type.[61] This concept is supported by a report illustrating the development of free-running type in patients with DSPT who were treated with chronotherapy.[29] Free-running type and DSPT may represent a continuum of the same CRSD.

Clinical Presentation

Patients with free-running type will typically present with periods of insomnia, hypersomnia, or both, which alternate with short asymptomatic periods. Because the circadian period is not aligned to the external 24-hour environment, symptoms will depend on when an individual tries to sleep in relation to the circadian rhythm of sleep propensity. Starting with the asymptomatic period when the patient's sleep phase is aligned to the external environment, sleep latency will gradually prolong and patients will complain of sleep-onset insomnia. As the sleep phase is shifted to daytime, patients will have trouble staying awake, and daytime sleepiness will be present until the sleep phase is realigned with the environment.

Epidemiology

The prevalence of free-running type in the general population is unknown. The disorder is most commonly seen in blind individuals and was first reported in a blind person in 1977.[62] The reported prevalence in blind individuals is 50%.[58,63] Cases in sighted individuals have been reported, with one report of free-running type developing after a car accident.[64–66]

Classification

The *ICSD-2* classifies this disorder as "circadian rhythm sleep disorder, free-running type," and it is also commonly called "nonentrained type" or "non–24-hour sleep–wake syndrome."[22] In the *DSM-IV-TR* this disorder is known as "circadian rhythm sleep disorder, unspecified type."[23] The ICD-9 code is 327.34.

Diagnostic Evaluation

Patients with free-running type will present with symptoms described in the preceding text. Sleep diary or actigraphy for an extended period will help confirm the free-running rhythm. Polysomnography is not essential for the diagnosis but can be useful in excluding other sleep disorders. When performed on a patient with free-running type, polysomnography should be normal for age if the recorded sleep time is at the patient's preferred sleep time.

Diagnosis

The diagnosis of free-running type can be established on the basis of the following:[22]

1. There is a complaint of insomnia or excessive sleepiness related to abnormal synchronization between the 24-hour light/dark cycle and the endogenous circadian rhythm of sleep and wake propensity.
2. Sleep log or actigraphy monitoring (at least 7 days) demonstrates a pattern of sleep and wake times that typically delays each day with a period longer than 24 hours.
3. The sleep disturbance is not better explained by any other disorder.

Differential Diagnosis

Patients with DSPT may display a similar progressive delay in sleep period for several days and this condition may be confused with the free-running type. Institutionalized patients with psychiatric disorders often become insensitive to social cues, which predisposes them to the development of free-running type.[9] As such, depressive symptoms and mood disorders are often comorbid conditions in patients with free-running type.

Management

Sleep hygiene education and structured exposure to social and physical activity cues can improve sleep and entrainment of circadian rhythms in individuals with free-running type.[67] When these behavioral approaches are insufficient, melatonin could be considered. Sack et al. demonstrated that melatonin 10 mg given 1 hour before the preferred bedtime for 3 to 9 weeks was an effective treatment in blind individuals with nonentrained rhythms.[68] A reduced dose of melatonin (0.5 to 4 mg per day) has also been shown to be effective in maintaining entrainment in blind subjects with free-running type.[69,70]

Oral vitamin B_{12} has proven efficacy in some cases of free-running type. Doses of 1.5 mg three times per day to 3 mg daily have been used with success.[28,42,65] The reason for the effectiveness of vitamin B_{12} is not clearly understood, and the patients did not have documented vitamin B_{12} deficiency.

In sighted individuals, melatonin and bright light therapy have showed promising results. A sighted patient with free-running type treated with melatonin and bright light was able to maintain a 24-hour schedule on melatonin maintenance therapy alone.[64,71]

Follow-up

If untreated, the sleep disturbance is chronic. Therefore, follow-up is often necessary. Patients should be encouraged to maintain a regular activity schedule. In blind individuals with free-running type who are taking melatonin or in sighted individuals on light therapy, treatment may need to be continued chronically with close follow-up.

General Approach to Evaluation and Treatment of Free-Running or Nonentrained Type

EVALUATION.

- Nonentrained type should be considered in patients in whom the major sleep period and sleep complaints change and cycle over time without evidence of stable entrainment to a 24-hour cycle.
- Careful attention should be paid to rule out other sleep disorders, as well as medical and psychiatric disorders.
- To confirm the diagnosis, sleep logs or actigraphy monitoring for at least 14 days is recommended.

MANAGEMENT.

- Enforcement of good sleep hygiene (avoidance of naps, regular sleep and wake times, and structured time for social and physical activities)
- In sighted patients, exposure to bright light during the day and avoidance of bright light in the evening
- If additional pharmacologic therapy is required, melatonin 10 mg an hour before bedtime for approximately 2 weeks, followed by a smaller maintenance dose that can range from as little as 0.5 mg to 1 mg 1 hour before bedtime
- Referral to a sleep specialist is appropriate when diagnosis is unclear or there are concerns about treatment.

Irregular Sleep–Wake Type

Irregular sleep–wake type is characterized by a lack of discernible sleep/wake circadian rhythm. There is no major sleep period, and sleep is fragmented into at least three periods during the 24-hour day. The etiology of this disorder is thought to be either related to changes in the hypothalamus and SCN, such as may be seen in Alzheimer disease, a population with a high prevalence of the disorder,[72] or a result of decreased exposure to environmental light and daytime activity that can be associated with low-amplitude circadian rhythms. Institutionalized patients are especially prone to such weak external entraining stimuli.

Clinical Presentation

Patients will present with insomnia or excessive sleepiness, depending on the time of day. Although sleep is usually fragmented, the longest sleep period tends to occur between 2 and 6 AM. On questioning, patients or caregivers report frequent naps through the day. It is important to note that the irregular sleep and wake pattern also affects the sleep quality of the caregiver and adds to the caregiver's burden.

Epidemiology

The prevalence of irregular sleep–wake type is unknown in the general population but is likely to be substantially lower than that of DSPT.[73] Originally described in cognitively intact individuals who had spent a large amount of time in bed because of prolonged illness, this disorder is most commonly associated with neurologic disorders such as dementia, mental retardation, and brain injury.[72, 74]

Classification

The *ICSD-2* classifies this disorder as "circadian rhythm sleep disorder, irregular sleep–wake type," and[22] in the *DSM-IV-TR* this disorder is known as "circadian rhythm sleep disorder, unspecified type".[23] The ICD-9 code is 327.33.

Diagnostic Evaluation

A detailed history will usually elucidate the presence of an irregular sleep pattern. Sleep diary or actigraphy will help confirm the lack of circadian rhythmicity in the sleep–wake pattern. A history of isolation or reclusion can often aid in diagnosis. Other sleep or psychiatric disorders that can cause fragmented sleep must also be excluded. Polysomnography for at least 24 hours will show normal total sleep time for age but loss of normal sleep–wake pattern. It can also help rule out an alternative diagnosis.

Diagnosis

Diagnosis of irregular sleep–wake type is based on *ICSD-2* criteria:[22]

1. There is a chronic complaint of insomnia, excessive sleepiness, or both.
2. Sleep log or actigraphy monitoring for at least 7 days demonstrates at least three irregular sleep bouts during a 24-hour period.
3. Total sleep time per 24-hour period is essentially normal for age.
4. The sleep disturbance is not better explained by another disorder.

Differential Diagnosis

Efforts should be made to distinguish irregular sleep–wake type from individuals who complain of insomnia and/or daytime sleepiness because of poor sleep hygiene or voluntary maintenance of irregular sleep schedules. Other causes of insomnia, whether initiation or maintenance in nature, as well as other causes of daytime sleepiness, including medical, neurologic, or psychiatric disorders, or medication-related causes, should also be kept in mind.

Management

Treatments for irregular sleep–wake type are aimed at consolidating the sleep–wake cycle. For institutionalized patients, increased daytime social interactions and light exposure have been shown to consolidate nighttime sleep.[75,76] Other strategies to consolidate sleep include scheduling physical activity, as well as minimizing nighttime light and noise.[77,78]

One study reported a 45% success rate by using a combination therapy of vitamin B_{12}, bright light, chronotherapy, and hypnotics.[43] Several small studies appear to support a role for melatonin. For example, treatment with melatonin 3 mg daily significantly increased nighttime sleep and sleep efficiency while reducing daytime sleep in children with psychomotor retardation and irregular sleep–wake type.[7] However, in a large multicenter study of Alzheimer disease, melatonin failed to improve sleep.[79]

A practical approach to the management of irregular sleep–wake disorder is to begin with behavioral and environmental strategies. These include bright light exposure, structured social and physical activities, and avoidance of naps during the day. During the sleep period, the environment should be conducive to sleep:

- Minimal noise
- Darkened room
- Comfortable room temperature
- Incontinence care
- The role of melatonin has not been established
- Hypnotic or sedating psychoactive medications should be used with caution in elderly patients with dementai

Follow-up

To ensure the success of therapy, caregivers should make certain that daytime activities are followed and that patients have limited napping opportunities during the day. Outpatients should be followed up to ensure adherence to therapy and for absence of any potential adverse effects of pharmacotherapy.

Shift-Work Sleep Disorder

Shift-work sleep disorder (SWSD) is characterized by a recurrent complaint of insomnia and excessive sleepiness that is related to a work schedule that overlaps with the usual sleep period. These patients typically complain of insomnia during the scheduled sleep time and excessive sleepiness at work. This condition is seen most frequently in night and early morning shift workers who have to work during their usual scheduled sleep period and sleep during their usual wake period. Factors that can influence the ability to deal with shift work include age, diurnal preference, domestic duties, and the presence of other sleep disorders.[49,80] Sleep in night-shift workers is usually shortened by 15% to 20% compared to daytime workers, averaging 4 to 6 hours versus 7 to 9 hours, respectively.[81] The sleep loss involves mostly stage 2 and rapid eye movement (REM) sleep.[82] Chronic sleep deprivation associated with shift work can lead to negative effects on job performance and social functioning. Decreased alertness can also lead to personal and public safety issues that should also be addressed.[81]

Clinical Presentation

Individuals with SWSD usually complain of difficulty falling asleep or maintaining sleep, unrefreshing sleep, and sleepiness at work. In addition to the sleep disturbance and excessive sleepiness, patients with SWSD can also present with gastrointestinal symptoms (e.g., dyspepsia, constipation, and diarrhea), alcohol or drug misuse or abuse, higher accident rates, and depression.[83,84] Shift work has been associated with increased incidence of breast cancer and medical disorders (e.g., gastrointestinal, cardiovascular, and reproductive diseases).[81]

Epidemiology

With an estimate of 20% of the workforce in industrialized countries employed in shift-work jobs, the potential for the development of this CRSD is quite high.[85] Although 40% to 80% of industrial night workers complain of problems sleeping, the number of clinically significant cases is unknown.[19] Recent data suggest that shift-work type affects approximately 5% to 10% of the population.[82,86]

Classification

This disorder is classified as "circadian rhythm sleep disorder, shift-work type" by the ICSD-2 and commonly referred to as "shift-work disorder."[22] The *DSM-IV-TR* subtypes this CRSD as "shift-work type." It carries an ICD-9 code of 327.36.[23]

Diagnostic Evaluation

The diagnosis can usually be made on the basis of clinical presentation and a history of shift work. Sleep diary or actigraphy may be useful in documenting the shift-work–related pattern of sleep/wake cycle. Polysomnography should be performed when excessive sleepiness is present and an underlying sleep-related breathing disorder is suspected. Polysomnography done at the patient's "shifted" sleep time may reveal prolonged sleep latency or shortened total sleep time, depending on the alignment between the sleep time and the internal circadian clock.[22]

Diagnosis

The diagnostic criteria proposed by the *ICSD-2* are:[22]

1. There is a complaint of insomnia or excessive sleepiness that is temporally associated with a recurring work schedule that overlaps with the usual time of sleep.
2. The symptoms are associated with the shift-work schedule over the course of at least 1 month.
3. Sleep log or actigraphy monitoring for at least 7 days demonstrates disturbed circadian rhythm and sleep-time misalignment.
4. The sleep disturbance is not better explained by another current disorder.

Differential Diagnosis

Other CRSDs that may have similar presentation must be excluded. Excessive daytime somnolence can also be caused by primary hypersomnia and sleep-related disordered breathing. It is prudent to consider primary and secondary insomnias, as well as medical, psychological, neurologic, and medication-related causes of sleepiness.

Management

Clinical management of SWSD should be aimed at realigning circadian rhythms with the sleep and work schedules, as well as improving sleep and alertness. Most of the strategies developed for adjustment to shift work have focused on the night-shift worker, in whom exposure to bright light has been shown to improve adaptation of circadian rhythms.[87,88] Most studies used light intensities between 1,200 and 10,000 lux for a period of 3 to 6 hours during the night shift.[89] More recently, intermittent bright light exposure (approximately 20 minutes per hour blocks) has also been shown to accelerate circadian adaptation to night-shift work.[90,91] Therefore, either continuous or intermittent bright light initiated early during the night shift and stopped approximately 2 hours before the end of the shift can be used in the workplace. Another complementary strategy is to facilitate realignment by avoiding exposure to morning bright light during the commute home.[90–92] In addition to its circadian phase resetting effects, light has acute alerting effects that can be useful during the work period.[93]

Melatonin has also been used to improve adjustment to shift work. A recent review of the role of melatonin indicates that when taken at bedtime after the night shift, it can improve daytime sleep duration, but had limited effects on alertness.[89] Melatonin is not approved by the FDA. Furthermore, potential adverse effects such as headaches, nausea, and exacerbation of cardiovascular disease should be considered.

Hypnotics have also been used to treat insomnia in patients with SWSD. Although hypnotic medications can improve sleep, they do not address the issue of circadian phase alignment and, therefore, if needed, should be used together with behavioral strategies to improve circadian adjustment. Stimulants such as caffeine can be used to help manage sleepiness. Recently, modafinil, a stimulant medication, was approved by the FDA to help manage excessive sleepiness associated with SWSD.

Family and social factors are important because they can impair adjustment to shift work. Family responsibilities such as childcare and household chores, as well as noise during the day, can decrease the amount and quality of sleep. Optimizing the sleep environment and attention to healthy sleep habits should be encouraged. Finally, patient, family, and employer education and support are essential for effective and successful management of SWSD.

Follow-up

Treatment must be individualized, and follow-up should be focused on establishing good sleep hygiene and constant reinforcement of these practices. Successful management requires a multimodal approach and support from the patient's physician, family, and employer.

General Approach to Evaluation and Treatment of Shift-Work Sleep Disorder

EVALUATION.

- SWSD should be suspected in any patient who complains of insomnia and/or EDS associated with work schedules.
- Careful attention should be paid to rule out other sleep disorders (primary insomnia, sleep apnea, restless legs), as well as medical and psychiatric disorders.
- To confirm the diagnosis, sleep logs or actigraphy monitoring for at least 7 days is recommended.

MANAGEMENT.

- Good sleep hygiene and optimized sleep environment (dark room, noise level)
- Provide time for relaxation and, if hungry, take a light snack before bedtime
- Bright light exposure during night shift—5 to 10,000 lux (either continuous or intermittent)—during the first half but no later than 2 hours before the end of shift
- Wear sunglasses to block exposure to bright light during the commute home
- If light therapy is not a practical option, melatonin 3 mg may be tried at bedtime (not FDA approved)
- For excessive sleepiness associated with shift work (despite attempts to optimize adjustment), consider stimulants (may depend on the type of work and safety concerns), caffeine or modafinil (200 mg), at the beginning of the shift.

Jet Lag

Jet lag type is characterized by misalignment of the endogenous circadian sleep–wake cycle with the external environment because of a change in time zone. The symptoms of jet lag (i.e., difficulty falling asleep at night and EDS) are caused by the inability of the individual's circadian rhythm to shift rapidly to accommodate the environmental cues of the destination time zone. Symptoms are often worse with increasing number of time zones crossed and on eastward- versus westward-bound flights.[94] Because the period of the endogenous circadian rhythm is slightly longer than 24 hours, adjustment to westward travel (requiring phase delay) is easier than that to eastward travel (requiring phase advance).

Clinical Presentation

Individuals who suffer from jet lag will have sleep-initiation or sleep-maintenance insomnia, daytime sleepiness, and decreased performance and alertness after arriving at the destination. Generalized malaise, gastrointestinal upset, and mood changes have also been reported.[95] The variability of symptom severity among individuals is likely attributable to age, diurnal preference, and other sleep disorders. Exacerbation of underlying psychiatric disorders has also been associated with jet lag.[96]

Epidemiology

Jet lag can affect individuals of all ages, but symptoms may be more severe in elderly patients. There are no known gender differences.

Classification

This disorder is classified as "circadian rhythm sleep disorder, jet lag type" by the ICSD-2 and commonly referred to as "jet lag disorder."[22] The *DSM-IV-TR* also subtypes this primary CRSD as "jet lag type." It has an ICD-9 code of 327.35.[23]

Diagnostic Evaluation

The diagnosis of jet lag disorder is made by the clinical history. Unless the history or physical examination suggests another sleep disorder, polysomnography is usually not indicated.

Diagnosis

The ICSD-2 has set forth the following criteria for the diagnosis of jet lag disorder:[22]

1. There is a complaint of insomnia or EDS associated with transmeridian jet travel across at least two time zones.
2. There is associated impairment of daytime function, general malaise, or somatic symptoms such as gastrointestinal disturbance within 1 to 2 days of travel.
3. The sleep disturbance is not better explained by another current disorder.

Differential Diagnosis

If symptoms of excessive sleepiness or insomnia persist or worsen after travel, another sleep disorder should be sought as the cause. Jet lag symptoms may also worsen with underlying obstructive sleep apnea, depression, or other sleep disorders, and they should be excluded. Generalized malaise and gastrointestinal symptoms may represent an underlying medical condition that warrants an evaluation.

Management

Treatment of jet lag disorder aims at synchronizing the endogenous circadian rhythm with the local time zone and at preventing sleep loss as soon as possible. A proactive approach to prevent the development of symptoms includes adequate hydration, avoidance of caffeine and alcohol, and static exercises on the plane.[94] Good sleep hygiene during travel is also very important.

Timed bright light exposure and avoidance of light at the wrong time of the day have been shown to be effective strategies in accelerating entrainment of circadian rhythms. The timing of light exposure depends on the direction of travel and the number of times zones crossed. For example, on an eastward flight, when arriving in the morning, one should avoid bright light early in the morning but get as much light as possible in the afternoon.[97] The avoidance of natural bright light may be the most practical strategy.

Even before departure, a strategy to phase advance the circadian rhythm before eastward flights with bright light therapy has been proposed, but this approach has not been widely adopted.[98] In summary, strategic exposure to light appears to be a safe and potentially beneficial therapy for air travelers who suffer from jet lag.[34,90,99]

Pharmacologic approaches include melatonin and hypnotic medications. Some studies have also shown that melatonin can help alleviate jet lag.[97] The general recommendation is melatonin 2 to 5 mg taken before bedtime on arrival at the destination and the dose may be repeated for up to 4 days as needed.[97,100] It is important to note that melatonin has not been approved by the FDA for the treatment of CRSDs. Furthermore, potential adverse effects such as headaches, nausea, and exacerbation of cardiovascular disease should be considered. The use of zolpidem 10 mg for the initial three nights after arrival has been shown to improve sleep quality and length.[101] If behavioral strategies such as bright light exposure and good sleep hygiene are not sufficient to alleviate jet lag, use of a short-acting hypnotic during the first few days of arrival is a reasonable approach.

Follow-up

Symptoms of jet lag disorder should resolve over time. Prolonged sleep-related symptoms should prompt a search for an underlying sleep, psychiatric, or neurologic disorder. Somatic complaints may indicate the presence of a medical illness.

REFERENCES

1. Czeisler CA, Duffy JF, Shanahan TL, et al. Stability, precision, and near-24-hour period of the human circadian pacemaker. *Science*. 1999;284(5423):2177–2181.
2. Moore RY, Eichler VB. Loss of a circadian adrenal corticosterone rhythm following suprachiasmatic lesions in the rat. *Brain Res*. 1972;42(1):201–206.
3. Moore RY. A clock for the ages. *Science*. 1999;284(5423):2102–2103.
4. Bellingham J, Foster RG. Opsins and mammalian photoentrainment. *Cell Tissue Res*. 2002;309(1):57–71.
5. Rajaratnam SM, Middleton B, Stone BM, et al. Melatonin advances the circadian timing of EEG sleep and directly facilitates sleep without altering its duration in extended sleep opportunities in humans. *J Physiol*. 2004;561(Pt 1):339–351.
6. Cajochen C, Krauchi K, Wirz-Justice A, et al. Role of melatonin in the regulation of human circadian rhythms and sleep. *J Neuroendocrinol*. 2003;15(4):432–437.
7. Pillar G, Shahar E, Peled N, et al. Melatonin improves sleep-wake patterns in psychomotor retarded children. *Pediatr Neurol*. 2000;23(3):225–228.
8. Weitzman ED, Czeisler CA, Coleman RM, et al. Delayed sleep phase syndrome. A chronobiological disorder with sleep-onset insomnia. *Arch Gen Psychiatry*. 1981;38(7):737–746.
9. Regestein QR, Monk TH. Delayed sleep phase syndrome: A review of its clinical aspects. *Am J Psychiatry*. 1995;152(4):602–608.
10. Aoki H, Ozaki Y, Yamada N. Hypersensitivity of melatonin suppression in response to light in patients with delayed sleep phase syndrome. *Chronobiol Int*. 2001;18(2):263–271.

11. Alvarez B, Dahlitz M, Vignau J. The delayed sleep phase syndrome: Clinical and investigative findings in 14 subjects. *J Neurol Neurosurg Psychiatry*. 1992;55:665–670.
12. Uchiyama M, Okawa M, Shibui K, et al. poor recovery sleep after sleep deprivation in delayed sleep phase syndrome. *Psychiatry Clin Neurosci*. 1999;53(2):195–197.
13. Iwase T, Kajimura N, Uchiyama M, et al. Mutation screening of the human Clock gene in circadian rhythm sleep disorders. *Psychiatry Res*. 2002;109(2):121–128.
14. Archer SN, Robilliard DL, Skene DJ, et al. A length polymorphism in the circadian clock gene Per3 is linked to delayed sleep phase syndrome and extreme diurnal preference. *Sleep*. 2003;26(4):413–415.
15. Hohjoh H, Takasu M, Shishikura K, et al. Significant association of the arylalkylamine N-acetyltransferase (AA-NAT) gene with delayed sleep phase syndrome. *Neurogenetics*. 2003;4(3): 151–153.
16. Takahashi Y, Hohjoh H, Matsuura K. Predisposing factors in delayed sleep phase syndrome. *Psychiatry Clin Neurosci*. 2000;54(3):356–358.
17. Horne JA, Ostberg O. A self-assessment questionnaire to determine morningness-eveningness in human circadian rhythms. *Int J Chronobiol*. 1976;4(2):97–110.
18. Thorpy MJ, Korman E, Spielman AJ, et al. Delayed sleep phase syndrome in adolescents. *J Adolesc Health Care*. 1988;9(1): 22–27.
19. Wagner DR. Disorders of the circadian sleep-wake cycle. *Neurol Clin*. 1996;14(3):651–670.
20. Schrader H, Bovim G, Sand T. The prevalence of delayed and advanced sleep phase syndromes. *J Sleep Res*. 1993;2(1):51–55.
21. Pelayo R, Thorpy MJ, Govinski P. Prevalence of delayed sleep phase syndrome among adolescents. *Sleep Res*. 1988;17:392.
22. American Academy of Sleep Medicine. *The international classification of sleep disorders: Diagnostic and coding manual*, 2nd ed. Westchester, IL: American Academy of Sleep Medicine; 2005.
23. American Psychiatric Association. *Diagnostic and statistical manual of mental disorders*, 4th ed, Text Revision. Washington, DC, American Psychiatric Association; 2000.
24. Kamei Y, Urata J, Uchiyaya M, et al. Clinical characteristics of circadian rhythm sleep disorders. *Psychiatry Clin Neurosci*. 1998;52(2):234–235.
25. Dagan Y, Stein D, Steinbock M, et al. Frequency of delayed sleep phase syndrome among hospitalized adolescent psychiatric patients. *J Psychosom Res*. 1998;45(1Spec No):15–20.
26. Shirayama M, Shirayama Y, Iida H, et al. The psychological aspects of patients with delayed sleep phase syndrome (DSPS). *Sleep Med*. 2003;4(5):427–433.
27. Czeisler CA, Richardson GS, Coleman RM, et al. Chronotherapy: Resetting the circadian clocks of patients with delayed sleep phase insomnia. *Sleep*. 1981;4(1):1–21.
28. Ohta T, Iwata T, Kayukawa Y, et al. Daily activity and persistent sleep-wake schedule disorders. *Prog Neuropsychopharmacol Biol Psychiatry*. 1992;16(4):529–537.

29. Oren DA, Wehr TA. Hypernyctohemeral syndrome after chronotherapy for delayed sleep phase syndrome. *N Engl J Med*. 1992;327(24):1762.

30. Minors DS, Waterhouse JM, Wirz-Justice A. A human phase-response curve to light. *Neurosci Lett*. 1991;133(1):36–40.

31. Czeisler CA, Kronauer RE, Allan JS, et al. Bright light induction of strong (type 0) resetting of the human circadian pacemaker. *Science*. 1989;244(4910):1328–1333.

32. Lewy AJ, Sack RL, Singer CM. Immediate and delayed effects of bright light on human melatonin production: Shifting "dawn" and "dusk" shifts the dim light melatonin onset (DLMO). *Ann N Y Acad Sci*. 1985;453:253–259.

33. Rosenthal NE, Joseph-Vanderpool JR, Levendosky AA, et al. Phase-shifting effects of bright morning light as treatment for delayed sleep phase syndrome. *Sleep*. 1990;13(4):354–361.

34. Chesson AL Jr, Littner M, Davila D, et al. Practice parameters for the use of light therapy in the treatment of sleep disorders. Standards of Practice Committee, American Academy of Sleep Medicine". *Sleep*. 1999;22(5):641–660.

35. Dahlitz M, Alvarez B, Vignau J, et al. Delayed sleep phase syndrome response to melatonin. *Lancet*. 1991;337(8750):1121–1124.

36. Nagtegaal JE, Laurant MW, Kerkhof GA, et al. Effects of melatonin on the quality of life in patients with delayed sleep phase syndrome. *J Psychosom Res*. 2000;48(1):45–50.

37. Kamei Y, Hayakawa T, Urata J, et al. Melatonin treatment for circadian rhythm sleep disorders. *Psychiatry Clin Neurosci*. 2000;54(3):381–382.

38. Oldani A, Ferini-Strambi L, Zucconi M, et al. Melatonin and delayed sleep phase syndrome: Ambulatory polygraphic evaluation. *Neuroreport*. 1994;6(1):132–134.

39. Nagtegaal JE, Kerkhof GA, Smits MG, et al. Delayed sleep phase syndrome: A placebo-controlled cross-over study on the effects of melatonin administered five hours before the individual dim light melatonin onset. *J Sleep Res*. 1998;7(2):135–143.

40. Mundey K, Benloucif S, Harsanyi K, et al. Phase-dependent treatment of delayed sleep phase syndrome with melatonin. *Sleep*. 2005;28(10):1271–1278.

41. Cavallo A, Omaye ST, Zee PC. Melatonin: Prototype monograph summary. In: Schneeman BO, ed. *Dietary supplements: A framework for evaluating safety*. Washington, DC: The National Academies Press; 2005:367–371.

42. Okawa M, Mishima K, Nanami T, et al. Vitamin B12 treatment for sleep-wake rhythm disorders. *Sleep*. 1990;13(1):15–23.

43. Yamadera H, Takahashi K, Okawa M. A multi-center study of sleep-wake rhythm disorders: Therapeutic effects of vitamin B12, bright light therapy, chronotherapy, and hypnotics. *Psychiatry Clin Neurosci*. 1996;50(4):203–209.

44. Okawa M, Takahashi K, Egashira K, et al. Vitamin B12 treatment for delayed sleep phase syndrome: A multi-center double-blind study. *Psychiatry Clin Neurosci*. 1997;51(5):275–279.

45. Ozaki N, Iwata T, Itoh A, et al. A treatment trial of delayed sleep phase syndrome with triazolam. *Jpn J Psychiatry Neurol*. 1989;43(1):51–55.

46. Okawa M, Uchiyama M, Ozaki S, et al. Circadian rhythm sleep disorders in adolescents: Clinical trials of combined treatments based on chronobiology. *Psychiatry Clin Neurosci*. 1998;52(5):483–490.

47. Jones CR, Campbell SS, Zone SE, et al. Familial advanced sleep-phase syndrome: A short-period circadian rhythm variant in humans. *Nat Med*. 1999;5(9):1062–1065.

48. Rufiange M, Dumont M, Lachapelle P. Correlating retinal function with melatonin secretion in subjects with an early or late circadian phase. *Invest Ophthalmol Vis Sci*. 2002;42(7):2491–2499.

49. Reid KJ, Chang AM, Zee PC. Circadian rhythm sleep disorders. *Med Clin North Am*. 2004;88(3):631–651,viii.

50. Toh KL, Jones CR, He Y, et al. An hPer2 phosphorylation site mutation in familial advanced sleep phase syndrome. *Science*. 2001;291(5506):1040–1043.

51. Reid KJ, Chang AM, Dubocovich ML, et al. Familial advanced sleep phase syndrome. *Arch Neurol*. 2001;58(7):1089–1094.

52. Ando K, Kripke DF, Ancoli-Israel S. Estimated prevalence of delayed and advanced sleep phase syndromes. *Sleep Res*. 1995;24:509.

53. Billiard M, Verge M, Aldaz C. A case of advanced sleep phase syndrome. *Sleep Res*. 1993;22:109.

54. Singer CM, Lewy AJ. Case report: Use of the dim light melatonin onset in the treatment of ASPS with bright light. *Sleep Res*. 1989;18:445.

55. Lack L, Wright H. The effect of evening bright light in delaying the circadian rhythms and lengthening the sleep of early morning awakening insomniacs. *Sleep*. 1993;16(5):436–443.

56. Campbell SS, Dawson D, Anderson MW. Alleviation of sleep maintenance insomnia with timed exposure to bright light. *J Am Geriatr Soc*. 1993;41(8):829–836.

57. Moldofsky H, Musisi S, Phillipson EA. Treatment of a case of advanced sleep phase syndrome by phase advance chronotherapy. *Sleep*. 1986;9(1):61–65.

58. Sack RL, Lewy AJ, Blood ML, et al. Circadian rhythm abnormalities in totally blind people: Incidence and clinical significance. *J Clin Endocrinol Metab*. 1992;75(1):127–134.

59. Czeisler CA, Shanahan TL, Klerman EB, et al. Suppression of melatonin secretion in some blind patients by exposure to bright light. *N Engl J Med*. 1995;332(1):6–11.

60. Aschoff J, Fatranska M, Giedke H, et al. Human circadian rhythms in continuous darkness: Entrainment by social cues. *Science*. 1971;171(967):213–215.

61. Uchiyama M, Shibui K, Hayakawa T, et al. Larger phase angle between sleep propensity and melatonin rhythms in sighted humans with non-24-hour sleep-wake syndrome. *Sleep*. 2002;25(1):83–88.

62. Miles LE, Raynal DM, Wilson MA. Blind man living in normal society has circadian rhythms of 24.9 hours. *Science*. 1977;198(4315):421–423.

63. Lewy AJ. Effects of light on human melatonin production and the human circadian system. *Prog Neuropsychopharmacol Biol Psychiatry*. 1983;7(4–6):551–556.

64. McArthur AJ, Lewy AJ, Sack RL. Non-24-hour sleep-wake syndrome in a sighted man: Circadian rhythm studies and efficacy of melatonin treatment. *Sleep*. 1996;19(7):544–553.

65. Kamgar-Parsi B, Wehr TA, Gillin JC. Successful treatment of human non-24-hour sleep-wake syndrome. *Sleep*. 1983;6(3):257–264.

66. Boivin DB, James FO, Santo JB, et al. Non-24-hour sleep-wake syndrome following a car accident. *Neurology*. 2003;60(11):1841–1843.

67. Weber AL, Cary MS, Connor N, et al. human non-24-hour sleep-wake cycles in an everyday environment. *Sleep*. 1980;2(3):347–354.

68. Sack RL, Brandes RW, Kendall AR, et al. Entrainment of free-running circadian rhythms by melatonin in blind people. *N Engl J Med*. 2000;343(15):1070–1077.

69. Palm L, Blennow G, Wetterberg L. Long-term melatonin treatment in blind children and young adults with circadian sleep-wake disturbances. *Dev Med Child Neurol*. 1997;39(5):319–325.

70. Lewy AJ, Bauer VK, Hasler BP, et al. Capturing the circadian rhythms of free-running blind people with 0.5 mg melatonin. *Brain Res*. 2001;918(1–2):96–100.

71. Hayakawa T, Kamei Y, Urata J, et al. Trials of bright light exposure and melatonin administration in a patient with non-24 hour sleep-wake syndrome. *Psychiatry Clin Neurosci*. 1998;52(2):261–262.

72. Hoogendijk WJ, van Someren EJ, Mirmiran M, et al. Circadian rhythm-related behavioral disturbances and structural hypothalamic changes in Alzheimer's disease. *Int Psychogeriatr*. 1996;8(Suppl 3):245–252. discussion 269–272.

73. Yamadera H, Takahashi K, Okawa M. A multicenter study of sleep-wake rhythm disorders: Clinical features of sleep-wake rhythm disorders. *Psychiatry Clin Neurosci*. 1996;50(4):195–201.

74. Witting W, Kwa IH, Eikelenboom P, et al. Alterations in the circadian rest-activity rhythm in aging and Alzheimer's disease. *Biol Psychiatry*. 1990;27(6):563–572.

75. Okawa M, Mishima K, Hishikawa Y, et al. Circadian rhythm disorders in sleep-waking and body temperature in elderly patients with dementia and their treatment. *Sleep*. 1991;14(6):478–485.

76. Ancoli-Israel S, Martin JL, Kripke DF, et al. Effect of light treatment on sleep and circadian rhythms in demented nursing home patients. *J Am Geriatr Soc*. 2002;50(2):282–289.

77. Schnelle JF, Cruise PA, Alessi CA, et al. Sleep hygiene in physically dependent nursing home residents: Behavioral and environmental intervention implications. *Sleep*. 1998;21(5):515–523.

78. Naylor E, Penev PD, Orbeta L, et al. Daily social and physical activity increases slow-wave sleep and daytime neuropsychological performance in the elderly. *Sleep*. 2000;23(1):87–95.

79. Singer C, Tractenberg RE, Kaye J, et al. A multicenter, placebo-controlled trial of melatonin for sleep disturbance in Alzheimer's disease. *Sleep*. 2003;26(7):893–901.

80. Dumont M, Benhaberou-Brun D, Paquet J. Profile of 24-h light exposure and circadian phase of melatonin secretion in night workers. *J Biol Rhythms*. 2001;16(5):502–511.
81. Scott AJ. Shift work and health. *Prim Care*. 2000;27(4):1057–1079.
82. Akerstedt T. Shift work and disturbed sleep/wakefulness. *Occup Med (Lond)*. 2003;53(2):89–94.
83. Moore-Ede MC, Richardson GS. Medical implications of shiftwork. *Annu Rev Med*. 1985;36:607–617.
84. Reinberg A, Vieux N, Andlauer P. Tolerance to shiftwork: A chronobiological approach. *Adv Biol Psychiatry*. 1983;11:35.
85. Presser HB. Towards a 24 Hour Economy. *Science*. 1999;284:1778–1779.
86. Drake CL, Roehrs T, Richardson G, et al. Shift work sleep disorder: Prevalence and consequences beyond that of symptomatic day workers. *Sleep*. 2004;27(8):1453–1462.
87. Dawson D, Campbell SS. Timed exposure to bright light improves sleep and alertness during simulated night shifts. *Sleep*. 1991;14(6):511–516.
88. Dawson D, Encel N, Lushington K. Improving adaptation to simulated night shift: Timed exposure to bright light versus daytime melatonin administration. *Sleep*. 1995;18(1):11–21.
89. Burgess HJ, Sharkey KM, Eastman CI. Bright light, dark and melatonin can promote circadian adaptation in night shift workers. *Sleep Med Rev*. 2002;6(5):407–420.
90. Boivin DB, James FO. Phase-dependent effect of room light exposure in a 5-h advance of the sleep-wake cycle: Implications for jet lag. *J Biol Rhythms*. 2002;17(3):266–276.
91. Crowley SJ, Lee C, Tseng CY, et al. Combinations of bright light, scheduled dark, sunglasses, and melatonin to facilitate circadian entrainment to night shift work. *J Biol Rhythms*. 2003;18(6):513–523.
92. Eastman CI, Stewart KT, Mahoney MP, et al. Dark goggles and bright light improve circadian rhythm adaptation to night-shift work. *Sleep*. 1994;17(6):535–543.
93. Campbell SS, Dijk DJ, Boulos Z, et al. Light treatment for sleep disorders: Consensus report. III. Alerting and activating effects. *J Biol Rhythms*. 1995;10(2):129–132.
94. Waterhouse J, Reilly T, Atkinson G. Jet-lag. *Lancet*. 1997;350(9091):1611–1616.
95. Winget CM, DeRoshia CW, Markley CL, et al. A review of human physiological and performance changes associated with desynchronosis of biological rhythms. *Aviat Space Environ Med*. 1984;55(12):1085–1096.
96. Katz G, Knobler HY, Laibel Z, et al. Time zone change and major psychiatric morbidity: The results of a 6-year study in Jerusalem. *Compr Psychiatry*. 2002;43(1):37–40.
97. Herxheimer A, Waterhouse J. The prevention and treatment of jet lag. *BMJ*. 2003;326(7384):296–297.
98. Burgess HJ, Crowley SJ, Gazda CJ, et al. Preflight adjustment to eastward travel: 3 days of advancing sleep with and without morning bright light. *J Biol Rhythms*. 2003;18(4):318–328.
99. Boulos Z, Campbell SS, Lewy AJ, et al. Light treatment for sleep disorders: Consensus report. VII. Jet lag. *J Biol Rhythms*. 1995;10(2):167–176.

100. Herxheimer A, Petrie KJ. Melatonin for the prevention and treatment of jet lag. *Cochrane Database Syst Rev* 2002;(2): CD001520.
101. Jamieson AO, Zammit GK, Rosenberg RS, et al. Zolpidem reduces the sleep disturbance of jet lag. *Sleep Med*. 2001;2(5): 423–430.

Sleep Disorders in Children

Judith Anne Owens and Katherine Finn Davis

INTRODUCTION

Sleep is one of the primary activities of growing children; by the time children reach their third birthday, they will have spent more time sleeping than in all waking activities combined. Although there appears to be considerable individual variability in sleep duration (and presumably in sleep needs), this substantial sleep requirement continues into the adolescent years, suggesting that sleep plays a vital biologic role in cognitive, physical, and psychological development across childhood. In the context of this increased need for sleep, the potential impact of insufficient and poor-quality sleep in the pediatric population is considerable. Children with sleep disturbances have been noted to exhibit poor conduct, hyperactivity, short attention spans, and poor academic performance. Furthermore, sleep disturbances in children are common, with approximately 25% of the pediatric population experiencing some type of sleep disturbance or problem, ranging from inadequate sleep hygiene to obstructive sleep apnea (OSA) syndrome.[1]

A basic understanding of the major normal developmental changes in sleep architecture, sleep patterns, and behaviors across childhood is necessary to fully appreciate the etiology and impact of sleep disorders on children and adolescents.[2] First, as children mature, they assume more adult sleep patterns (i.e., shorter sleep duration, longer sleep cycles, and less daytime sleep). Second, a striking decrease in the amount of rapid eye movement (REM) sleep occurs from birth (50% of time spent in sleep) through early childhood into adulthood (25% to 30% of time spent in sleep). The nocturnal alternating or "ultradian" rhythm of non-REM and REM sleep in infancy usually lasts approximately 50 minutes and gradually increases in duration through childhood to approximately 90- to 110-minute cycles in adulthood. Finally, the initial preponderance of slow-wave sleep that is highest in early childhood has an abrupt drop-off after puberty and then declines over the lifespan.[3]

DEVELOPMENTAL SLEEP DIFFERENCES

Newborns (0 to 2 Months)

Newborns generally sleep for approximately 16 to 20 hours per 24 hours, which is acquired in 1- to 4-hour sleep periods followed by wake periods lasting 1 to 2 hours. This sleep is equally distributed during the nocturnal and diurnal periods. During this early developmental stage, sleep–wake periods are chiefly dependent on hunger and satiety because circadian sleep–wake rhythms are not fully developed until 2 to 4 months, and environmental cues play a relatively small role. For example, bottle-fed newborns typically sleep longer periods than breast-fed infants

(3 to 5 vs. 2 to 3 hours). Newborns have three basic sleep states as defined by electroencephalogram (EEG) patterns, eye movements, and muscle tone—active ("REM-like"; 50% of sleep), quiet ("non–REM-like"), and "indeterminate" sleep states (with features of both). Unlike older children and adults, newborns enter sleep through active or "REM-like" sleep. Because this active sleep state is behaviorally characterized by grimaces, smiles, sucking, twitching, and jerking, it is sometimes interpreted by parents as disrupted or restless sleep.

Most sleep issues that are perceived as "problematic" at this age actually represent a discrepancy between these developmentally appropriate sleep behaviors and parental expectations about sleep patterns. Newborns who are noted to be excessively "fussy" and difficult to console may have causal medical issues such as gastroesophageal reflux, colic, or formula intolerance due to food allergies (e.g., milk protein).

Infants (2 to 12 Months)

Infants typically sleep 9 to 12 hours at night and 2 to 4.5 hours during the day (comprised of one to four naps, each lasting 30 minutes to 2 hours). It should be noted that the greatest individual variability in sleep amount appears to occur in the first year of life. The longest nighttime sleep period during the first 3 months is approximately 3 to 4 hours long and lengthens to 6 to 8 hours at 4 to 6 months of age. In terms of sleep architecture, the amount of active/REM sleep declines and three distinct stages of non-REM sleep (stage 1, 2, and slow-wave sleep) emerge by around 6 months of age. The ultradian sleep cycle lasts approximately 50 minutes, and each cycle frequently ends with a brief arousal (approximately 7 to 10 times per night at 2 months to 4 to 6 times at 12 months).

Many physical, cognitive, and social developmental issues can influence sleep during this time. Two key developmental "milestones" of infant sleep are referred to as *sleep consolidation* and *sleep regulation*. Sleep consolidation is defined as the ability to sleep for a continuous period of time, concentrated during the nocturnal period, which is supplemented in young children by shorter periods of diurnal sleep (naps). This is commonly referred to as *sleeping through the night*. Infants first develop the ability to consolidate sleep in the first 8 to 12 weeks of life; by 9 months of age, approximately 70% to 80% of infants will have achieved this milestone. Sleep regulation, or the ability of the infant to "self soothe," begins to develop in the first 3 months of life and is defined as the ability to master the sleep–wake transition at sleep onset, as well as to return to sleep independently after normal night arousals/awakenings. In addition, other developmental milestones including the emergence of gross motor skills such as rolling over and crawling may temporarily interfere with sleep. Cognitively, the development of object permanence, and therefore of separation anxiety, can cause increased bedtime resistance and problematic night waking; bedtime rituals and transitional objects (e.g., pacifier, doll, or blanket) are commonly used strategies to reduce these separation problems.

Both transient and chronic sleep problems are common in infancy; approximately 25% to 50% of 6- to 12-month-olds and

30% of 1-year-olds have problematic night wakings and approximately 50% of 1-year-olds have sleep-onset or settling difficulties. The identified risk factors for the persistence of sleep problems include "difficult" temperament, maternal depression, family stress, and medical conditions in the infant. Common sleep disorders in infants include the behavioral insomnias of childhood, particularly sleep-onset association disorder, and rhythmic movement disorders (head banging, body rolling, and body rocking are discussed in Chapter 5).

Toddlers (12 Months to 3 Years)

Toddlers sleep approximately 12 to 13 hours in a 24-hour period. Napping continues to be an important source of sleep; most toddlers abandon the morning nap by 18 months but continue to nap in the afternoon (usually for 1.5 to 3.5 hours).

Many developmental changes occur in toddlers, and sleep issues at this stage often reflect these changes. For example, toddlers develop gross motor skills, which allow them increased mobility to climb out of their crib or bed at night, and therefore, the timing of the transition from the crib to bed typically becomes an important concern between 2 and 3 years of age. Cognitively, a toddler's vast learning ability and achievement of new skills may interfere with nighttime settling. Fortunately, the child's developing comprehension of cause and effect allows basic behavioral interventions to be useful. Development of imagination and fantasy may lead to nighttime fears, and social and emotional development of autonomy and independence can lead to increased bedtime resistance. Separation anxiety peaks at about 18 to 24 months and may lead to increased night wakings, and, as the symbolic meaning of objects develops, transitional objects remain important at naptime and bedtime to help reduce this anxiety. Finally, regression in sleep behavior is a typical response to stress at this age and may increase the likelihood of "reactive" (in response to a sleep problem) cosleeping.

Sleep problems are very common, occurring in approximately 25% to 30% of toddlers; bedtime resistance is reported in 10% to 15% of toddlers and night wakings in 15% to 20%.[4] Common sleep disorders in toddlers include the behavioral insomnias of childhood (sleep-onset association disorder and limit-setting sleep disorder/bedtime resistance) and rhythmic movement disorders (head banging, body rolling, and body rocking).

Preschoolers (3 to 5 Years)

Preschoolers need approximately 11 to 12 hours of sleep in a 24-hour period. Naps are still important because 92% of children nap at 3 years of age, 57% at 4 years—of age, and 27% at 5 years—of age. However, the duration of the naps decrease and are eventually given up completely by 5 years of age. Sleep cycles occur at approximately 90-minute intervals, similar to the 90- to 110-minute typical cycle in adults, and sleep architecture is still distinguished by a relatively high proportion of both REM and slow-wave sleep.

It is very important for preschoolers to maintain a routine and to normalize sleep–wake patterns, including a consistent bedtime and wake time along with a regular daytime routine.

The developing language and cognitive skills at this age gives children the ability to express their needs and may lead to increased limit-setting problems and bedtime resistance. Developing imagination and fantasy can lead to nighttime fears. A so-called second-wind phenomenon is often seen in preschoolers and is due to the late-day circadian-mediated peak in alertness that occurs in all humans but may be amplified or delayed in some children and often results in bedtime resistance.

Data suggest that 15% to 30% of preschoolers experience night wakings and difficulty falling asleep, both sometimes coexisting in the same child, and that sleep problems if not addressed tend to become chronic. Common sleep disorders in preschoolers include nighttime fears, nightmares, behavioral insomnias of childhood (i.e., sleep-onset association disorder/night wakings and limit-setting sleep disorder/bedtime resistance), OSA syndrome, sleep-disordered breathing, and partial arousal parasomnias (sleepwalking and sleep terrors—see Chapter 5).

School-aged Children (6 to 12 Years)

School-aged children need approximately 10 to 11 hours of sleep in a 24-hour period. The sleep architecture at this age more closely resembles the distribution of sleep stages in adults. School-aged children normally have a high physiologic level of alertness, and naps are typically infrequent at this age; therefore, any reports of daytime sleepiness are highly suggestive of inadequate and disrupted nocturnal sleep.

During this period of growth and development, children begin to assume more responsibility for self-care, and therefore, it is a critical time to instill healthy sleep habits. Common sleep issues are irregular sleep–wake schedules (discrepancy between school and non–school night bedtimes and wake times) and increased caffeine use. Extracurricular activities, peer relationships, and media/electronics (e.g., television, computers, and video games) are increasingly important and compete for sleep time. Nighttime worries may increase as the child becomes more cognitively aware of real dangers (e.g., fires and burglars) and have also been associated with increased pressure to excel academically.

Until recently, sleep problems in middle childhood were considered rare, but current studies report an overall prevalence of parent-reported sleep problems in as many as one third of children in this age-group. Common sleep disorders in school-aged children include nightmares, anxiety-related sleep-onset delay, partial arousal parasomnias, and OSA syndrome, sleep-disordered breathing, behaviorally induced insufficient sleep syndrome, and inadequate sleep hygiene.

Adolescents (12 to 18 Years)

Experimental data suggest that adolescents generally require approximately 9 to 9.25 hours of sleep; however, a number of survey studies suggest that many average only 7 to 7.25 hours. Adolescence is a period of dramatic, biologically driven changes in sleep.[5] At onset of puberty, adolescents develop an approximate 2-hour, physiologically based phase delay (later sleep onset and wake times) as a result of pubertal/hormonal influences in circadian sleep–wake cycles and melatonin secretion. This often results in a substantial discrepancy between the circadian-based preference of the adolescent for both a late sleep-onset time and wake time and the demands of the average adolescent's schedule, which may require awakening for school at 5 or 6 AM.

These physiologic changes are accompanied by increased social, occupational, and academic demands, which also tend to delay sleep onset. Parents are also less likely to supervise bedtimes and enforce adequate sleep hygiene as adolescents mature. The result is often chronic insufficient sleep and the accumulation of a substantial sleep debt. In addition, there is an increasing discrepancy between weekday and weekend bedtime and wake time schedules, with "weekend oversleep" in an attempt to make up for restricted sleep during the week. Finally, adolescents have a physiologic predisposition to experience decreased daytime alertness in mid-to-late puberty. All these factors contribute to a high level of daytime sleepiness in this age-group, with related impairments in mood, attention, memory, behavioral control, and academic performance.

In addition to the widespread problem of insufficient sleep, the prevalence of sleep problems in this age-group is as high as 20%, and certain groups, such as those with chronic medical or psychological problems, may be at higher risk. Common sleep disorders in adolescence include behaviorally induced insufficient sleep syndrome, inadequate sleep hygiene, insomnia, delayed sleep phase syndrome, restless legs syndrome (RLS), periodic limb movement disorder (PLMD), and narcolepsy.

SLEEP DISORDERS

Adequate sleep is necessary for optimal functioning; consequently, sleep disorders in children have a pervasive impact on many aspects of health and development. Health outcomes related to inadequate sleep range from an increase in unintentional injuries to possible harmful effects on the cardiovascular, immune, and metabolic systems. A child's physical, emotional, cognitive, and social developments are negatively affected as well. Children with daytime sleepiness related to sleep disorders can experience significant mood dysfunction, leading to poor academic and sports performance. Children who are sleep deprived have also been reported to exhibit poor impulse control, impaired verbal and cognitive abilities, decreased creativity, and short attention spans. Furthermore, children classified as "poor sleepers" by teachers and parents are more likely to have behavioral and mood problems.

In general, younger children respond differently to inadequate sleep than older children and adolescents do. An overtired toddler or preschooler may manifest paradoxical hyperactivity, irritability, and impulsivity, whereas older children display typical signs and symptoms of daytime sleepiness similar to adults such as yawning, low energy, and drowsiness.

However, children of all ages who experience inadequate or disrupted sleep as a result of sleep disorders can exhibit the following nonspecific signs and symptoms:

- Mood changes and negative sense of well-being
- Excessive daytime sleepiness (EDS) with drowsiness and unscheduled naps
- Fatigue and somatic complaints
- Cognitive impairment and poor school performance related to excessive sleepiness, negative mood, and fatigue

The sleep disorders that are either unique to or found largely in infancy and childhood or that have a substantially different clinical presentation and/or etiology in children compared to adults are discussed in the subsequent text.

Behavioral Insomnia of Childhood

Behavioral insomnia of childhood is characterized by difficulty falling asleep, staying asleep, or both, which are usually a result of either inappropriate sleep-onset associations or limit setting.

Limit-Setting Sleep Type

Limit-setting sleep disorder is a disorder in which parents or caregivers are unable or unwilling to establish appropriate sleep behaviors and enforce bedtime limits.

CLINICAL PRESENTATION.   The associated signs and symptoms are similar to those resulting from other sleep disorders that lead to inadequate sleep. Children often exhibit the following characteristics:

- *Noncompliant behavior*: Including verbal protests in response to parental requests to get ready for bed (e.g., change into pajamas or brush teeth).
- *Bedtime resistance*: Including stalling or refusal to go to bed or requiring a parent to be present at bedtime.
- *"Curtain calls"*: Typified by repeated demands for parental attention (another story, drink of water, or trip to bathroom) after bedtime.
- *Delayed sleep onset*: Usually 30 minutes or more after the scheduled bedtime.
- *Frequent night wakings*: Resulting from lack of limit-setting or sleep associations that have developed (e.g., parent present at bedtime).
- Daytime behavior problems due to insufficient sleep.

EPIDEMIOLOGY.   The limit-setting type is most common in preschool and early school-aged children. The prevalence is approximately 10% to 30% in toddlers and preschoolers and about 15% in school-aged children. Limit setting may coexist with sleep-onset association disorder. Without intervention, it often becomes a chronic problem.

DIAGNOSTIC EVALUATION.   Evaluation requires a medical history and physical examination. Although the medical history and examination are usually benign, an evaluation is necessary because children with contributory acute or chronic medical conditions are prone to bedtime resistance. Diagnostic tests are not indicated.

A comprehensive evaluation should include:

- Review of medication use for potential contributory factors

- *Developmental history*: Children with developmental delays or sensory integration issues may have more problems with self-soothing at bedtime
- *Family history*: This involves assessment of parenting skills and limit-setting abilities
- *Behavioral assessment*: A history of more global behavior issues such as oppositional defiant disorder (ODD), attention deficit-hyperactivity disorder (ADHD), and noncompliance may be present.

DIAGNOSIS. Diagnostic criteria include difficulty initiating or maintaining sleep, manifested by stalling and/or refusal behavior at bedtime or following night wakings as a result of inadequate or inappropriate limit setting by the caregiver(s).

DIFFERENTIAL DIAGNOSIS. Limit-setting type should be distinguished from:

- *Inappropriate sleep schedules*: This involves inconsistent bedtimes and wake times, late napping (after 4 PM), significant discrepancy between weekday and weekend sleep schedules.
- *Delayed sleep phase syndrome*: Difficulty falling asleep occurs only when the individual attempts to go to bed earlier than his/her "preferred" (later) bedtime.
- *Nighttime fears*: This is usually suspected when anxiety is seen as a large component of bedtime resistance. This resistance disappears when the parents remain with the child at bedtime and sleep onset is not delayed.
- *Transient insomnia*: This is usually seen in response to illness, stress, unfamiliar sleeping environment, and so on, in a child who was previously sleeping normally.
- *Periodic limb movements / restless legs*: This can result in difficulty falling asleep or in fragmented sleep, but usually there is a history of increased symptoms at rest and/or restless sleep and nocturnal leg kicks (See Chapter 5 for further description of PLMD and RLS).

MANAGEMENT. Successful management should include three components: Establishment of appropriate sleep habits, development of a sleep schedule that matches the child's circadian rhythm, and appropriate and consistent limit-setting by parents. Strategies include:

- Establishing a consistent bedtime—that matches the child's natural sleep-onset tendency.
  - Instituting a bedtime routine—a 20- to 45-minute set routine involving quiet activities (e.g., bath and reading)
  - Ignoring any complaints or protests at bedtime
  - Checking on the child briefly (if upset or crying)
  - Returning the child to bed or room if necessary
  - Providing a transitional object—such as a doll, blanket, or stuffed animal
- Maintaining a good sleep hygiene practices—avoid caffeine after lunchtime, get regular exercise (but not too close to bedtime), and set a consistent meal schedule.
- Evaluating daytime sleep habits—such as inappropriate napping (after 4 PM).

- Reinforcing good behavior—Star charts and small rewards for achieving goals such as staying in bed all night.

FOLLOW-UP.   Any toddler or young child with limit-setting sleep disorder who does not respond to simple behavioral management tactics or is causing family discord should be referred to a mental health professional for evaluation and treatment. If there is a concern about the presence of an underlying sleep disorder or medical problem, appropriate referral is necessary. Collaboration with a behavioral therapist in complex situations is recommended.

Sleep-Onset Association Type

Sleep-onset association is a sleep disorder characterized by the child learning to fall asleep only under particular circumstances or associations and, consequently, not developing the ability to "self soothe."

CLINICAL PRESENTATION.   Associated signs and symptoms are similar to those resulting from other sleep disorders that result in inadequate sleep. The presenting issue is usually prolonged night waking resulting in insufficient sleep (for both parent and child). Clinical features include the following:

- The child falls asleep only under certain conditions or in the presence of specific sleep associations (e.g., feeding, rocking, and lights-on), which are readily available at bedtime.
- When the child experiences the brief arousal that normally occurs at the end of each ultradian sleep cycle (every 60 to 90 minutes) or awakens for other reasons, he/she is not able to get back to sleep ("self soothe") unless those same conditions are present.
- The child "signals" the parent by crying (or coming into the parents' bedroom if the child is not confined to a crib) until the necessary associations are provided.

EPIDEMIOLOGY.   Sleep-onset association type is usually seen in infants and young children. The prevalence of sleep-onset association disorder in 6- to 12-month olds is 25% to 50%, 1-year olds is 30%, and toddlers is 15% to 20%. As mentioned earlier, this condition may coexist with limit-setting sleep disorder.

DIAGNOSTIC EVALUATION.   Although the medical history and physical examination are usually normal, an evaluation is necessary because chronic medical conditions may contribute to sleep-onset association insomnia. Diagnostic tests are usually not indicated. Evaluation should also include:

- *Medical history*: Typically benign, but should include an evaluation for other possible causes such as reflux or pain.
- *Developmental history*: Typically normal, although developmentally delayed children can have sleep problems that are more representative of their developmental age (younger) than their chronologic age.
- *Family history*: May be positive for psychopathology, particularly maternal depression.
- *Night waking history*: Parents often recognize the sleep association that works to get their child to fall asleep or return to sleep (e.g., breast-feeding or rocking).

- *Behavioral assessment*: Children with behavioral problems are at higher risk for sleep disturbances.
- *Physical examination*: Is generally noncontributory.
- *Diagnostic tests*: Not indicated.

DIAGNOSIS. An essential feature of the diagnostic criteria is that sleep onset involves a prolonged process that requires special conditions that are problematic and/or demanding (being rocked, held, fed, etc.). If the conditions are absent, sleep onset is significantly delayed. Similarly, night wakings are prolonged and the child often requires parental intervention to return to sleep.

DIFFERENTIAL DIAGNOSIS. Sleep-onset association insomnia should be distinguished from the following conditions:

- *Underlying sleep disorders such as OSA and RLS*: These sleep disorders are associated with physical signs and symptoms such as snoring or nocturnal leg kicking.
- *Poor limit-setting*: This usually involves the inability to fall asleep rather than night wakings and is associated with poor parental limit setting.
- *Inadequate sleep*: Not having enough sleep can *increase* arousals during sleep.
- *Transient sleep disturbances*: These may occur because of illness, jet lag, and stress but are usually self-resolving.
- *Inadequate sleep hygiene*: Such as caffeine use after lunchtime, inconsistent sleep schedules, and rough or stimulating play near bedtime.
- *Environmental issues*: The presence of excessive noise, uncomfortable temperature (too cold or hot), or excessive light can cause the child to have trouble falling asleep and returning to sleep after a nighttime waking. Symptoms of sleep-onset association disorder will continue even with improvement of environmental issues.

MANAGEMENT. The initial intervention strategy should be chosen on the basis of the child's temperament and parental tolerance and individualized as much as possible to increase the likelihood of success. Additionally, the key to both short- and long-term successful management of sleep-onset association disorder is establishing good sleep habits at an early age. Specific interventions include:

- *Extinction ("crying it out")*: Involves putting the child to bed at a preset bedtime and then systematically ignoring the child until a set time the next morning.
- *Gradual extinction*: Involves putting the child to bed when he/she is drowsy but awake and waiting for progressively longer periods, typically in 5-minute increments, before checking on the child. On each subsequent night, the initial waiting period before checking on the child is increased by the same number of minutes. When parents check on the child, the interaction should be brief (1 to 2 minutes) and non-reinforcing (a brief touch rather than cuddling).
- *Fading of adult intervention*: Involves a strategy for the parents to gradually eliminate intervention. The parent may begin by first sitting on the bed while the child falls asleep, and on each successive night the parent moves farther away

from the bed until eventually they are outside of the bedroom door. A goal must be agreed upon (e.g., child falling asleep independently) and successive steps to attaining this goal explicitly outlined.

- *Institution of a regular bedtime routine*: Engaging in quiet activities for approximately 20 minutes before bedtime (e.g., reading, bathing, or singing).
- *Maintenance of daytime naps*: Sleep deprivation *increases* likelihood of sleep problems.
- *Introduction of transitional objects*: Such as blankets, dolls, and stuffed animals.
- *Discontinuation of nighttime feedings after 6 months of age*: continuation may lead to "learned hunger."
- *Anticipation of an "extinction burst"*: An increase in the severity and frequency of the problem before improvement occurs.

FOLLOW-UP. Any child with sleep-onset association disorder who does not respond to simple behavioral management tactics or is causing family discord should be referred to a sleep specialist or a behavior management professional. If there is a concern about the presence of an underlying sleep disorder or medical problem, appropriate referral is necessary.

Obstructive Sleep Apnea in Childhood

OSA is at one end of a spectrum of sleep-disordered breathing in childhood, whereas benign or primary snoring (without ventilatory abnormalities) is at the other end.[6] In contrast to adults, partial obstructive hypoventilation, characterized by hypopneas (30% to 50% reduction in airflow), is the most common pattern of pathologic sleep-disordered breathing in children. A fourth entity, upper airway resistance syndrome (UARS), is characterized by paradoxical chest and abdominal wall movement and increasingly more negative intrathoracic pressure swings; polysomnography (PSG) generally reveals increased arousals in the absence of apneic/hypopneic events and helps make a diagnosis.

In general terms, OSA in childhood and adolescence, as in adults, is usually related to some combination of decreased upper airway patency (upper airway obstruction), or reduced capacity to maintain airway patency (decreased upper airway diameter and muscle tone), and decreased drive to breathe in the face of reduced upper airway patency (reduced central ventilatory drive). In addition to adenotonsillar hypertrophy, airway obstruction may also be related to allergies, asthma, gastroesophageal reflux (due to pharyngeal edema), and velopharyngeal flap cleft palate repair. Other factors that may influence patency of the upper airway include:

- Obesity (including syndromes associated with obesity such as Prader-Willi syndrome); neuromuscular disorders, including hypotonic cerebral palsy and muscular dystrophies; and hypothyroidism.
- Conditions that may be associated with reduction in central ventilatory drive including Arnold-Chiari II malformation, myelomeningocele, and brain stem injury or masses.

In some children, a combination of risk factors exists; Down syndrome is a classic example in which multiple risk factors for OSA are commonly present (e.g., hypotonia, glossoptosis [posterior tongue displacement], obesity, midface hypoplasia, increased risk of lower respiratory tract anomalies, and hypothyroidism).

Clinical Presentation

The most common *nocturnal* presenting complaints in childhood OSA are:

- Loud continuous nightly snoring (OSA is unlikely in the absence of habitual snoring, although many children who snore do not have OSA)
- Apneic pauses (although more commonly, parents may describe episodic choking, gasping, and snorting during the night)
- Paradoxical movement of chest wall and abdomen during breathing
- Restless sleep and increased body movements
- Nocturnal diaphoresis
- Abnormal sleeping position, such as sleeping with the neck hyperextended.

Common *daytime* symptoms include:

- Mouth breathing, due to adenoidal hypertrophy, and dry mouth
- Chronic nasal congestion/rhinorrhea
- Hyponasal speech
- Symptoms of EDS, which may include difficulty waking in the morning and falling asleep in school or at inappropriate times
- Mood changes, such as irritability, low frustration tolerance, impatience, depression/anxiety, and social withdrawal
- Acting-out behaviors, including aggression and hyperactivity
- Inattention, poor concentration, and distractibility
- ADHD-like symptoms
- Academic problems.
  Associated symptoms may include:
- Enuresis (especially secondary), due to alterations in antidiuretic hormone (ADH) secretion related to disturbed sleep
- Growth failure (in severe cases, failure to thrive) that may be related to some combination of decreased food intake, increased metabolic needs from increased work of breathing, and alterations in normal nocturnal growth hormone secretion patterns
- Increase in partial arousal parasomnias (e.g., sleepwalking and sleep terrors) in susceptible children, related to sleep fragmentation and increased slow-wave sleep.

Epidemiology

OSA occurs in 1% to 3% of children of preschool age; there is little prevalence data available for other ages. In contrast, primary snoring occurs occasionally in 20% of children, and habitually (nightly) in 10% (range—3% to 12%). The peak age of occurrence of OSA is between 2 and 6 years, coinciding with the peak age of lymphoid hyperplasia and adenotonsillar hypertrophy. A second peak occurs during adolescence, which more closely resembles "adult" OSA in terms of risk factors (e.g., obesity) and clinical presentation (e.g., snoring, apnea, and hypersomnolence). OSA has an equal gender distribution in prepubertal children, although some studies have suggested a male preponderance even in younger children. Some data suggest that African American children may have a higher risk.[7] A family history of OSA or disruptive snoring is found in a significant percentage of children with OSA symptoms.

Diagnostic Evaluation

Evaluation should begin with a detailed medical, developmental, and social history and physical examination:

- *Medical history*: Medical risk factors for and medical sequelae of OSA may be present. The history may be positive for both upper airway (chronic sinusitis) and lower airway (asthma) diseases, allergies, and frequent upper respiratory infections. There may be a history of frequent episodes of streptococcal pharyngitis/tonsillitis, as well as symptoms suggestive of gastroesophageal reflux (heartburn, vomiting).
- Developmental history frequently reveals significant academic concerns and attentional and learning problems.
- Family history is often positive for diagnosed OSA, as well as loud snoring.
- Behavioral assessment should include evaluation of behavioral and mood concerns.
- Physical examination may reveal overweight and obesity or, alternatively, especially in younger children, failure to thrive. HEENT (head, eyes, ears, nose, and throat) examination may show "adenoidal facies," midface hypoplasia, retrognathia and micrognathia, chronic nasal congestion and swollen turbinates, deviated septum, and very frequently, increased tonsillar tissue. Hyponasality may indicate the presence of enlarged adenoids. Children with OSA often have signs of atopy, including "allergic shiners," nasal crease ("allergic salute"), and eczema, and are frequently mouth breathers. In very severe cases, cardiac examination may show signs of pulmonary hypertension and resulting cor pulmonale; fortunately, these signs of severe OSA are now rarely seen. Systemic hypertension is much less common in children than in adults.

Diagnostic Tests

- An upright lateral neck x-ray may be warranted to evaluate for hypertrophy of the tonsils/adenoids and to assess the upper airway patency. Cephalometric radiographs may be helpful in assessing the upper airway structure in children with craniofacial anomalies but are generally not necessary in healthy children.
- In cases of severe OSA, electrocardiogram (ECG) may show evidence of right ventricular enlargement.
- Laboratory tests such as complete blood count (polycythemia) and blood gases (hypoxemia, respiratory acidosis) are rarely indicated.

At the present time, the only way to make a definitive diagnosis of OSA in children is with overnight PSG. Other "screening" studies thus far appear to have limited utility in children (home audio/videotaping, overnight oximetry) as do shortened PSG or "nap" studies because they are likely to underestimate the presence and severity of disease, and the American Academy of Pediatrics recommends that overnight PSG be performed in all children with suspected OSA.[8]

Transesophageal balloon manometry is performed in some sleep labs to detect UARS, especially in the face of significant OSA symptoms with a normal sleep study but is currently not widely available.

The indications of the American Thoracic Society for cardiopulmonary sleep studies in children include:

- Differentiation of benign snoring from snoring associated with sleep-disordered breathing
- Assessment of the severity of OSA
- Clarification of diagnosis when symptoms and risk factors are discordant
- Screening of children at high risk for OSA (e.g., trisomy 21, and achondroplasia)
- Delineation of severity of OSA in children at risk for peri- and postoperative symptoms
- Titration of continuous positive airway pressure (CPAP) in children with diagnosed OSA.

It should be noted that currently there are no universally accepted polysomnographic parameters for diagnosing OSA in children, and it is still unclear as to which parameters predict morbidity; however, most pediatric pulmonologists consider an apnea index >1 to be abnormal. In cases in which the apnea–hypopnea index is between one and five obstructive events per hour, clinical judgment must be exercised about risk factors for OSA and evidence of daytime sequelae. Other currently accepted diagnostic PSG criteria in children include oxygen desaturation nadir $<92\%$, change in nadir oxygen from baseline $>4\%$, maximum end-tidal carbon $>53\%$, and increase in end-tidal carbon dioxide $>45\%$ for $>60\%$ of total sleep time (TST).

Differential Diagnosis

Other factors and conditions that may accompany or cause respiratory disturbances, excessive sleepiness, or both in children include:

- Clinical features of EDS, which can result from other sleep disorders, including narcolepsy, insufficient sleep syndrome, and PLMD
- Respiratory disturbance, which can be due to central sleep apnea, primary snoring, paroxysm, or asthma
- Increased nocturnal movements, as well as respiratory disturbances associated with nocturnal seizures, which may mimic OSA-related gasping and arousals.

Management

The decision of whether and how to treat OSA depends on the severity (symptoms, sleep study results, and complications), duration, and the underlying etiologic factors in a given child. Most pediatric sleep experts believe that any child with an apnea index >5 and/or oxygen desaturation <85% should be treated. The decision to treat is based on the presence or absence of other clinical sequelae for an apnea index between 1 and 5; however, because studies suggest that there may be long-term neurobehavioral consequences of even mild untreated childhood OSA,[5] a more aggressive approach may be warranted. Therapies include:

- Adenotonsillectomy is the most common and the first-line treatment in any child with significant adenotonsillar hypertrophy even in the presence of additional risk factors such as obesity and generally results in complete resolution of symptoms. Although the procedure is generally well-tolerated, there appear to be certain groups that are at higher risk for perioperative complications, which include children with age <2 years, severe OSA, significant clinical sequelae of OSA (e.g., failure to thrive), and associated medical conditions, such as craniofacial syndrome and morbid obesity.
- There are little data on the utility of other surgical procedures, such as nasal septoplasty or uvulopharyngopalatoplasty in children.
- CPAP (or bilevel positive airway pressure [BiPAP]) can be used successfully in children and adolescents. CPAP may be used if adenotonsillectomy is not indicated or contraindicated or fails to completely resolve symptoms; it can also be used as a preoperative stabilizing measure in children with severe OSA.
- Weight management, including nutritional, exercise, and behavioral components, is indicated for all children with OSA who are overweight or obese.
- Oral appliances such as mandibular advancing devices and tongue retainers are occasionally used in older children and adolescents; referral to an orthodontist specializing in these devices is indicated in this situation.

Follow-up

Following adenotonsillectomy, OSA symptoms may take up to 8 weeks to resolve completely. All patients should be reevaluated postoperatively, and if there are significant residual risk factors or continued symptoms, a follow-up sleep study at least 6 weeks postoperatively may be indicated.

Overall, studies suggest that in most children, symptoms of OSA, including academic and behavior problems, resolve completely with appropriate treatment. Chronicity and severity of OSA, as well as individual factors (e.g., age and developmental level), are likely to play important roles in determining long-term effects.[9] It should also be noted that children with OSA may also be predisposed to redevelop OSA as adults, although no long-term prospective studies have yet been done.

Partial Arousal Parasomnias (also see Chapter 5)

Partial arousal parasomnias are episodic nocturnal phenomena most commonly seen in childhood (sleepwalking and sleep terrors) and are similar in etiology and clinical presentation. They share the characteristics of autonomic or skeletal muscle disturbances, autonomic behaviors, and disorientation.[10] Sleep-walking and sleep terrors occur almost exclusively during delta sleep and therefore usually occur within 1 to 2 hours of sleep onset. Episodes typically last from a few minutes (sleep terrors) to up to an hour (sleepwalking); some children may have multiple episodes in a single night. During an episode, children or adolescents have the appearance of being awake but are often agitated and incoherent and have no memory of the event the next day. Both disorders are exacerbated in susceptible individuals by factors that increase arousals during sleep (e.g., OSA and intercurrent illness) or increase the percentage of delta sleep (e.g., sleep deprivation and medications); environmental conditions (e.g., noise) that increase arousals, especially during slow-wave sleep, may also trigger events. In many cases, there seems to be a genetic predisposition; there is an 80% to 90% likelihood that a child with sleepwalking or sleep terrors has an affected first-degree relative. Although sleepwalking and sleep terrors can occur at any age from infancy through adulthood, most individuals will outgrow these behaviors by adolescence.

Clinical Presentation

During sleepwalking, the child may appear confused or dazed, mumble or give inappropriate answers to questions, appear clumsy, and perform bizarre or strange actions, such as urinating in a closet or leaving the house. Sleep terrors usually have a sudden onset and are usually much more dramatic in presentation. The child often appears extremely agitated, frightened, and confused and may cry out or scream. Extreme physiologic arousal (e.g., hyperventilation, tachycardia, diaphoresis, and dilated pupils) is common. Sleep terrors, however, may be much milder (sometimes described as a confusional arousal), with the child simply appearing agitated.

Epidemiology

Between 15% and 40% of children sleepwalk on at least one occasion; 3% to 4% have more frequent (weekly, monthly) episodes. Onset of episodes is usually between 4 and 6 years; peak occurrence is between 4 and 8 years. Approximately 10% of sleepwalkers will continue to sleepwalk for 10 years. Approximately 3% of children experiences sleep terrors, and the age of onset is usually between 4 and 12 years. The frequency of episodes is often highest at the onset and tends to be higher with younger age of onset. Because of the common genetic predisposition, the prevalence of sleep terrors in children who sleepwalk is higher, approximately 10%.

Diagnostic Evaluation

Evaluation requires a detailed medical history and physical and neurologic examination:

- Medical history may reveal evidence suggestive of a sleep disorder that results in disrupted and/or insufficient sleep, such as OSA and RLS/PLMD. The medical history may also suggest the need to rule out a seizure disorder; possible risk

factors include a history of seizures, and unusual characteristics of the episodes themselves such as stereotypic features,
multiple nightly occurrences, and late onset (adolescence).
- Developmental history and behavioral assessment are generally noncontributory, although in some children episodes
may be triggered by stress or anxiety. Symptoms suggestive
of EDS are rare.
- Family history is often positive for partial arousal parasomnias.
- Physical and neurologic examination is usually normal.

Diagnostic Tests

Because these are generally episodic events and the clinical
presentation is usually clear, overnight PSG is not routinely
indicated for the evaluation of partial arousal parasomnias.
They may not be captured on a single night study. However,
if there is a concern about another underlying sleep disorder
(e.g., sleep-disordered breathing and PLMD) or if there are unusual features that raise a suspicion of a seizure disorder, an
overnight sleep study with full seizure montage may be appropriate. Home videotaping of an episode may be helpful in assessing
atypical presentations (e.g., stereotypies).

Differential Diagnosis

Nocturnal seizures are not uncommon in children and adolescents and may be confused with partial arousal parasomnias (see
the preceding text). Nocturnal panic attacks are uncommon in
children but may present with similar features as sleep terrors.

Management

Management of partial arousal parasomnias should first include
reassurance and education of the child and family about the
benign and self-limited nature of the disorder and about the
child's safety.

Because sleepwalking and sleep terrors can result in physical
harm resulting from falling down the stairs, walking out into
traffic, or attempts to escape, ensuring safety (bedroom window
locks, safety gates, alarm systems, etc.) should be one of the primary concerns when dealing with partial arousal parasomnias.
Successful management requires a multimodal approach:

- Trigger/exacerbating factors should be minimized or avoided.
- Sleep hygiene and behavioral management of the episodes
should be reviewed. Parents should avoid awakening the child
during an episode because attempts to awaken a child during
a parasomnia will typical increase agitation and prolong the
event.
- Scheduled awakening is a behavioral technique that is most
likely to be successful in situations in which partial arousal
episodes occur on a nightly basis, where the parent wakes the
child approximately 15 to 30 minutes before the time of night
that the first parasomnia episode typically occurs.
- Pharmacologic management is seldom indicated except in
cases of frequent or severe episodes, high risk of injury, violent behavior, or serious disruption to the family. The primary
pharmacologic agents used are short-acting benzodiazepines

given as a small dose at bedtime (e.g., clonazepam [Klonopin] for 3 to 6 months [until episodes are totally suppressed]); tricyclic antidepressants (e.g., clomipramine, desipramine, and imipramine) at bedtime have also been used in patients who are nonresponsive to benzodiazepines. Abrupt discontinuation may result in rebound, increased slow-wave sleep, so it is best to taper medication slowly over several weeks.

Follow-up

Most children naturally stop sleepwalking or experiencing sleep terrors through childhood. By midchildhood, half of the children with sleepwalking/terrors no longer experience parasomnias, and most resolve spontaneously in adolescence.

Other Sleep Disorders in Children

Other sleep disorders in children include rhythmic movement disorders, sleep enuresis, and sudden infant death syndrome (SIDS).

Rhythmic Movement Disorders

Rhythmic movement disorders (body rocking, head banging, and body rolling) involve repetitive and stereotypic movements of large muscles and occur primarily during sleep–wake transitions, especially at bedtime.[11] In almost all cases, rhythmic movement behaviors are benign and occur in normally developing children, although further evaluation for developmental delays in a child with persistent rhythmic behaviors, especially if they also occur during the day, may be warranted. Significant injury is rare. Approximately two thirds of 9-month-old infants engage in some type of rhythmic behavior, and it is estimated that 3% to 15% of children have significant head banging. Most children who engage in these behaviors have an onset before 1 year of age, with body rocking starting at an earlier age than head banging. Less than half of the children continue to have these behaviors at 18 months, and only 8% show this behavior at 4 years of age. There is a male preponderance, with the male-to-female ratio being 4:1. Usually, the most important aspect in the management of head banging or body rocking is reassurance to the family that this behavior is normal, common, benign, and self-limited; parents should also avoid reinforcing the behaviors with attention. Any underlying sleep disorder (e.g., OSA) should be treated or avoided. Additional pharmacologic treatment is rarely needed; benzodiazepines, hydroxyzine, and tricyclic antidepressants have been used for severe cases.

SLEEP ENURESIS. Nocturnal enuresis is defined as repeated voiding of urine in the bed at least twice per week for at least 3 consecutive months in a child ≥5 years old. The child may be considered to have enuresis even if this criterion is not met but if significant distress or functional impairment is involved. Enuresis is more common in children whose parents have enuresis and in the male gender and African American children. Nocturnal incontinence occurs in 12% to 25% of 4-year-olds, 7% to 10% of 8-year-olds, and 2% to 3% of 12-year-olds.[12]

Differential diagnosis includes urinary tract infection, fecal impaction, diabetes mellitus or insipidus, chronic renal failure, neurologic anomalies, and obstructive uropathy.[13] While managing enuresis, treatment is not recommended in children younger than 6 years because of highly spontaneous cure rates. The most common treatments are counseling, enuresis alarms, desmopressin acetate, and imipramine.[13]

SUDDEN INFANT DEATH SYNDROME.   SIDS is defined as the unexpected death of an infant <12 months of age, the cause of which remains unexplained after an autopsy, investigation of the death scene, and review of clinical history.[14] Since the widespread recommendation of the supine sleeping position for infants 10 years ago, its incidence in the United States has been falling and is currently 0.74 per 1,000 live births. SIDS rates are highest in male infants, during winter months, in low birth weight or premature infants, in infants whose mothers abused drugs or smoked cigarettes, and in infants of young, impoverished mothers. SIDS seldom occurs during the first month of life; most deaths occur between 1 and 6 months of age and is the most common cause of death in infants younger than 6 months.[15] The American Academy of Pediatrics has recently recommended against bed-sharing in the first year of life, as a potential risk factor for SIDS.[16]

The diagnosis of SIDS is one of exclusion. Although many mechanisms have been suggested, none have been proved. Leading hypotheses include cellular brain stem abnormalities and maturational delay in association with neural or cardiorespiratory control.[13] SIDS deaths have also been associated with carbon dioxide rebreathing as a result of lying facedown, especially in soft bedding.

SLEEP IN SPECIAL POPULATIONS

Sleep problems have been found to occur at higher rates in children with special health care needs.[13] This includes children with chronic medical problems, behavior and mood disorders, and developmental disabilities. As a result, it is particularly important to screen for sleep problems in these populations. In general, the types of sleep problems affecting children with special health care needs are not unique to them *per se* but are more frequent and severe forms of those that affect the general population.

Sleep in Children with Chronic Medical Conditions

The relationship between sleep problems and chronic medical conditions has only recently been investigated in children and adolescents. This is a complicated task because chronic medical conditions involve complex underlying disease processes, emotional and family responses, hospitalization and medications, and related secondary symptoms, such as pain—all of which can impact sleep. Nevertheless, the studies that have been conducted to date have focused on examining sleep in different chronic illness subgroups. These include asthma, burns, cystic fibrosis, rheumatologic disorders, and sickle cell disease.[14]

Sleep in Children with Behavioral and Mood Disorders

There is also an important relationship between sleep problems and behavioral or mood disorders—behavior and mood difficulties often emerge as resultant functional impairments of sleep problems. Also, preexisting behavior and mood disorders may be exacerbated in children who experience sleep problems and vice versa. A good example of this is the relationship between sleep problems and ADHD. Empiric evidence has demonstrated that the central nervous system regions that regulate sleep and attention/arousal are definitely linked. Studies have suggested that a substantial proportion of children diagnosed with ADHD (up to 25%)[15] actually have a primary sleep disorder (most notably OSA, RLS, PLMD, or narcolepsy) that accounts for at least a portion of their behavioral disorder. In addition, children diagnosed with ADHD often experience sleep problems (predominantly sleep-onset delay and restless sleep) that may be intrinsic to ADHD or may be related to comorbid psychiatric conditions (depression or ODD) or concomitant psychotropic medications that directly affect sleep.

Sleep in Children with Developmental Disabilities

For years, children with developmental disabilities have been noted to experience a high frequency of sleep problems. For example, research estimates that 30% to 80% of children with severe mental retardation, >50% of the children with severe cognitive impairment, and approximately 50% to 70% of children with pervasive developmental delay and autism experience significant sleep problems.[17] This high prevalence of sleep problems may be associated with a number of different factors including intrinsic abnormalities in sleep regulation and circadian rhythms, medications used to treat associated symptoms, cognitive delays, sensory deficits, and increased parental stress.

REFERENCES

1. Carskadon, MA. The second decade. In: Guilleminault C, ed. *Sleeping and waking disorders: Indications and techniques.* Menlo Park, CA: Addison Wesley; 1982.
2. Mindell JA, Carskadon MA, Owens JA. Developmental features of sleep. *Child Adolesc Psychiatr Clin N Am.* 1999;8(4): 695–725.
3. Fritz G, Rockney R, Bernet W, et al. Practice parameter for the assessment and treatment of children and adolescents with enuresis. *J Am Acad Child Adolesc Psychiatry.* 2004;43(12):1540–1550.
4. Kuhn BR, Weidinger D. Interventions for infant and toddler sleep disturbance: A review. *Child & Fam Behav Ther.* 2000;22(2): 33–50.
5. Millman RP. Excessive sleepiness in adolescents and young adults: Causes, consequences, and treatment strategies. *Pediatrics.* 2005;115(6):1774–1786.
6. Marcus CL. Sleep-disordered breathing in children. *Am J Respir Crit Care Med.* 2001;164(1):16–30.
7. Redline S, Tishler PV, Schluchter M, et al. Risk factors for sleep disordered breathing in children: Associations with obesity, race, and respiratory problems. *Am J Respir Crit Care Med.* 1999;159:1527–1532.
8. AAP Clinical Practice Guideline. Diagnosis and management of childhood obstructive sleep apnea. *Pediatrics.* 2002;9(4):704–712.

9. Gozal D, Pope D. Snoring during early childhood and academic performance at ages thirteen to fourteen years. *Pediatrics.* 2001;107(6):1394–1399.

10. Mindell JA, Owens JA. *A clinical guide to pediatric sleep: Diagnosis and management of sleep problems.* Philadelphia, PA: Lippincott Williams & Wilkins; 2003:88–96; Chapter 10: Sleepwalking and sleep terrors.

11. Mindell JA, Owens JA. *A clinical guide to pediatric sleep: Diagnosis and management of sleep problems.* Philadelphia, PA: Lippincott Williams & Wilkins; 2003:97–101,Chapter 11: Headbanging and bodyrocking.

12. Kercsmar CM. The respiratory system. In: Behrman RE, Kliegman RM, eds. *Nelson essentials of pediatrics,* 4th ed. Philadelphia, PA: WB Saunders; 2002.

13. Quine L. Sleep problems in primary school children: Comparison between mainstream and special school children. *Child: Health and development.* 2001;27:201–220.

14. Owens JA, Witmans M. Sleep problems. *Curr Probl Pediatr Adolesc Health Care.* 2004;34:154–179.

15. Chervin RD, Archbold KH, Dillon JE, et al. Inattention, hyperactivity, and symptoms of sleep-disordered breathing. *Pediatrics.* 2002;109(3):449–456.

16. AAP. Task force on sudden infant death syndrome. The changing concept of sudden infant death syndrome: Diagnostic coding shifts, controversies regarding the sleeping environment, and new variables to consider in reducing risk. *Pediatrics.* 2005;116:1245–1255.

17. Johnson C. Sleep problems in children with mental retardation and autism. *Child Adolesc Psychiatr Clin N Am.* 1996;5(3): 673–681.

Appendix A.   The Epworth Sleepiness Scale

How likely are you to doze off or fall asleep in the following situations, in contrast to feeling just tired? This refers in your usual way of life in recent times. Even if you have not done some of these things recently try to work out how they would have affected you. Use the following scale to choose the most appropriate number for each situation:

0 = no chance of dozing
1 = slight chance of dozing
2 = moderate chance of dozing
3 = high chance of dozing

SITUATION	CHANCE OF DOZING
Sitting and reading	
Watching TV	
Sitting inactive in a public place (e.g. a theater or a meeting)	
As a passenger in a car for an hour without a break	
Lying down to rest in the afternoon when circumstances permit	
Sitting and talking to someone	
Sitting quietly after a lunch without alcohol	
In a car, while stopped for a few minutes in traffic	
Total Score=	

From Johns, MW. A new method for measuring daytime sleepiness: the Epworth sleepiness scale, *Sleep.* 1991;14(6):540–545. With permission.

185

Appendix B. Body Mass Index

	Normal						Overweight					Obese										Extreme obesity														
BMI	19	20	21	22	23	24	25	26	27	28	29	30	31	32	33	34	35	36	37	38	39	40	41	42	43	44	45	46	47	48	49	50	51	52	53	54
Height (inches)	Body weight (pounds)																																			
58	91	96	100	105	110	115	119	124	129	134	138	143	148	153	158	162	167	172	177	181	186	191	196	201	205	210	215	220	224	229	234	239	244	248	253	258
59	94	99	104	109	114	119	124	128	133	138	143	148	153	158	163	168	173	178	183	188	193	198	203	208	212	217	222	227	232	237	242	247	252	257	262	267
60	97	102	107	112	118	123	128	133	138	143	148	153	158	163	168	174	179	184	189	194	199	204	209	215	220	225	230	235	240	245	250	255	261	266	271	276
61	100	106	111	116	122	127	132	137	143	148	153	158	164	169	174	180	185	190	195	201	206	211	217	222	227	232	238	243	248	254	259	264	269	275	280	285
62	104	109	115	120	126	131	136	142	147	153	158	164	169	175	180	186	191	196	202	207	213	218	224	229	235	240	246	251	256	262	267	273	278	284	289	295
63	107	113	118	124	130	135	141	146	152	158	163	169	175	180	186	191	197	203	208	214	220	225	231	237	242	248	254	259	265	270	278	282	287	293	299	304
64	110	116	122	128	134	140	145	151	157	163	169	174	180	186	192	197	204	209	215	221	227	232	238	244	250	256	262	267	273	279	285	291	296	302	308	314
65	114	120	126	132	138	144	150	156	162	168	174	180	186	192	198	204	210	216	222	228	234	240	246	252	258	264	270	276	282	288	294	300	306	312	318	324
66	118	124	130	136	142	148	155	161	167	173	179	186	192	198	204	210	216	223	229	235	241	247	253	260	266	272	278	284	291	297	303	309	315	322	328	334
67	121	127	134	140	146	153	159	166	172	178	185	191	198	204	211	217	223	230	236	242	249	255	261	268	274	280	287	293	299	306	312	319	325	331	338	344
68	125	131	138	144	151	158	164	171	177	184	190	197	203	210	216	223	230	236	243	249	256	262	269	276	282	289	295	302	308	315	322	328	335	341	348	354
69	128	135	142	149	155	162	169	176	182	189	196	203	209	216	223	230	236	243	250	257	263	270	277	284	291	297	304	311	318	324	331	338	345	351	358	365
70	132	139	146	153	160	167	174	181	188	195	202	209	216	222	229	236	243	250	257	264	271	278	285	292	299	306	313	320	327	334	341	348	355	362	369	376
71	136	143	150	157	165	172	179	186	193	200	208	215	222	229	236	243	250	257	265	272	279	286	293	301	308	315	322	329	338	343	351	358	365	372	379	386
72	140	147	154	162	169	177	184	191	199	206	213	221	228	235	242	250	258	265	272	279	287	294	302	309	316	324	331	338	346	353	361	368	375	383	390	397
73	144	151	159	166	174	182	189	197	204	212	219	227	235	242	250	257	265	272	280	288	295	302	310	318	325	333	340	348	355	363	371	378	386	393	401	408
74	148	155	163	171	179	186	194	202	210	218	225	233	241	249	256	264	272	280	287	295	303	311	319	326	334	342	350	358	365	373	381	389	396	404	412	420
75	152	160	168	176	184	192	200	208	216	224	232	240	248	256	264	272	279	287	295	303	311	319	327	335	343	351	359	367	375	383	391	399	407	415	423	431
76	156	164	172	180	189	197	205	213	221	230	238	246	254	263	271	279	287	295	304	312	320	328	336	344	353	361	369	377	385	394	402	410	418	426	435	443

Adapted from National Institutes of Health. *Clinical guidelines on the identification, evaluation, and treatment of overweight and obesity in adults: The evidence report.* National Institutes of Health; NIH Publication No. 98-4083. September 1998:139–140.

Appendix C

Interpretation of the Polysomnogram and the Multiple Sleep Latency Testing

POLYSOMNOGRAPHY

Sleep disorders such as obstructive sleep apnea, motor disorders of sleep, narcolepsy, and nocturnal seizures sometimes require formal evaluation in the sleep laboratory. The most commonly utilized techniques for recording and evaluating sleep disorders include the polysomnogram (PSG), the multiple sleep latency test (MSLT), and sometimes, the maintenance of wakefulness test (MWT). The accurate interpretation of these studies requires a comprehensive sleep and medical history. PSG is an electrographic recording of simultaneous physiologic parameters during sleep and wakefulness. It describes the interaction of multiple organ systems (i.e., nervous, respiratory, and sometimes genitourinary systems) during sleep and wakefulness. PSG is utilized in the evaluation of abnormalities of sleep and sleep–wake transition, excessive daytime sleepiness (EDS), excessive nocturnal awakenings, and abnormal behavioral events during sleep, and to assess the efficacy of treatments of various sleep disorders.[1]

International standards require PSG to include four neurophysiologic channels at a minimum.

1. One electroencephalography (EEG) channel (central with an ear reference provides the best amplitude) to monitor sleep staging
2. Two electrooculogram (EOG) channels to monitor both horizontal and vertical eye movements (electrodes are placed at the right and left outer canthi, 1 cm above and 1 cm below the horizontal eye axis)
3. One electromyography (EMG) channel (usually chin or mentalis and/or submentalis) to record atonia of rapid eye movement (REM) sleep

On the basis of the clinical indication, extended montages incorporating additional physiologic parameters are sometimes added. Examples include the following:

1. Additional EEG channels, particularly in patients with sleep-related epilepsy
2. Additional EMG channels, particularly anterior tibialis, to detect periodic limb movements of sleep and parasomnias such as REM-sleep behavior disorder (RBD)
3. Airflow
4. Electrocardiography
5. Pulse oximetry
6. Abdominal and thoracic respiratory efforts
7. Snorogram—sound recordings to measure snoring

8. Patient position—monitored utilizing position sensors or direct observation by the technologist

Optional parameters include the following:

1. Continuous video monitoring of unusual nocturnal events or seizures
2. Esophageal pressure (Pes) monitoring for the evaluation of upper airway resistance syndrome (UARS). Esophageal manometry—measurement of Pes, providing a reflection of intrathoracic pressure fluctuations associated with breathing efforts
3. Nasal cannula pressure (NPRE) transducer systems—increasingly popular in sleep laboratories, allowing for the detection of increased respiratory effort by its effects on the inspiratory airflow wave contour
4. Nocturnal penile tumescence (NPT)—for the assessment of erectile dysfunction
5. Esophageal–gastric pH at various esophageal levels
6. Carbon dioxide (CO_2) monitoring utilizing transcutaneous CO_2 or end-tidal CO_2 techniques for the assessment of sleep-related hypoventilation and for the evaluation of sleep-related breathing disorders in pediatric patients

Overnight parameters (e.g., times of lights-on/off, total time in bed, and total sleep time [TST]) are collected and stored. The standard paper speed for recording and interpreting PSG is 10 mm per second, resulting in 30-second epoch length. The standard EEG, EMG, and EOG recordings are evaluated, and the predominant stage of sleep, according to the manual by Rechtschaffen and Kales,[2] is subsequently assigned to the entire epoch (See Appendix K). Electrodes are applied on the basis of the 10–20 system of the International Federation of Societies for Electroencephalography and Clinical Neurophysiology.[3] The TST and the relative proportion of the night spent in each of the sleep stages are calculated. Latencies to sleep, REM-sleep, and slow-wave sleep (SWS) are reported.

Definition of basic sleep architecture terms:

- Lights-out: The beginning of sleep recording
- Lights-on: The end of sleep recording
- Recorded time or total bedtime (TBT): Time from lights-out to lights-on
- TST: Sum of all recorded sleep time in minutes
- Sleep efficiency: [(TST/TBT) × 100]
- WASO: Wake after sleep onset
- Sleep latency: Time from lights-out to the first epoch of recorded sleep
- REM latency: Time from the first epoch of sleep to the first epoch of REM sleep.

Figure C-1 demonstrates the proper EEG electrode placement according to the 10–20 system. Figure C-2 is a typical recording from the nocturnal PSG demonstrating snoring during SWS.

Special neurophysiologic events (e.g., epileptic events, *alpha* intrusion into sleep, and periodic activity of tibialis anterior) are

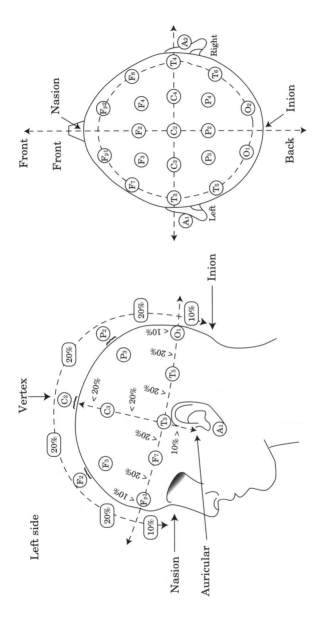

Figure C-1. *Continued*

reported. Respiratory activity (e.g., apneic or hypopneic episodes and oxygen saturation) is correlated with sleep stages. Other parameters such as body position, gastroesophageal reflux, bruxism, and penile tumescence are recorded.

If sleep apnea syndrome is diagnosed, a trial and titration of continuous positive airway pressure/bilevel positive airway pressure (CPAP/BiPAP) or a trial of an oral appliance may be undertaken, either in a split-night protocol or in a second-night PSG recording.

PSG is performed in the sleep laboratory under constant supervision by a trained technologist, and its quality therefore depends on the quality and the expertise of the performing technologist. Another limitation arises from the fact that recording conditions may not exactly translate to what happens during a regular night in the patient's home. Although diagnosing a sleep problem on the basis of a recording over a single night is common practice, some authorities caution that more than one night of recording may be necessary so that the patient may become comfortable with unfamiliar surroundings and sleep more naturally. This effect is greatest on the first night in the sleep laboratory ("first night effect").[4] The night-to-night variability is sometimes encountered in patients in whom sleep-disordered breathing varies according to sleep stage or position and can result in a false-negative study. From one night to another, the severity of apnea may vary, resulting in a false-negative study in subjects with mild disease.[5,6] Therefore, subjects with an initial negative PSG in which the clinical suspicion for sleep apnea is high may benefit from having a repeat PSG. Also in the evaluation of patients with sporadic nocturnal events, consecutive studies may be ordered because these events may be missed on a single-night PSG. External factors and anxiety that disturb the subject's sleep may be present in the home environment but absent from the controlled environment of the sleep lab.[7,8] This is termed *the reverse first night effect*.

Patient preparation is important so that the patient sleeps naturally. Before sleep testing, patients are instructed to maintain a regular sleep–wake schedule and avoid hypnotics, nicotine, alcohol, drugs acting on the central nervous system (including

Figure C-1.   The internationally standardized *10–20 system* is usually employed to record the spontaneous electroencephalogram (EEG). The letters used are: "F", frontal lobe; "T", temporal lobe; "C", central lobe; "P", parietal lobe; "O", occipital lobe; "A", ear. Even electrode numbers (2, 4, 6, and 8) refer to the right hemisphere and odd electrode numbers (1, 3, 5, and 7) refer to the left hemisphere. "Z" refers to an electrode placed on the midline. The smaller the number, the closer the position to the midline. "Fp" stands for Front polar. "Nasion" is the point between the forehead and nose. "Inion" is the most prominent projecting point of the occipital bone at the base of the skull. The "10" and "20" (10–20 system) refer to the 10% and 20% interelectrode distance. When recording a more detailed EEG with more electrodes, extra electrodes are added utilizing the spaces in between the existing 10–20 system. (Modified from: BrainMaster Technologies, Inc. http://www.brainmaster.com/index.html.)

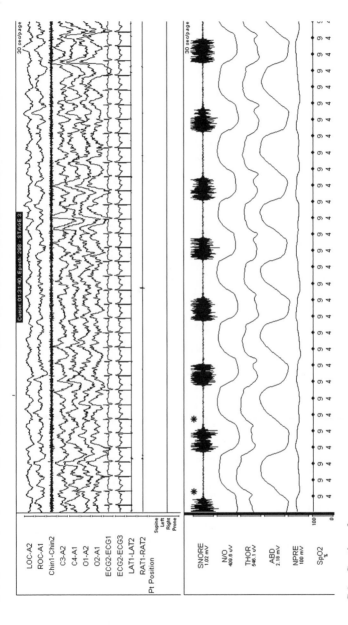

Figure C-2. *Continued*

those for the treatment of narcolepsy), and strenuous exercise on the day of PSG testing.

A typical PSG report is demonstrated in Figure C-3.

MULTIPLE SLEEP LATENCY TEST AND THE MAINTENANCE OF WAKEFULNESS TEST

It is suggested that the assessment of sleepiness or wakefulness involve a comprehensive integration of findings from the clinical history, along with objective data from the MSLT or the MWT. Absence of sleepiness on these tests should not be interpreted as the absence of sleepiness in the patient.

Multiple Sleep Latency Test

Indications for Use of the Multiple Sleep Latency Test

1. In patients with suspected narcolepsy, it confirms the diagnosis of narcolepsy
2. In patients with suspected idiopathic hypersomnia, it helps differentiate idiopathic hypersomnia from narcolepsy[9]
3. It is not typically needed for the diagnosis of obstructive sleep apnea or for the assessment of sleepiness in medical and neurologic disorders (other than narcolepsy), insomnia, or circadian rhythm abnormalities[9]
4. Repeat MSLT testing may be indicated in circumstances in which an initial test might have been affected by extraneous factors or when appropriate study conditions were not present during initial testing, when ambiguous or uninterpretable findings were present, or when the patient was suspected to have narcolepsy but earlier tests did not provide polygraphic confirmation.[9]

Recommendations for the Multiple Sleep Latency Test Protocol

The MSLT is a series of four or five naps taken at 2-hour intervals, starting in the morning the day after a PSG recording

←

Figure C-2. **Polysomnography snoring during the stage slow-wave sleep.** Illustrated in this figure is a 30-second epoch from a diagnostic polysomnogram of a 43-year-old man with a history of snoring and hypersomnia. The epoch demonstrates snoring during slow-wave sleep. The typical channels include:

- Two electrooculogram channels (left: LOC-A2, right: ROC-A1)
- Chin electromyogram (EMG) channel
- Electroencephalogram (left central, right central, left occipital, and right occipital)
- Two electrocardiogram, channels
- Two Limb EMG channels (left leg and right leg)
- Position channel (supine, left, right, and prone)
- Snoring channel (snoring is depicted by *)
- Nasal–oral airflow
- Respiratory effort (thoracic, abdominal)
- Nasal pressure
- Oxygen desaturation.

(From: BrainMaster Technologies, Inc. 2005; [cited 2005 Nov 11]. Available from: http://www.brainmaster.com/index.html.)

SAMPLE POLYSOMNOGRAM REPORT

Name: _____
Reg. #: _____
DOB: _____
Date: _____

UNIVERSITY OF MICHIGAN HOSPITALS
DEPARTMENT OF NEUROLOGY
SLEEP DISORDERS CENTER

Physician requesting evaluation: _____
Indication: Possible obstructive sleep apnea
Test Description: PSG

Procedure: Central & occipital EEG, EOG, submentalis EMG, thermocouple, nasal pressure, ECG, thoracoabdominal motion, anterior tibialis EMG, snore sensor, and pulse oximetry were monitored. The tracing was scored in 30 sec. epochs. The attending physician below participated in the review and interpretation of the study and in the preparation of this report.

Sleep Architecture			Minutes	% of TST
Recording time (min)	441.5	Wake Time	52.0	
Total Sleep Time (min)	377.0	Stage 1 sleep	94.5	25.1
Latency to sleep (min)	11.5	Stage 2 sleep	183.5	48.7
REM Latency (min)	86.0	Stage 3/4 sleep	0.0	0.0
# of Stage Shifts	138	Stage REM sleep	99.0	26.3
% Sleep Efficiency	85.4%	Total NREM sleep	278.0	

EEG and Sleep Stage Analysis: Stage 1 is increased. No slow wave sleep was recorded.

Figure C-3. *Continued*

Respiratory Analysis:	Total
# of apneic episodes	58
Total sleep time (min)	377.0
Apnea/hypopnea index (AHI)	9.3
NREM AHI	3.5
REM AHI	25.5
AHI (hypopneas w/4% desat)	1.1
Baseline % SaO2	93
Min % SaO2	88

Number of events	NREM	REM	Position	Prone	Supine	Left	Right
Obstructive apneas	0	0	# of events	0	37	21	0
Mixed apneas	0	0	TST/pos. (min)	0	157	220	0
Central apneas	0	1	# events/hr	0.0	14.1	5.7	0.0
Hypopneas (total)	16	41					
Hypopneas w/4% desats	-	4	Snoring: rare moderate				
Wake apneas	0		Arousals: frequent				

EKG Analysis: The usual heart rate/min was 68-76 in NREM sleep and 60-72 in REM sleep. PVC's and PAC's were recorded intermittently throughout the study.

Leg movement analysis: There were 37.9 periodic leg movements per hour of sleep; 5.4 per hour were associated with arousals. There were 24.2 periodic leg movements per hour of wakefulness.

Interpretation: This is a baseline polysomnogram. The findings are consistent with obstructive sleep apnea, nearly exclusively in the form of hypopneas, more prominent in the supine position and during supine-REM sleep. In addition to the scored events, snoring was noted, at times crescendo in pattern. Periodic limb movements were noted, occasionally associated with arousals.

ICSD code: A8, A11

during the individual's major sleep period. The test is used in the objective characterization of excessive sleepiness. Sleep logs may be obtained for 1 week before the MSLT is performed to assess sleep–wake schedules.[10] The MSLT is indicated as part of the evaluation of patients with hypersomnia and suspected narcolepsy and may be useful in the evaluation of patients with suspected idiopathic hypersomnia.[11] The sleep environment should be dark and quiet during testing and stimulants, stimulant-like medications, and REM-suppressing medications should ideally be avoided 2 weeks before testing.[10] Subjects should avoid tobacco, vigorous physical activity, unusual exposures to bright sunlight, and caffeinated beverages.[10]

The conventional recording montage for the MSLT includes central EEG (C3-A2, C4-A1) and occipital (O1-A2, O2-A1) derivations, left and right eye EOGs, mental/submental EMG, and electrocardiogram (ECG), as demonstrated in Figure C-4.

Sleep onset is determined by the time from lights-out to the first epoch of any sleep stage and is defined as the first epoch of >15 seconds of cumulative sleep in a 30-second epoch. The absence of sleep on a nap opportunity is recorded as a sleep latency of 20 minutes, which is included in the calculation of mean sleep latency (MSL).[10] REM-sleep latency is defined as the time of the first epoch of sleep to the beginning of the first epoch of REM sleep regardless of the intervening stages of sleep or wakefulness. The MSLT report (Figure C-6) should include the start and end times of each nap or nap opportunity, latency from lights-out to the first epoch of sleep, MSL (arithmetic mean of all

---

←

Figure C-3. A typical polysomnogram report from the Michael S. Aldrich Sleep Disorders Laboratory at the University of Michigan Health System. Most reports consist of the following information:

1. Patient identification (i.e., name, date of birth, and medical record number)
2. Date of testing
3. Name of the requesting physician
4. Indication for the procedure (obstructive sleep apnea, hypersomnia, parasomnia, etc.)
5. Description of the procedure completed (and when appropriate, instrumentation and masks utilized)
6. Electroencephalogram (EEG) and sleep-stage analysis (percentage spent in each stage and discussion of abnormal EEG findings)
7. Respiratory analysis (apnea–hypopnea index, minimum oxygen saturation according to sleep stage, etc.)
8. Number of events (i.e., obstructive, mixed, and central hypopneas)
9. Electrocardiogram analysis (i.e., heart rate, range in rapid eye movement [REM], non-REM, and description of arrhythmias)
10. Leg movement analysis (i.e., periodic limb movements, index, and whether associated with arousals)
11. Interpretation, and when appropriate, suggestions for follow-up or recommendations
12. Code (ICSD, ICD-9)
13. Signature of the interpreting physician.

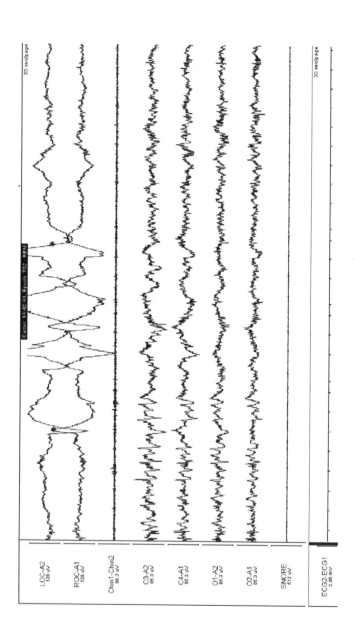

naps or nap opportunities), and total number of sleep-onset REM periods (SOREM). Any events that represent deviation from the standard protocol (e.g., patient smoking or drinking caffeinated beverage during the break) or conditions (e.g., unusual noise in the laboratory and fire alarms) should be documented by the sleep technologist for review by the interpreting sleep physician.[10]

Maintenance of Wakefulness Test

Indications for Use of the Maintenance of Wakefulness Test

1. The MWT may be used in the assessment of an individual's ability to remain awake when his or her inability to to do so constitutes a public or personal safety issue.[11]
2. The MWT may be indicated in patients with excessive sleepiness to assess response to treatment.[11]

The reader should be advised that there is little evidence linking the MSL on the MWT with risk of accidents in real-world situations; therefore, it is advised that the sleep physician should not rely solely on MSL as a single indicator of impairment or potential risk for accidents but should also rely on clinical judgment.[11]

←

Figure C-4.   Multiple sleep latency test—sleep-onset rapid eye movement period (SOREM). Illustrated in this figure is a 30-second epoch from an MSLT of a 19-year-old woman with a history of severe daytime sleepiness. The epoch demonstrates SOREM (SOREM is indicated by *). The typical channels include:

1. Two electrooculogram channels (left: LOC-A2, right: ROC-A1)
2. Chin electromyogram (EMG) channel
3. Electroencephalogram (EEG) (left central, right central, left occipital, and right occipital)
4. Snoring channel
5. An electrocardiogram channel.

→

Figure C-5.   A typical MSLT report from the Michael S. Aldrich Sleep Disorders Laboratory at the University of Michigan Health System. Most reports consist of the following information:

1. Patient identification (i.e., name, date of birth, and medical record number)
2. Date of testing
3. Name of the requesting physician
4. Indication for the procedure (i.e., obstructive sleep apnea, hypersomnia, and parasomnia)
5. Description of the procedure completed (and when appropriate, instrumentation and masks utilized)
6. Tabulation of the time in bed, sleep latencies for each of the naps, documentation of the presence or lack of sleep-onset rapid eye movement periods, and tabulation of the calculated mean sleep latency
7. Interpretation, and when appropriate, suggestions for follow-up or recommendations.
8. Code (ICSD, ICD-9)
9. Signature of the interpreting physician.

SAMPLE MSLT REPORT

UNIVERSITY OF MICHIGAN HOSPITALS
DEPARTMENT OF NEUROLOGY
SLEEP DISORDERS CENTER

Name: _____
Reg. #: _____
DOB: _____
Date: _____

Procedure: Multiple Sleep Latency Test

Physician requesting evaluation_____

Indication:

Description: Four fifteen to thirty-five minute nap test periods were recorded and the patient was allowed to sleep for up to fifteen minutes after the onset of sleep. EEG (C3-A2, C4-A1), mentalis EMG, EOG, ECG and snoring were monitored throughout each recording. The tracing was scored using 30-second epochs. The attending physician below participated in the review and interpretation of the study and in the preparation of this report.

RESULTS:	NAP 1	NAP 2	NAP 3	NAP 4	MEAN
Time test began	08:05	10:07	12:14	14:02	
Time in bed (min.)	20.0	20.0	20.0	20.5	
Latencies to (min.)					
First sleep epoch	20.0	20.0	20.0	20.0	20.0
REM sleep	-	-	-	-	
Number of REM periods = 0					

INTERPRETATION:

This multiple sleep latency test does not demonstrate excessive daytime sleepiness. No amount of sleep was observed. In conjunction with the clinical evaluation and the nocturnal polysomnogram, the results do not suggest an intrinsic sleep disorder such as monosymptomatic narcolepsy or idiopathic hypersomnia.

ICSD code:

Recommendations for the Maintenance of Wakefulness Test Protocol

Unlike the MSLT, subjects undergoing the MWT are asked to attempt to remain awake. The MWT is performed at 2-hour intervals and consists of four trials lasting 40 minutes in duration.[12] The first trial begins at approximately 1.5 to 3 hours after the patient's usual wake-up time. Performance of PSG before MWT is left to the discretion of the clinician on the basis of the clinical circumstances. As for the MSLT protocol, the room should be maximally insulated from external light and noise, and the use of tobacco, caffeine, and other medications by the patient before and during MWT should be addressed by the sleep clinician before the test. The subject should be seated in bed and asked to remain awake for a period of 20 to 40 minutes. The conventional recording montage for the MWT includes central EEG (C3-A2, C4-A1) and occipital (O1-A2, O2-A1) derivations, left and right eye EOGs, mental/submental EMG, and ECG.[12] Sleep onset is defined as the first epoch of >15 seconds of cumulative sleep in a 30-second epoch. The test is repeated four to five times during the day, and the MSL is determined. Each trial lasts 20 to 40 minutes (if no sleep is recorded). The following data should be recorded: Start and stop times for each trial, sleep latency, TST, stages of sleep achieved for each trial, and the MSL (the arithmetic mean of the four trials). Events that represent deviation from the standard protocol or conditions should be documented by the sleep technologist for review by the sleep specialist. On the basis of normative data (based on a review by the MSLT and MWT Task Force of the Standards of Practice Committee of the American Academy of Sleep Medicine), an MSL <8 minutes on the 40-minute MWT is abnormal. Scores between 8 and 40 are of uncertain significance. The strongest evidence for an individual's ability to maintain wakefulness is provided by a capacity to remain awake throughout all trials of the 40-minute MWT (which is the upper limit of the 95% confidence interval).[9] A major problem with the MWT relates to the wide variety of protocols used, the absence of consensus about the length of the session, and the lack of normative data.

SLEEP HYPNOGRAM

Shown in Figure C-6 is a sample sleep hypnogram. On the vertical axis, the graph depicts the sleep stages (wake, stage 1, 2, slow-wave, REM, awakenings), respiratory data (number of obstructive, central, and mixed apneas; hypopneas; and oxygen desaturations), the patient's position during the night, and periodic leg movements, all against the horizontal axis depicting time (usually in 1-hour intervals). Integration of digital analysis in sleep medicine has enabled this graphic illustration.[13,14] It is advantageous as a visual aid, depicting multiple data against time and allowing the clinician easy visualization of multiple and simultaneous physiologic sleep variables recording.

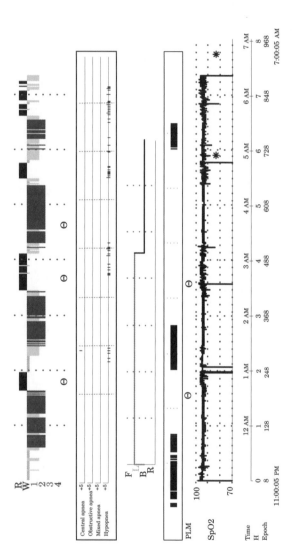

Figure C-6.   Sample hypnogram. This is from a patient with possible obstructive sleep apnea. The graph depicts the sleep stages (i.e., wake, stage 1, slow-wave, rapid eye movement [REM], and awakenings), respiratory data (i.e., number of central, obstructive, and mixed apneas, and hypopneas), periodic leg movements (PLMs), and the patient's position during the night. The horizontal axis depicts time from 11:00:05 PM to 7:00:05 AM in 1-hour intervals. The (✱) demonstrates episodes of hypopneas occurring mostly during REM sleep and associated with oxygen desaturations.

REFERENCES

1. Polysomnography Task Force, American Sleep Disor ciation Standards of Practice Committee. Practice pa for the indications for polysomnography and related proc *Sleep*. 1997;20(6):406–422.

2. Rechtschaffen A, Kales A. *A manual of standardized terminolo techniques and scoring system for sleep stages of human subject* Washington, DC: U.S. Government Printing Office; 1968.

3. Jasper HH. The 10–20 electrode system of the International Federation. *Electroencephalogr Clin Neurophysiol*. 1958;10:370–375.

4. Agnew HW, Webb WB, Williams RL. The first-night effect: An EEG study of sleep. *Psychophysiology*. 1966;2:263–266.

5. Meyer TJ, Eveloff SE, Kline LR, et al. One negative polysomnogram does not exclude obstructive sleep apnea. *Chest*. 1993;103: 756–760.

6. Le Bon O, Hoffmann G, Tecco J, et al. Mild to moderate sleep respiratory events: One negative night may not be enough. *Chest*. 2000;118:353–359.

7. Hauri PJ, Olmstead EM. Reverse first night effect in insomnia. *Sleep*. 1989;12(2):97–105.

8. Riedel BW, Winfield CF, Lichstein KL. First night effect and reverse first night effect in older adults with primary insomnia: Does anxiety play a role? *Sleep Med*. 2001;2(2):125–133.

9. Arand D, Bonnet M, Hurwitz T, et al. The clinical use of the MSLT and MWT. *Sleep*. 2005;28(1):123–144.

10. Carskadon MA, Dement WC, Mitler MM, et al. Guidelines for the multiple sleep latency test (MSLT): A standard measure of sleepiness. *Sleep*. 1986;9(4):519–524.

11. Littner MR, Kushida C, Wise M, et al. Practice parameters for clinical use of the multiple sleep latency test and the maintenance of wakefulness test. *Sleep*. 2005;28(1):113–121.

12. Doghramji K, Mitler MM, Sangal RB, et al. A normative study of the maintenance of wakefulness test (MWT). *Electroencephalogr Clin Neurophysiol*. 1997;103(5):554–562.

13. Gath I, Bar-on E. Computerized method for scoring of polygraphic sleep recordings. *Comput Programs Biomed*. 1980;11(3):217–223.

14. King C. Sleep hypnogram and sleep analysis: A rapid, inexpensive procedure. *Sleep*. 1980;3(1):93–94.

Appendix D. Continuous Positive Airway Pressure Compliance Issues Unique to Sleep Medicine

Complication	Possible Cause	Possible Corrective Measu
Mask leaks	Incorrect mask size Strap adjustment too loose or too tight	Readjust headgear straps Refit mask
Skin breakdown	Use of mole-skin, or other form of adhesive pads applied to the skin in an effort to prevent blisters. Use of water-based lubricant.	Nasal pillows or full-face ma better fit
Pressure sores, blisters, or cellulitis	Strap adjustment too loose or too tight Incorrect mask size Worn-out mask Dirty mask	Inspect mask for cracks or breaks and replace mask as indicated Wash mask daily
Dry nose and throat Nasal congestion	Mask leaks, lack of humidification, nasal allergies, dry air	Nasal saline spray or nasal saline irrigation (q.d., b.i.d.) Heated humidification
Allergic rhinitis Epistaxis	Allergens gaining access through machine	Intranasal steroid preparation or antihistamines Particulate filter can be added to some units Consult ENT physician if symptoms persist

Dry mouth	Shunt development, air leaking from mouth, sleeping with mouth open	Chin strap
		Consider alternative mask size or model, or full-face mask
		Heated humidification
Conjunctivitis: Irritable, dry, or swollen eyes	Mask leaks toward eyes	Readjust the mask on the face
	Mask too tight	Readjust headgear straps
		Inspect mask for cracks or breaks; replace mask as indicated
Rhinorrhea	Dry air	Nasal saline spray to be used before bedtime
	Mouth or mask leaks	Nasal steroid preparation or ipratropium bromide at bedtime
		Heated humidification
Difficulty exhaling	Pressure too low or too high	Add C-flex to CPAP; consider testing and attempting BiPAP for comfort
Aerophagia		

(Continued)

Appendix D. *Continued*

Complication	Possible Cause	Possible Corrective Measures
Noisy CPAP unit	Faulty equipment Blocked air intake	Evaluate equipment Make sure that air filter is clean and not blocked by outside items
	Too close to sleeping area	Increase the length of hose and place unit farther away; consider special suitcases to house the CPAP unit
Bed partner intolerance	Multifactorial (noise, anxiety)	Promote education of the patient and bed partner; assess for possible reasons for insomnia in the bed partner; encourage use of earplugs; recommend attending a patient support group (i.e., A.W.A.K.E. Network of the American Sleep Apnea Association).
Claustrophobia	Anxiety with use of mask	Use smaller mask specifically applied to the nasal orifice, desensitization.

ENT, ear, nose, and throat; CPAP, continuous positive airway pressure; BiPAP, Bilevel positive airway pressure; A.W.A.K.E., alert, well, and keeping energetic.

Modified from Zozula, R. and R. Rosen. Compliance with continuous positive airway pressure therapy: Assessing and improving treatment outcomes. Curr Opin Pulm Med, 2001;7(6):391–398.

Sleep Hygiene

Practicing good sleep habits can be useful in the treatment of many sleep disorders. In patients with insomnia and circadian rhythm sleep disorders, increasing the drive for nocturnal sleep and improving the regularity of the sleep and wake cycle are essential components of behavioral therapy. The subsequent text provides some useful tips for better sleep.

Increase Drive for Sleep at Night (Sleep Homeostatic Factors)
- Avoid naps, except for a brief duration (30 minutes) during the day, but check with your physician first because in some sleep disorders naps can be beneficial.
- Avoid spending too much time awake in bed.
- Get regular exercise each day, preferably 40 minutes each day. It is best to complete exercise at least 3 to 4 hours before bedtime.
- Take a hot bath 2 hours before bedtime.

Increase Regularity of Sleep–Wake Schedule (Circadian Factors)
- Keep a regular bedtime and wake time 7 days a week (do not deviate by >1 hour).
- Do not expose yourself to bright light if you have to get up at night.
- Increase exposure to bright light during the day.
- Exercise at a regular time each day.

Medication and Drug Effects
- Do not smoke after 7 PM. Give up smoking entirely, if possible.
- Avoid caffeine after 10 AM. Limit intake of caffeinated beverages and food.
- Restrict alcoholic beverage consumption. Alcohol can fragment sleep over the second half of sleep.
- Review with your doctor the medications that could be stimulating or sedating.

Optimize in Sleep Setting
- Keep the clock face turned away, and do not find out what time it is when you wake up at night.
- Avoid strenuous exercise after 6 PM.
- Do not eat or drink heavily for 3 hours before bedtime. A light bedtime snack may help.
- If you have trouble with heart burn, be especially careful to avoid heavy meals and spices in the evening.
- Do not retire too hungry or too full.
- Keep your room dark, quiet, well ventilated, and at a comfortable temperature throughout the night.
- Use a bedtime ritual. Reading before lights-out may be helpful if it is relaxing.
- Set aside a worry time; make a list of problems for the following day.

Most of the time	Some of the time	Never	N/A	
				ID:_____
				Date:_____

Homeostatic Drive for Sleep

Most of the time	Some of the time	Never	N/A	
				Avoid naps, except for a brief 10-to 15-minute nap 8 hours after arising
				Restrict sleep period to the average number of hours you have actually slept in the preceding week
				Get regular exercise each day, preferably 40 minutes each day of an activity that causes sweating
				A warm non–caffeine containing drink to help you relax as well as warm you

Circadian Factors

				Keep a regular time out of bed 7 days a week
				Do not expose yourself to bright light if you have to get up at night
				Get at least one half hour of sunlight within 30 minutes of your out-of-bed time

Drug Effects

				Do not smoke to get yourself back to sleep
				Do not smoke after 7:00 pm, or give up smoking entirely
				Limit caffeine use to no more than three cups no later than 10:00 am
				Avoid alcoholic beverages after 7 PM

Arousal in Sleep Setting

				Keep clock face turned away, and do not find out what time it is when you wake up at night
				Avoid strenuous exercise after 7 pm
				Do not eat or drink heavily for three hours before bedtime
				If you have trouble with regurgitation, avoid heavy meals and spices in the evening
				Keep your room dark, quiet, well ventilated, and at a comfortable temperature throughout the night
				Use a bedtime ritual such as reading before lights-out
				List problems and one-sentence next step for the following day
				Avoid unfamiliar sleep environments
				Use bedroom only for sleep and sex, do not do other activities that lead to prolonged arousal

"I encourage you to follow the sleep hygiene instructions, especially the areas that were discussed today. We'll see you in two weeks. If you have any questions don't hesitate to call me."

Interviewer:_____

Sleep hygiene biweekly follow-up.

- Learn simple relaxation skills to use if you wake up at night.
- Use stress management in the daytime.
- Avoid unfamiliar sleep environments.
- Be sure that the mattress is not too soft or too firm and that the pillow is of proper height and firmness.
- Use bedroom for sleep and sex only; do not work or do other activities that lead to prolonged arousal.

Appendix F. Insomnia Algorithm

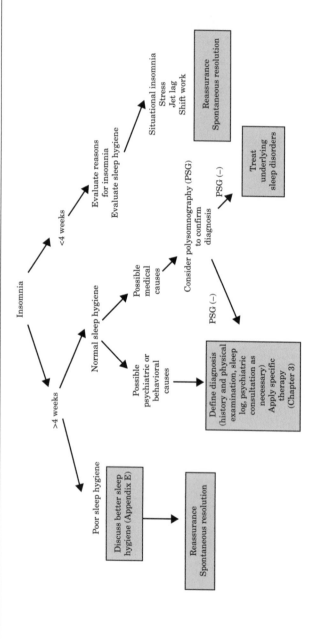

208

Appendix G. Hypersomnia Algorithm

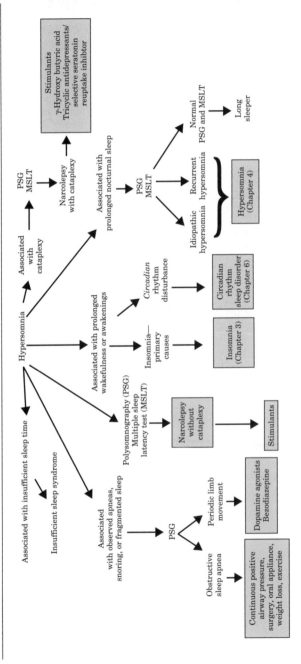

Stanford Sleepiness Scale

This 7-point rating scale consists of seven numbered statements describing subjective levels of sleepiness or alertness.

The Stanford Sleepiness Scale (SSS) rates the patient's perception of feeling sleepy during the day on a scale from 1 to 7. Sleepiness may be rated at different times of the day. This scale may be used to help establish a pattern of sleepiness and to monitor changes in sleepiness.

AN INTROSPECTIVE MEASURE OF SLEEPINESS

The Stanford Sleepiness Scale (SSS)

Degree of Sleepiness	Scale Rating
Feeling active, vital, alert, or wide awake	1
Functioning at high levels, but not at peak; able to concentrate	2
Awake, but relaxed; responsive but not fully alert	3
Somewhat foggy, let down	4
Foggy; losing interest in remaining awake; slowed down	5
Sleepy, woozy, fighting sleep; prefer to lie down	6
No longer fighting sleep, sleep onset soon; having dream-like thoughts	7
Asleep	X

From Hoddes E, Dement WC, Zarcone V: The development and use of the Stanford Sleepiness Scale (SSS). Psychophysiology. 1972;9:150. With permission.

Appendix I. Motor Disorders Algorithm

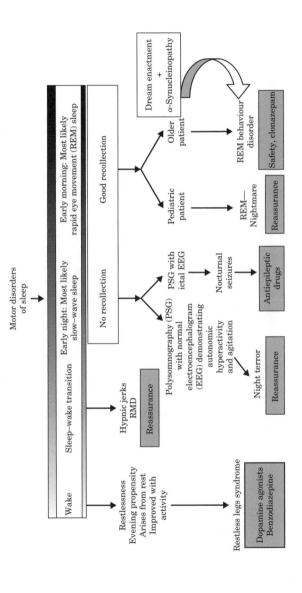

International Classification of Sleep Disorders (ICSD-2)

The most current version of the *International Classification of Sleep Disorders* (*ICSD-2*) describes and provides diagnostic criteria for all the recognized adult and pediatric sleep and arousal disorders. To facilitate its use in clinical practice as much as possible, the diagnoses in the ICSD are compatible with ICD-9 (the numbers given within parenthesis). An outline of the more common ICSD-2 diagnoses and compatibility with the ICD-9 codes is provided in this appendix. Specific descriptions for the major categories of sleep disorders and their diagnostic criteria are provided within each of the relevant chapters.

I. **Insomnias**
    A. Adjustment insomnia (307.41)
    B. Psychophysiological insomnia (307.42)
    C. Paradoxical insomnia (307.42)
    D. Idiopathic insomnia (307.42)
    E. Physiological insomnia, unspecified (327.00)
    F. Insomnia due to medical disorder (327.01)
    G. Insomnia due to mental condition (327.02)
    H. Insomnia due to drug or substance (292.85) or alcohol (292.82)
    I. Physiological condition, unspecified (780.52)
II. **Sleep-Related Breathing Disorders**
    A. Central sleep apnea
        1. Primary central sleep apnea (327.21)
        2. High-altitude periodic breathing (327.22)
        3. Central apnea due to medical condition, non–Cheyne-Stokes (327.28)
        4. Central apnea due to drug or substance (327.29)
        5. Central apnea due to Cheyne-Stokes breathing pattern (786.04)
        6. Primary sleep apnea of infancy (770.81)
    B. Obstructive sleep apnea, adult and pediatric (327.23)
    C. Sleep-related hypoventilation/hypoxemia
        1. Nonobstructive alveolar hypoventilation, idiopathic (327.24)
        2. Central alveolar hypoventilation, congenital (327.25)
        3. Sleep-related hypoventilation/hypoxemia due to medical condition (327.27) (includes pulmonary parenchymal or vascular pathology, lower airway obstruction, and neuromuscular and chest wall disorders)
        4. Other sleep apnea/sleep-related breathing disorders, unspecified (327.20)
III. **Hypersomnias**
    A. Narcolepsy
        1. Narcolepsy without cataplexy (347.00)
        2. Narcolepsy with cataplexy (347.01)

        3. Narcolepsy due to medical condition without cataplexy (347.10)
        4. Narcolepsy due to medical condition with cataplexy (347.11)
        5. Narcolepsy, unspecified (347.00)
  B. Recurrent hypersomnias
        1. Kleine-Levin syndrome (327.13)
        2. Menstrual-related hypersomnia (327.13)
  C. Idiopathic hypersomnia with long sleep (327.11)
  D. Idiopathic hypersomnia without long sleep (327.12)
  E. Hypersomnia due to medical condition (327.14)
  F. Hypersomnia not due to substance or physiological condition (327.15)
  G. Physiological hypersomnia, unspecified (327.10)
  H. Hypersomnia due to drug or substance (292.85) or alcohol (292.82)
  I. Behaviorally induced insufficient sleep syndrome (307.44)

IV. Circadian Rhythm Sleep Disorders
  A. Delayed sleep phase type (327.31)
  B. Advanced sleep phase type (327.32)
  C. Irregular sleep–wake type (327.33)
  D. Nonentrained type (327.34)
  E. Jet lag type (327.35)
  F. Shift-work type (327.36)
  G. Due to medical condition (327.37)

V. Parasomnia
  A. Confusional arousals (327.41)
  B. REM sleep behavior disorder (327.42)
  C. Recurrent isolated sleep paralysis (327.43)
  D. Parasomnia due to medical condition (327.44)
  E. Sleep-related groaning (catathrenia) (327.49)
  F. Exploding head syndrome (327.49)
  G. Sleep-related eating disorder (327.49)
  H. Sleepwalking (307.46)
  I. Sleep terrors (307.46)
  J. Nightmare disorder (307.47)
  K. Sleep-related dissociative disorders (300.15)
  L. Sleep enuresis (788.36)

VI. Sleep-Related Movement Disorders
  A. Restless legs syndrome (333.99)
  B. Periodic limb movement disorder (327.52)
  C. Sleep-related leg cramps (327.53)
  D. Sleep-related bruxism (327.54)
  E. Sleep-related rhythmic movement disorder (327.59)
  F. Sleep-related movement disorder (unspecified, due to medical condition, due to drug or substance) (327.59)

Sleep-Stage Scoring

Sleep-stage scoring is based on the criteria derived from several physiologic signals, usually as outlined by Rechtschaffen and Kales (R-K) (1968).[1] The R-K method divides sleep into five stages: Nonrapid eye movement (NREM)—stages 1, 2, 3, and 4—and stage rapid eye movement (REM) sleep; physiologic signals of interest are generated from the cerebral cortex (electroencephalogram [EEG]), eye movements (electrooculogram [EOG]), and the muscles of the face (chin electromyogram [EMG]). Table K-1 summarizes sleep stages according to the R-K criteria.

This appendix includes a discussion of the specific parameters required for staging sleep. Unless otherwise stated, all polysomnography (PSG) samples are recorded at a paper speed of 10 mm per second, where one page equates to 30 seconds and is defined as one epoch.

Abbreviations used in the PSG samples provided here include:

LOC-A2, ROC-A1	Left and right electrooculogram referred to right and left mastoid leads
LOC-AVG	Left and electrooculogram referred to an average reference electrode
Chin1-Chin2	Chin EMG electrode
EEG Monitoring	The position of the exploring reference electrode (e.g., F3, F4, C3, C4, O1, and O2) is chosen on the opposite side of the head from the mastoid electrode (A1, A2) or average (AVG)
LAT1-LAT2, RAT1-RAT2	Leg (anterior tibialis) EMG electrode (L, left; R, right)
ORAL-NASAL (N/O)	Oral/nasal airflow channel
THOR1-THOR2	Thoracic effort channel
ABD1-ABD2	Abdominal effort channel
NPRE	Nasal Pressure
SpO_2	Oxygen saturation (%)
SNORE	Snore sensor

Parameters for Staging Human Sleep

The following three physiologic parameters are universal to all PSG monitoring:

- EOG leads—left eye and right eye
- EEG leads—a minimum of one central EEG lead and one occipital EEG lead
- EMG lead—one submental EMG channel

Table K-1. Synopsis of sleep stages according to the Rechtschaffen and Kales criteria

Properties	Stage Wake (W)	Stage 1	Stage 2	Stage 3 and 4 Sleep	Stage-REM Sleep
Duration	—	10 min	20 min	30–45 min	The first REM period is very short, (lasting ~5 min), the second is ~10 min, and the third is ~15 min; The final REM period usually lasts for 30 min (but can last up to 1 h)
%TST	2%–5%	44%–55%	3%–8%	10%–15%	20%–25%
EEG	Eyes open: Low voltage, mixed frequency; *alpha* activity attenuates Eyes closed: Low voltage, high frequency; more than 50% *alpha* activity	Low voltage, mixed frequency; *theta activity; vertex sharp waves*	Low voltage, mixed frequency; at least one *K complex/sleep spindle*	**Stage 3:** 20%–50% high-amplitude delta activity **Stage 4:** >50% high-amplitude delta activity	Low voltage, mixed frequency Presence of *sawtooth waves Desynchronized EEG* (in all other stages, the EEG is *synchronized*)
EOG	Eye blinks, voluntary control, *SREM* when drowsy	*SREM*	Occasional *SREM*	Mirrors EEG	P-REM

(*Continued*)

Table K-1. *Continued*

Properties	Stage Wake (W)	Stage 1	Stage 2	Stage 3 and 4 Sleep	Stage-REM Sleep
EMG	Tonic activity High EMG activity Under voluntary control	Tonic activity High–medium EMG activity	Tonic activity Low EMG activity	Tonic activity Low EMG activity	*T-REM:* Relatively reduced *P-REM:* Episodic EMG twitching
Arousal threshold	—	Lowest	Lower	Highest	Low
Physiologic changes	—	Progressive reduction of physiologic activity and blood pressure; heart rate decreases			*T-REM:* Muscle paralysis, increased cerebral blood flow *P-REM :* Irregular breathing, variable heart rate, REM, phasic muscle twitching
Dreaming	—	—	—	Diffuse dreams	Vivid, bizarre, and detailed dreams
Parasomnias	Hypnic jerks—during transition to stage 1	Hypnic jerks	Confusional arousals, somniloquy	Sleepwalking, night terrors	REM-sleep behavior disorder, REM nightmares

For Stage MT (Movement Time) please see text.
REM, rapid eye movement; TST, total sleep time; EEG, electroencephalography; EOG, electrooculography; SREM, slow rolling eye movements; EMG, electromyography; T-REM, tonic-REM; P-REM, phasic-REM.

Source: Adapted from Chokroverty S, Thomas R, Bhatt M. *Atlas of sleep medicine.* Philadelphia, PA: Elsevier, Butterworth-Heinemann; 2005.
Adapted from Rechtschaffen A, Kales A, eds. *A manual of standardised terminology, techniques, and scoring system for sleep stages of human subjects.* Los Angeles, CA: Brain Information service/Brain Research Institute; 1968.

Electrooculogram Recording

- The EOG signals measure changes in the electric potential of the (+) anterior aspect of the eye (the cornea) relative to the (−) posterior aspect (the retina).
- EOG voltages are higher than the EEG signal. Because the eye is outside the skull structure, there is no bone to attenuate the signal.
- Cornea (front) has a positive polarity. The retina (back) has a negative polarity.
- EOG placement (LOC and ROC) is on the outer canthus of the eye—offset 1 cm below (LOC) and 1 cm above (ROC) the horizon.
- EOG picks up the inherent voltage of the eye. During eyes-open wakefulness, sharp deflections in the EOG tracing may indicate the presence of eye blinks.

Electroencephalogram Recording Criterion

- Wakefulness and sleep are determined by the characteristic patterns of the scalp EEG signals and are of fundamental importance in interpreting PSG studies.
- EEG is a record of the electric potentials generated by the cortex but can reflect the influence of deeper brain structures, such as the thalamus.
- Two centrocephalic and two occipital cortical channels are recorded: The PSG references the left and right centrocephalic electrodes (C3, C4) or the left and right occipital electrodes (O1, O4) to the electrodes on the opposite right and left ears (A2, A1).
- Measurement of the EEG signal is possible because of the relative difference in potential between the two recording electrodes.
- A (−) discharge, by convention, is represented by an upwardly deflecting wave.
- A minimum paper speed of 10 mm per second is recommended. One page equates to 30 seconds and is defined as one epoch.
- A time constant (TC) of 0.3 seconds or a low frequency filter (LFF) of 0.3 Hz is recommended.
- Pen deflections of 7.5 to 10 mm for 50 μV are recommended.
- Electrode impedances should not exceed 10 KΩ.

Electromyographic Recording

- The EMG signals are muscle twitch potentials that are used in PSG to distinguish between sleep stages on the basis of the fact that EMG activity diminishes during sleep.
- Mental, submental, and masseter placements are acceptable. This is a mandatory recording parameter for staging sleep.
- They are used to detect muscle tone changes for scoring rapid eye movement (REM) versus NREM sleep.
- Muscle tone is high during wakefulness and NREM sleep. It is lower in NREM sleep, progressively lower in slow-wave sleep (SWS), and lowest in REM sleep.
- Submental EMG records muscle tone.

Electroencephalographic Activity during Wakefulness and Sleep

Cortical activities can be characterized by their specific frequencies. Frequency is noted in cycles per second (i.e., Hertz [Hz]). EEG activity has been divided into four bands on the basis of the frequency and amplitude of the waveform and these bands are assigned Greek letters (alpha, beta, theta, delta). The EEG frequencies are defined in a slightly different manner according to the reference used.

Beta Activity

- Beta EEG—defined as a waveform of 14 to 30 Hz
- Originates in the frontal and central regions
- Present during wakefulness and drowsiness
- May become persistent during drowsiness, diminish during SWS, and reemerge during REM sleep
- Enhanced or persistent activity suggests use of sedative-hypnotic medications

Alpha Activity

- Alpha EEG—defined as a waveform of 8 to 14 Hz
- Originates in the parietooccipital regions bilaterally
- A normal alpha rhythm is synchronous and symmetric over the cerebral hemispheres
- Seen during quite alertness with eyes closed
- Eye opening—causes the alpha waves to "react" or decrease in amplitude
- Has a crescendo–decrescendo appearance
- Has diminished frequency with aging

Theta Activity

- Theta frequency defined as a waveform of 4 to 8 Hz
- Originates in the central vertex region
- Lacks an amplitude criteria for theta
- The most common sleep frequency

Sleep Spindles

- Defined as a waveform of 12 to 14 Hz
- Originates in the central vertex region
- Has a duration criterion of 0.5 to 2–3 seconds
- Typically occurs in stage-2 sleep but can be seen in other stages

K Complexes

- Defined as sharp, slow waves, with a biphasic morphology (first negative and then positive deflection)
- Predominantly central vertex in origin
- Duration must be at least 0.5 seconds
- Lacks an amplitude criteria
- Indicative of stage-2 sleep

Delta Activity

- Defined as a waveform of 0.5 to 2 Hz
- Seen predominantly in the frontal region
- Delta activity has an amplitude criterion of ≥ 75 μV

- Lacks a duration criterion
- Stage-3 sleep defined when 20% to 50% of the epoch is scored as delta activity
- Stage-4 sleep defined when >50% of the epoch is scored as delta activity

Stages of Sleep

Stage Wake

- Typically, the first several minutes of the record will consist of wake (W) stage (see Figure K-1).
- Stage W is recorded when >50% of the epoch has scorable alpha EEG activity.
- The EEG will show mixed beta and alpha activities as the eyes open and close, and predominantly alpha activity when the eyes remain closed.
- Submental EMG is relatively high tone and will reflect the high-amplitude muscle contractions and movement artifacts.
- The EOG channels will show eye blinking and rapid movement. The record will slow in frequency and amplitude as the subject stops moving and becomes drowsy.
- As the patient becomes drowsy, with the eyes closed, the EEG will show predominant alpha activity, although the EMG activity will become less prominent.

Stage-1 Non–Rapid Eye Movement Sleep

- Stage-1 sleep is scored when >15 seconds ($\geq$50%) of the epoch is made up of theta activity (3 to 7 Hz), sometimes intermixed with low-amplitude delta activity replacing the alpha activity of wakefulness (see Figures K-2 and K-3).
- This stage is characterized by low-voltage fast EEG activity with an amplitude of <50 to 75 μV.
- The alpha activity in the EEG drops to <50%.
- Vertex sharp waves may occur toward the end of stage-1 sleep. They are characterized by high-voltage sharp surface-negative followed by surface-positive components and are maximal over the Cz electrode.
- Sleep spindles or K complexes are never a part of stage-1 vertex waves.
- The EMG shows less activity than in the wake stage.
- The arousals are defined by paroxysms of EEG activity (typically to a faster alpha or theta activity) lasting 3 seconds but <15 seconds. If an arousal occurs in stage-1 sleep and if the burst results in alpha activity for >50% of the record, then the epoch is scored as stage W.
- The eyes begin to show slow rolling eye movements (SREM).
- The time spent in stage 1 may increase with age.

Stage-2 Non–Rapid Eye Movement

- Characterized by predominant theta activity and minimal alpha activity, stage-2 NREM accounts for the bulk of a typical PSG recording (up to 50% in adult patients) (see Figure K-4).

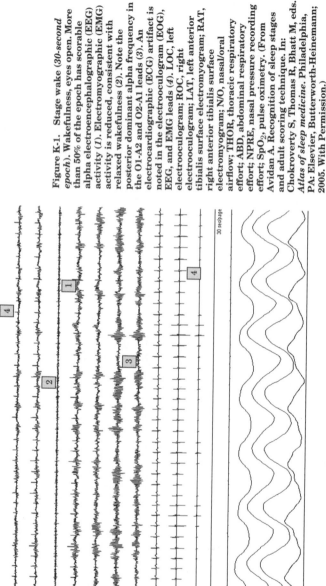

Figure K-1. Stage wake (*30-second epoch*). Wakefulness, eyes open. More than 50% of the epoch has scorable alpha electroencephalographic (EEG) activity (*1*). Electromyographic (EMG) activity is reduced, consistent with relaxed wakefulness (*2*). Note the posterior dominant alpha frequency in the O1-A2 and O2-A1 leads (*3*). An electrocardiographic (ECG) artifact is noted in the electrooculogram (EOG), EEG, and EMG leads (*4*). LOC, left electrooculogram; ROC, right electrooculogram; LAT, left anterior tibialis surface electromyogram; RAT, right anterior tibialis surface electromyogram; N/O, nasal/oral airflow; THOR, thoracic respiratory effort; ABD, abdominal respiratory effort; NPRE, nasal pressure recording effort; SpO$_2$, pulse oximetry. (From Avidan A. Recognition of sleep stages and adult scoring technique. In: Chokroverty S, Thomas R, Bhatt M, eds. *Atlas of sleep medicine.* Philadelphia, PA: Elsevier, Butterworth-Heinemann; 2005. With Permission.)

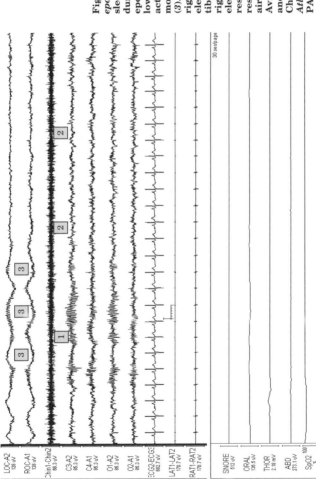

Figure K-2. Stage-1 Sleep (*30-second epoch*). The record depicts stage-1 sleep. Alpha activity (*1*) is present during the initial 10 seconds of the epoch and is gradually replaced by low-voltage, mixed-frequency theta activity (*2*). Slow rolling eye movements become more prominent (*3*). LOC, left electrooculogram; ROC, right electrooculogram; ECG, electrocardiogram; LAT, left anterior tibialis surface electromyogram; RAT, right anterior tibialis surface electromyogram; THOR, thoracic respiratory effort; ABD, abdominal respiratory effort; N/O, nasal/oral airflow; SpO₂, pulse oximetry. (From Avidan A. Recognition of sleep stages and adult scoring technique. In: Chokroverty S, Thomas R, Bhatt M, eds. *Atlas of sleep medicine.* Philadelphia, PA: Elsevier, Butterworth-Heinemann; 2005. With Permission.)

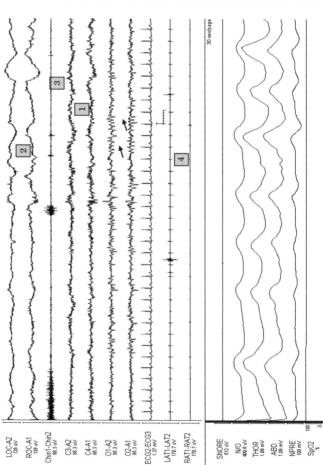

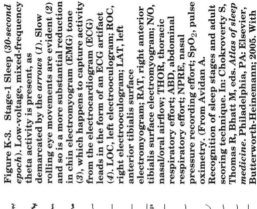

Figure K-3.   Stage-1 Sleep (*30-second epoch*). Low-voltage, mixed-frequency theta activity is present, as demarcated by the *arrows (1)*. Slow rolling eye movements are evident *(2)* and so is a more substantial reduction in chin electromyogram (EMG) tone *(3)*, which happens to capture activity from the electrocardiogram (ECG) leads in the form of an ECG artifact *(4)*. LOC, left electrooculogram; ROC, right electrooculogram; LAT, left anterior tibialis surface electromyogram; RAT, right anterior tibialis surface electromyogram; N/O, nasal/oral airflow; THOR, thoracic respiratory effort; ABD, abdominal respiratory effort; NPRE, nasal pressure recording effort; SpO₂, pulse oximetry. (From Avidan A. Recognition of sleep stages and adult scoring technique. In: Chokroverty S, Thomas R, Bhatt M, eds. *Atlas of sleep medicine*. Philadelphia, PA: Elsevier, Butterworth-Heinemann; 2005. With Permission.)

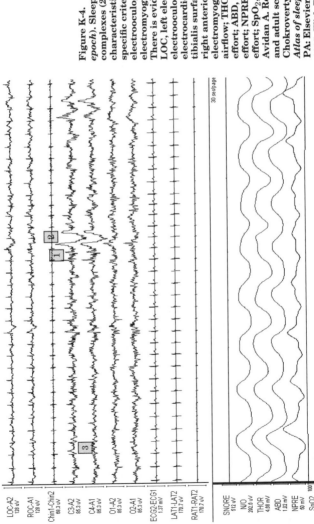

Figure K-4. Stage-2 sleep (*30-second epoch*). Sleep spindles (*1*) and K complexes (*2*) are the defining characteristics of this sleep stage. No specific criteria exist for electrooculogram (EOG) and electromyogram (EMG) in this stage. There is evidence of theta activity (*3*). LOC, left electrooculogram; ROC, right electrooculogram; ECG, electrocardiogram; LAT, left anterior tibialis surface electromyogram; RAT, right anterior tibialis surface electromyogram; N/O, nasal/oral airflow; THOR, thoracic respiratory effort; ABD, abdominal respiratory effort; NPRE, nasal pressure recording effort; SpO₂, pulse oximetry. (From Avidan A. Recognition of sleep stages and adult scoring technique. In: Chokroverty S, Thomas R, Bhatt M, eds. *Atlas of sleep medicine*. Philadelphia, PA: Elsevier, Butterworth-Heinemann; 2005. With Permission.)

- K complexes and sleep spindles occur for the first time and are typically episodic.
- Predominantly central vertex in origin, K complexes are sharp, biphasic slow waves, with a sharply negative (upward) deflection followed by a slower positive (downward) deflection. They characteristically stand out from the rest of the background.
- K complexes have a duration criterion of at least 0.5 seconds but lack an amplitude criterion.
- K complexes, even without the presence of sleep spindles, are sufficient for scoring stage-2 sleep.
- The EOG leads mirror EEG activity.
- Submental EMG activity is tonically low.
- Delta activity is only allowed to occur for <19% of the epoch. The threshold triggering slow-wave sleep scoring is reached if 20% of the epoch is comprised of delta activity.
- Excessive spindle activity may indicate the presence of medications (such as benzodiazepines).
- Sleep spindles are 12 to 14 Hz sinusoidal EEG activity in the central vertex region and must persist for at least 0.5 seconds. They are generated in the midline thalamic nuclei and represent an inhibitory activity.
- Central nervous system (CNS)-depressant drugs (i.e., benzodiazepines) often increase the frequency of the spindle activity in the record, whereas advancing age often diminishes the frequency.

Stages 3 and 4 Non–Rapid Eye Movement Sleep

- Stages 3 and 4 NREM sleep may also be termed *deep sleep, SWS,* or *delta sleep.* Traditional R-K scoring classifies stages 3 and 4 separately, but many sleep laboratories classify these stages together and do not make this distinction.
- SWS is marked by high-amplitude slow waves.
- SWS tends to diminish with age.

Stage-3 Non–Rapid Eye Movement Sleep

- Stage-3 NREM sleep marks the beginning of slow-wave (deep) sleep, occurring about 30 to 45 minutes after sleep onset (see Figure K-5).
- It is characterized by slow, large-amplitude EEG activity (at the rate of 0.5 to 4 per second—delta wave) with peak-to-peak amplitudes >75 μV between 20% and 50% of the epoch.

Stage-4 Non–Rapid Eye Movement Sleep

- Stage-4 NREM is characterized by delta activity of 4 Hz or slower activity, with peak-to-peak amplitudes >75 μV for at least 50% of the epoch (see Figure K-6).

Stage Rapid Eye Movement Sleep

- REM sleep typically occurs 90 to 120 minutes after sleep onset and occupies 20% to 25% of the night (see Figures K-7, K-8).
- The EEG activity of REM sleep is characterized by relatively low-amplitude, mixed-frequency EEG theta waves,

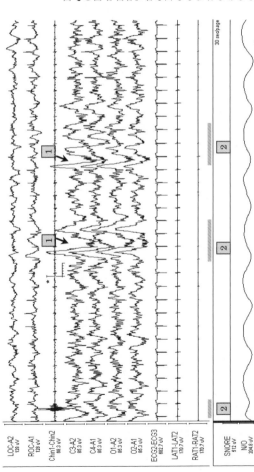

Figure K.5. **Stage-3 sleep** (*30-second epoch*). Stage-3 nonrapid eye movement (NREM) sleep is characterized by slow large-amplitude delta activity (*1*) at the rate of 0.5 to 4 per second with peak-to-peak amplitudes >75 μV. The ruler provided (*) is at 1 second and 75 μV units. Delta activity should occur for >20% but <50% of the epoch, as demarcated by the *patterned lines* (*2*). LOC, left electrooculogram; ROC, right electrooculogram; ECG, electrocardiogram; LAT, left anterior tibialis surface electromyogram; RAT, right anterior tibialis surface electromyogram; N/O, nasal/oral airflow; THOR, thoracic respiratory effort; ABD, abdominal respiratory effort; NPRE, nasal pressure recording effort; SpO₂, pulse oximetry. (From Avidan A. Recognition of sleep stages and adult scoring technique. In: Chokroverty S, Thomas R, Bhatt M, eds. *Atlas of sleep medicine*. Philadelphia, PA: Elsevier, Butterworth-Heinemann; 2005. With Permission.)

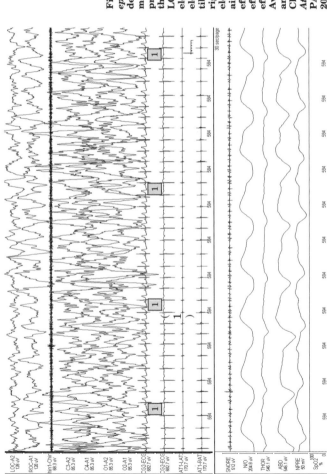

Figure K-6.   Stage-4 sleep (*30-second epoch*). This is a 30-second epoch depicting stage-4 nonrapid eye movement (NREM) sleep. The predominate feature in this epoch is the high-amplitude delta activity (*1*). LOC, left electrooculogram; ROC, right electrooculogram; ECG, electrocardiogram; LAT, left anterior tibialis surface electromyogram; RAT, right anterior tibialis surface electromyogram; N/O, nasal/oral airflow; THOR, thoracic respiratory effort; ABD, abdominal respiratory effort; NPRE, nasal pressure recording effort; SpO₂, pulse oximetry. (From Avidan A. Recognition of sleep stages and adult scoring technique. In: Chokroverty S, Thomas R, Bhatt M, eds. *Atlas of sleep medicine.* Philadelphia, PA: Elsevier, Butterworth-Heinemann; 2005. With Permission.)

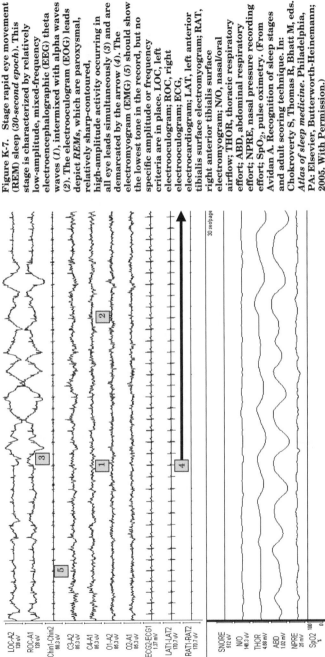

Figure K-7. Stage rapid eye movement (REM) sleep (*30-second epoch*). This stage is characterized by relatively low-amplitude, mixed-frequency electroencephalographic (EEG) theta waves (*1*), intermixed with alpha waves (*2*). The electrooculogram (EOG) leads depict *REMs*, which are paroxysmal, relatively sharp-contoured, high-amplitude activity occurring in all eye leads simultaneously (*3*) and are demarcated by the arrow (*4*). The electromyogram (EMG) (*5*) should show the lowest tone in the record, but no specific amplitude or frequency criteria are in place. LOC, left electrooculogram; ROC, right electrooculogram; ECG, electrocardiogram; LAT, left anterior tibialis surface electromyogram; RAT, right anterior tibialis surface electromyogram; N/O, nasal/oral airflow; THOR, thoracic respiratory effort; ABD, abdominal respiratory effort; NPRE, nasal pressure recording effort; SpO$_2$, pulse oximetry. (From Avidan A. Recognition of sleep stages and adult scoring technique. In: Chokroverty S, Thomas R, Bhatt M, eds. *Atlas of sleep medicine*. Philadelphia, PA: Elsevier, Butterworth-Heinemann; 2005. With Permission.)

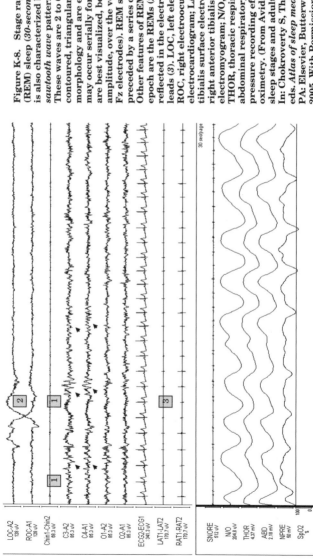

Figure K-8.   Stage rapid eye movement (REM) sleep *(30-second epoch)*. This stage is also characterized by the unique *sawtooth wave* pattern *(1, arrowheads)*. These waves are 2 to 6 Hz, sharply contoured, triangular, and jagged-like in morphology and are evenly spaced. They may occur serially for a few seconds and are best visualized, because of its highest amplitude, over the vertex region (Cz and Fz electrodes). REM sleep may be preceded by a series of *sawtooth waves.* Other features of REM sleep shown in this epoch are the REMs (2) and muscle atonia reflected in the electromyogram (EMG) leads (3). LOC, left electrooculogram; ROC, right electrooculogram; ECG, electrocardiogram; LAT, left anterior tibialis surface electromyogram; RAT, right anterior tibialis surface electromyogram; N/O, nasal/oral airflow; THOR, thoracic respiratory effort; ABD, abdominal respiratory effort; NPRE, nasal pressure recording effort; SpO₂, pulse oximetry. (From Avidan A. Recognition of sleep stages and adult scoring technique. In: Chokroverty S, Thomas R, Bhatt M, eds. *Atlas of sleep medicine.* Philadelphia, PA: Elsevier, Butterworth-Heinemann; 2005. With Permission.)

intermixed with some alpha waves, usually 1 to 2 Hz slower than that during the waking state. It resembles the waking state more than the sleeping state.
- The EMG should show the lowest tone in the record, but no specific amplitude or frequency criteria are in place.
- The EOG of REM shows paroxysms of conjugate high-amplitude activity that has a relatively sharp contour and occurs in all eye leads simultaneously.
- The EOG activity is not needed to mark the start of an REM period; REM epochs may be recognized by EEG activity before EOG movements start.
- Any two of the previous three criteria (mixed frequency EEG, minimal EMG tone, and rapid eye movements) must be present to score REM sleep.
- The first REM period is typically brief, with subsequent REM periods becoming progressively more robust.
- The *sawtooth wave* pattern characterizes stage-REM sleep. The waves are 4 to 7 Hz (theta rhythm), sharply contoured, triangular, and jagged-like in morphology and are evenly formed.
- These waves may occur serially for a few seconds and are highest in amplitude over the vertex region (Cz and Fz electrodes). REM sleep may be preceded by a series of sawtooth waves.
- REM sleep is sometimes divided into *phasic* (P) and *tonic* (T) components.
  - Phasic-REM (P-REM) sleep is characterized by phasic twitching in the EMG channel occurring concurrently with bursts of REMs, suggestively correlated with dream content. The phasic EMG twitching in this stage involves very short muscle twitches that may occur in the middle ear muscles, genioglossal muscle, and facial muscles.
  - Tonic-REM (T-REM) sleep generally consists of low-voltage activated EEG and is characterized by a marked decrease in skeletal muscle electromyographic activity, without obvious EOG activity. T-REM appears to be mediated by areas near the locus coeruleus.

Stage Movement Time
- Movement time (MT) is a scorable sleep stage identified by amplifier blocking or excessive EMG activity that obscures the EEG and EOG tracing in >50% of the epoch (see Figure K-9).
- Scorable stage of sleep must occur before and after stage MT.
- The duration of MT is generally >15 seconds but <1 minute. When the MT is immediately preceded and followed by stage W, the epoch is scored as stage W, rather than stage MT.

Electroencephalogram Arousals, Random Body Movements, or Movement Arousal
- Arousals are paroxysms of activity lasting 3 seconds or longer, but for <15 seconds of the record. Sleep must be maintained before and after the arousal (Figure K-10).
- If an arousal obscures the record for >15 seconds, than the epoch is scored as MT.

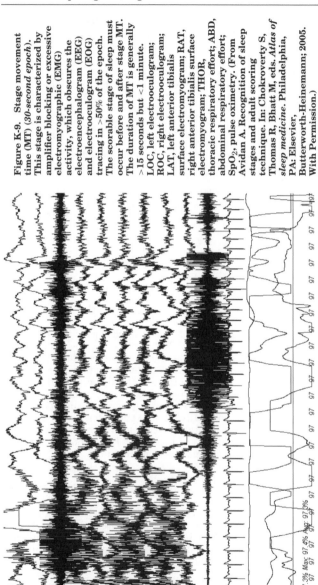

Figure K-9. Stage movement time (MT) (*30-second epoch*). This stage is characterized by amplifier blocking or excessive electromyographic (EMG) activity, which obscures the electroencephalogram (EEG) and electrooculogram (EOG) tracing in >50% of the epoch. The scorable stage of sleep must occur before and after stage MT. The duration of MT is generally >15 seconds but <1 minute.
LOC, left electrooculogram; ROC, right electrooculogram; LAT, left anterior tibialis surface electromyogram; RAT, right anterior tibialis surface electromyogram; THOR, thoracic respiratory effort; ABD, abdominal respiratory effort; SpO₂, pulse oximetry. (From Avidan A. Recognition of sleep stages and adult scoring technique. In: Chokroverty S, Thomas R, Bhatt M, eds. *Atlas of sleep medicine*. Philadelphia, PA: Elsevier, Butterworth-Heinemann; 2005. With Permission.)

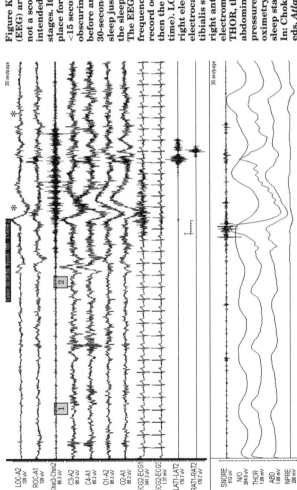

Figure K-10. Electroencephalographic (EEG) arousal (*30-second epoch*). This is not a scorable epoch of sleep but is intended as an aid in the scoring of sleep stages. Its duration is short and must take place for longer than 3 seconds but <15 seconds. There should be no EEG obscuring. Sleep must be maintained before and after the arousal. In this 30-second epoch, the patient was in stage-2 sleep just before arousal (*), as noted by the sleep spindles (*1*) and K complex (*2*). The EEG leads show a shift to a higher frequency. If an arousal obscuring the record occurs for more than 15 seconds, then the epoch is scored as MT (movement time). LOC, left electrooculogram; ROC, right electrooculogram; ECG, electrocardiogram; LAT, left anterior tibialis surface electromyogram; RAT, right anterior tibialis surface electromyogram; N/O, nasal/oral airflow; THOR, thoracic respiratory effort; ABD, abdominal respiratory effort; NPRE, nasal pressure recording effort; SpO₂, pulse oximetry. (From Avidan A. Recognition of sleep stages and adult scoring technique. In: Chokroverty S, Thomas R, Bhatt M, eds. *Atlas of sleep medicine.* Philadelphia, PA: Elsevier, Butterworth-Heinemann; 2005. With Permission.)

- The minimum arousal is simply a paroxysmal burst in the EEG channel to a faster alpha or theta activity. If the burst results in alpha activity for >50% of the record, then the epoch is scored as wake.

REFERENCE

1. Rechtschaffen A, Kales A. *Manual of standardised terminology, techniques, and scoring system for sleep stages of human subjects.* US Department of Health: Education, and Welfare Public Health Service - NIH/NIND; 1968.

SELECTED READINGS

1. Aldrich MS. *Sleep Medicine.* Vol. 53. New York: Oxford University Press; 1999.
2. Avidan AY, Recognition of sleep stages including scoring techniques. In: Chokroverty S, Thomas R, Bhatt, M, eds. *Atlas of sleep medicine.* Philadelphia, PA: Elsevier, 2005:95–121.
3. Berry RB. *Sleep medicine pearls.* Philadelphia, PA: Hanley & Belfus; 1999.
4. Brown CC. A proposed standard nomenclature for psychophysiologic measures. *Psychophysiology.* 1967;4:260–264.
5. Butkov N. *Atlas of clinical polysomnography (volume II).* Ashland, Oregon: Synapse Media; 1996:330–362.
6. Geyer JD, Payne TA, Carney PR, et al. *Atlas of digital polysomnography.* Philadelphia, PA: Lippincott Williams & Wilkins; 2000.
7. Jasper HH. The ten twenty electrode system of the International Federation Committee Chairman. *Electroencephalogr Clin Neurophysiol.* 1958;10:371–375.
8. McCarley RW. Sleep neurophysiology of: Basic mechanisms underlying control of wakefulness and sleep. In: Chokroverty S, ed. *Sleep disorders medicine,* (2nd ed). Boston, MA: Butterworth-Heinemann; 1999.
9. Pampiglione G, Remond A, Storm van Leeuwen W, et al. Preliminary proposal for an EEG terminology by the Terminology Committee of the International Federation for Electroencephalography and Clinical Neurophysiology. *Electroencephalogr Clin Neurophysiol.* 1961;3(1):646–650.
10. Pressman MR. *Primer of polysomnogram interpretation.* Boston, MA: Butterworth & Heineman; 2002.
11. Shepard JW. *Atlas of sleep medicine.* Armonk, NY: Futura Publishing; 1991.
12. Walczak T, Chokroverty, S. Electroencephalography, electromyography and electrooculography: General principles and basic technology. In: Chokroverty S, ed. *Sleep disorders medicine,* (2nd ed). Boston, MA: Butterworth-Heinemann; 1999.

Valuable Resources

PROFESSIONAL SLEEP ASSOCIATIONS AND SOCIETIES

1. **American Academy of Sleep Medicine (AASM)**
   One Westbrook Corporate Center, Suite 920,
   Westchester, IL 60154
   Phone: 708-492-0930
   Fax: 708-492-0943
   Web address: http://www.aasmnet.org
2. **American Board of Sleep Medicine (ABSM)**
   Examination Coordinator
   One Westbrook Corporate Center, Suite 920
   Westchester, IL 60154
   Phone: 708-492-1290
   Fax: 708-492-0943
   Web address: http://www.absm.org/about.htm
3. **Sleep Research Society**
   6301 Bandel Road; Suite 101
   Rochester, MN 55901
   Phone: 507-285-4384
   Fax: 507-287-6008
   Web address: http://www.sleepresearchsociety.org/
4. **American Insomnia Association**
   One Westbrook Corporate Center, Suite 920
   Westchester, IL 60154
   Phone: 708-492-0930
   Fax: 708-492-0943
   Web address: http://www.americaninsomniaassociation.
   org/home.asp
5. **National Sleep Foundation**
   1522 K Street, NW, Suite 500
   Washington, DC 20005
   Phone: 202-347-3471
   Fax: 202-347-3472
   Web address: http://www.sleepfoundation.org/about/index.php
6. **Associated Professional Sleep Societies (APSS)**
   One Westbrook Corporate Center, Suite 920
   Westchester, IL 60154
   Phone: 708-492-0930
   Fax: 708-273-9354
   Academy of Dental Sleep Medicine
   One Westbrook Corporate Center, Suite 920,
   Westchester, IL 60154
   Phone: 708-273-9366
   Fax: 708-492-0943
   Web address: http://www.dentalsleepmed.org

PATIENT EDUCATIONAL RESOURCES

1. American Sleep Apnea Association: www.sleepapnea.org
2. Narcolepsy Network: http://www.narcolepsynetwork.org/

3.   Restless Legs Syndrome Foundation: www.rls.org
4.   National Heart, Lung and Blood Institute at
      http://www.nhlbi.nih.gov/

SLEEP JOURNALS

1.   SLEEP: http://www.journalsleep.org
2.   Sleep Medicine: http://www.elsevier.com/wps/find/
      journaldescription.cws_home/620282/description#description
3.   Journal of Clinical Sleep Medicine: http://www.aasmnet.org/
      JCSM.aspx
4.   Journal of Sleep Research: http://www.blackwellpublishing.
      com/journal.asp?ref=0962-1105&site=1
5.   Sleep Medicine Reviews: http://www.sciencedirect.com/
      science/journal/10870792
6.   Sleep Research Online: http://www.sro.org/sropastissues.htm

Subject Index

Page numbers followed by 'f' indicate figures; those followed by 't' indicate tables

A

Actigraphy, 150, 154
Adenotonsillectomy, 178
ADHD. *see* Attention deficit-hyperactivity disorder (ADHD)
Adjustable oral appliances, 18
Advanced Sleep Phase Type (ASPT), 146–149
AHI. *see* Apnea–hypopnea index (AHI)
Alcohol, and snoring, 14, 15t, 17t, 18, 19t, 22t, 23, 33
Allergic salute, 176
Allergic shiners, 176
Alzheimer disease (AD), 5–6
Amitriptyline, 61
Anhedonia, 73
Anterograde amnesia, 55
Antidepressants, 61–62, 114
Antihistamines, 62, 114
Apnea, 20
Apnea–hypopnea index (AHI), 20, 21
Arousal disorders, 99–104
Arthritis, 6
Asphyxia, 19
Asthma, 29–32
  classification of, 29–31
  clinical presentation of, 29
  diagnostic evaluation of, 31
  differential diagnosis of, 31–32
  epidemiology of, 31
  follow-up, 32
  management of, 32
Attention deficit-hyperactivity disorder (ADHD), 171, 183
Automatic behavior, 72, 74

B

Behavioral insomnia, of childhood, 170–174
  limit-setting sleep type, 170–172
    clinical presentation of, 170
    diagnosis of, 171
    diagnostic evaluation of, 170–171
    differential diagnosis of, 171
    epidemiology of, 170
    follow-up, 172
    management of, 171–172
  sleep-onset association type, 172–174
    clinical presentation of, 172
    diagnosis of, 173
    diagnostic evaluation of, 172–173
    differential diagnosis of, 173
    epidemiology of, 172
    management of, 173–174
Benign neonatal sleep myoclonus, 125
Benzodiazepine receptor agonists (BzRAs), 52t, 50–61
Benzodiazepines, 5, 180
Berlin questionnaire, 79
Body mass index, 186
Brief epileptic myoclonus, 125
Bright light therapy, 143
Bronchitis, 32
Bronchodilators, 3
Bruxism, sleep related, 121–122
  clinical presentation of, 121–122
  diagnostic evaluation of, 122
  differential diagnosis of, 122
  management of, 122
  polysomnographic features of, 122
BzRAs. *see* Benzodiazepine receptor agonists (BzRAs)

C

C-reactive protein (CRP), 2
Carbamazepine, 5, 111
Cardiopulmonary sleep studies
  American Thoracic Society indications for, 177

Cardiovascular disease, 2
Cataplexy, 5, 72, 74
  medications for, 86t
Catathrenia. see Sleep-related
      expiratory groaning
Central sleep apnea, 13, 23,
      25–29, 31f
  classification of, 27
  clinical manifestation of, 27
  clinical presentation of, 27
  compared to obstructive
      apnea, 28t
  diagnostic evaluation of,
      27–28
  differential diagnosis of, 28
  epidemiology of, 27
  follow-up, 29
  management of, 29
  polysomnographic features of,
      28
Cerebrovascular accident
      (CVA), 107
Cheyne-Stokes respiration. see
      Central sleep apnea
CHF. see Congestive heart
      failure (CHF)
Chloral hydrate, 102
Chronic dyspnea, 3
Chronic obstructive pulmonary
      disease (COPD), 2, 3
Chronic pain, 6
Chronic pulmonary obstructive
      disease (CPOD), 32–33
  classification of, 32–33
  clinical presentation of, 32
  diagnostic evaluation of, 33
  differential diagnosis of, 33
    multiple sleep latency test
      (MSLT), 33, 187–199
  epidemiology of, 33
  follow-up, 33
  management of, 33
  types of, 32
Chronotherapy, 143, 148
Circadian periodicity, 3
Circadian rhythm, 45
Circadian rhythm sleep
      disorders (CRSDs),
      137–158
  advanced sleep phase type
      (ASPT), 146–149
    classification of, 147
    clinical presentation of, 146
    diagnosis of, ICDS-2
      criteria for, 147

diagnostic evaluation of,
    147
differential diagnosis of,
    147
epidemiology of, 146–147
evaluation of, 148
follow-up, 148
management of, 147–149
pathogenesis of, 146
bright light therapy for, 144f
delayed sleep phase type
    (DSPT), 140–146
  bright light therapy,
      143–144
  chronotherapy for, 143
  classification of, 142
  clinical presentation of,
      140–141
  diagnosis of, 142–143
  diagnostic evaluation of,
      142
  differential diagnosis of,
      142–143
  epidemiology of, 141
  evaluation of, 145
  follow-up, 145
  management of, 143–146
  pharmacotherapy for,
      143–145
free-running (nonentrained)
    type, 149–151
  classification of, 150
  clinical presentation of, 149
  diagnosis of, 150
  diagnostic evaluation of,
      150
  differential diagnosis of,
      150
  epidemiology of, 149
  evaluation of, 151
  follow-up, 151
  management of, 150–151
irregular sleep–wake type,
    151–153
  classification of, 152
  clinical presentation of, 151
  diagnosis of, 152
  diagnostic evaluation of,
      152
  differential diagnosis of,
      152
  epidemiology of, 152
  follow-up, 153
  management of, 153
jet lag type, 156–158

classification of, 157
clinical presentation of, 156
diagnosis of, ICSD-2 criteria for, 157
diagnostic evaluation of, 157
differential diagnosis of, 157
epidemiology of, 157
follow-up, 158
management of, 157–158
presentation of, 138*t*
shift-work sleep disorder (SWSD), 153–156
  classification of, 154
  clinical presentation of, 154
  diagnosis of, ICSD-2 criteria for, 154
  diagnostic evaluation of, 154
  differential diagnosis of, 155
  epidemiology of, 154
  evaluation of, 156
  follow-up, 155
  management of, 155–156
treatment of, 138*t*
types of, 141*f*
Claustrophobia, 23
Clomipramine, 91, 102
Clonazepam, 111
Coffin-Lowry syndrome, 75
Cognitive behavior therapy (CBT), 47
Confusional arousals, 99
  clinical manifestations of, 99
  diagnostic evaluation of, 99
  differential diagnosis of, 102
  epidemiology of, 99
  management of, 102
  organic causes of, 99
Congestive heart failure (CHF), 2
Continuous positive airway pressure (CPAP), 18, 23, 177, 178
COPD. *see* Chronic obstructive pulmonary disease (COPD)
CPAP. *see* Continuous positive airway pressure (CPAP)
CRP. *see* C-reactive protein (CRP)

D

Daytime somnolence, 6
Delayed Sleep Phase Type (DSPT), 140–146
Dementia, 5–6
Desipramine, 102
Dextroamphetamine, 90
Diabetic peripheral neuropathy, 3
Diaphoresis, 31
Diffuse Lewy body disease (DLBD), 107
Dopamine antagonists, 114
Down syndrome, 175
Dysautonomia, 6
Dyspepsia, 4
Dyspnea, 32

E

Eczema, 176
Emphysema, 32
End-stage renal disease (ESRD), 4
Enuresis, 127, 181
  primary, 127
  secondary, 127
Epilepsy, 4–5
Estazolam, 51
Eszopiclone, 51
Excessive daytime sleepiness (EDS), 4, 2, 137, 170
Excessive fragmentary myoclonus, 126
  clinical manifestations of, 126
  diagnostic features of, 126
  differential diagnosis of, 126
  epidemiology of, 126
  management of, 126

F

Fibromyalgia, 2, 6
Fluoxetine, 91
Flurazepam, 51
Forced vital capacity (FVC), 31
Fragmentary myoclonus, 125
Functional outcomes of sleep questionnaire, 79
Functional residual capacity, 32

G

Gabapentin, 5
Gastritis, 3

Gastroesophageal reflux disease
(GERD), 2, 3, 32
Gastrointestinal disorders, 2, 3
GERD. *see* Gastroesophageal
reflux disease (GERD)

H
Humidifiers, 23
Hypercarbia, 27, 29
Hyperphagia, 73
Hypersexuality, 73
Hypersomnia, 4, 70–92
algorithm for, 209, 210*f*
classification of, 73–77
clinical characteristics of,
70–92
clinical presentation of, 70–73
automatic behavior, 72
hypnagogic hallucinations,
71
hypnopompic
hallucinations, 71
periodic limb movement
disorder (PLMD), 71
restless legs syndrome
(RLS), 71
sleep paralysis, 72
diagnosis of, 81
diagnostic evaluation of,
78–81
Epworth sleepiness scale,
79, 185
multiple sleep latency test
(MSLT), 79, 187–199
sleep diary, 78
Stanford sleepiness scale
(SSS), 79
differential diagnosis of,
81–85
due to drug or substance, 76
epidemiology/demographics
of, 77–78
follow-up, 92
ICSD-2 classification for, 73*t*
ICSD-2 diagnostic criteria for,
82*t*
idiopathic, 75
management of, 90–92
menstrual-associated, 75
due to medical condition, 76
nonpharmacologic treatment
of, 90
physiologic (organic), 77
recurrent, 75, 78, 85
Hypersomnia, unspecified, 77

Hypertension, 2
Hypnagogic hallucinations, 71,
74
Hypnic jerks, 124–126
clinical manifestations of, 125
diagnostic features of, 125
differential diagnosis of, 125
epidemiology of, 124
management of, 126
Hypnogram, 27*f*
Hypnopompic hallucination, 71
Hypochondriasis, 143
Hypocretin-1, 81
Hyponasality, 176
Hypopnea, 20, *See also*
Obstructive apnea, 22
Hypoxemia, 20, 22, 29, 32
sleep-related, 3

I
Idiopathic hypersomnia, 85, 90
with long sleep time, 75
without long sleep time, 75
mean sleep latency, 80
Imipramine, 91, 111
Indiplon, 63, 64
Insomnia, 1, 3–5, 36–65
algorithm for, 209*f*
and depression, 40
chronic, 37
classification of, 36–38
based on duration, 36
based on etiology, 37
clinical presentation of, 36–41
diagnostic assessment of, 43*t*
diagnostic evaluation of,
41–43
Epworth sleepiness scale,
43, 185
epidemiology of, 38–41
management of, 45–65
using antidepressants for,
56*t*
behavioral treatment for,
45–47
cognitive therapy for, 49
follow-up, 64–65
relaxation therapy for, 49
stimulus control
instructions for, 48*t*
stimulus control therapy
for, 47–49
medical disorders associated
with, 38*t*

medications associated with, 39*t*

nonpharmacologic vs pharmacologic treatment, 64

nonpharmacological treatment for, 45–49

pharmacologic treatment for, 49–63

  antidepressants, 61–62

  antihistamines, 62

  antipsychotic medications, 62

  benzodiazepine receptor agonists (BzRAs), 51–61

  melatonin, 63

  over-the-counter agents, 62

pharmacotherapy

  treatment considerations for, 63–64

psychiatric disorders associated with, 38*t*

research diagnostic criteria (RDC) for, 36, 37*t*

short-term, 37

sleep disorders associated with, 38*t*

Insufficient sleep syndrome, behaviorally induced, 76, 90

diagnosis of, 85

mean sleep latency, 80

International classification of sleep disorders (ICSD), 73

International classification of sleep disorders (ICSD-2), 212–213

Irritable bowel syndrome, 4

K

Kleine-Levin syndrome, 73, 75, 78, 81

L

Laser-assisted uvulopalatoplasty (LAUP), 18

Levodopa, 111

Limit-setting sleep disorder, 170

M

Maintenance of wakefulness test (MWT), 80

Mallampati classification, 15, 16*f*

Mandibular-advancement devices, 18, 178

Melatonin, 63, 146, 150, 155, 158

Menopause

and sleep quality, 1–2

Menstrual-associated hypersomnia, 75

Metabolic disorders, 2–3

Methylphenidate, 90

Mirtazapine, 61, 62

Modafinil, 90, 91, 155

side effects of, 91

Monoamine oxidase inhibitor (MAOI), 107

Motor disorders

algorithm for, 211*f*

MSLT. *see* Multiple sleep latency test (MSLT)

Multicomponent therapy, *see* Multifaceted CBT

Multifaceted CBT, 49

Multiple sclerosis (MS), 5

Multiple sleep latency test (MSLT), 33, 77, 79

interpretation of, 187–199

Multiple system atrophy (MSA), 6, 107

Myoclonic epilepsy, 120

Myoclonic jerks, 119

Myotonic dystrophy, 76

N

Narcolepsy, 5, 70–92

with cataplexy, 74

without cataplexy, 74–75

classification of, 70–92

clinical characteristics of, 70–92

clinical presentation of, 70–73

  automatic behavior, 72

  hypnagogic hallucinations, 71

  hypnopompic hallucinations, 71

  periodic limb movement disorder (PLMD), 71

  restless legs syndrome (RLS), 71

  sleep paralysis, 72

diagnosis of, 81

diagnostic evaluation of, 78–81

Narcolepsy, *(contd.)*
Epworth sleepiness scale,
79, 185
multiple sleep latency test
(MSLT), 79, 187–199
sleep diary, 78
Stanford sleepiness scale
(SSS), 79, 210
differential diagnosis of,
81–85
epidemiology/demographics
of, 77–78
follow-up, 92
ICSD-2 diagnostic criteria for,
82*t*
management of, 90–92
mean sleep latency, 80
due to medical condition, 75
unspecified, 75
Niemann-Pick disease, 75
Nightmares, 104–105
clinical manifestations of,
104–105
diagnostic evaluation of, 105
epidemiology of, 104
management of, 105
Nocturnal dyspnea, 2
Nocturnal oxygen
supplementation, 3
Nocturnal paroxysmal dystonia
(NPD), 127–128
clinical forms of, 127
diagnostic features of, 128
differential diagnosis of, 128
management of, 128
Nocturnal polysomnography,
22–23, 79
polysomnographic features of
obstructive apnea,
22–23
procedure for, 22
Nocturnal wheezing, 31, 32
Nonorganic hypersomnia,
77
Nonrapid eye movement
(NREM) sleep, 98

O

Obesity, and snoring, 14, 15*t*,
17, 19*t*, 21, 22*t*, 23
Obstructive apnea
polysomnographic features of,
22–23
vs central sleep apnea, 28*t*

Obstructive sleep apnea (OSA),
2, 3, 25*f*, 71, 85, 90, 99
in childhood, 174–178
clinical presentation of, 175
diagnostic evaluation of,
176
diagnostic tests for,
176–177
differential diagnosis of,
177
epidemiology of, 175–176
follow-up, 178
management of, 177–178
hypnogram, 27*f*
Obstructive sleep
apnea–hypopnea
syndrome (OSAHS), 13,
19–25
apnea–hypopnea index (AHI),
20, 21
classification of, 20
clinical presentation of, 20
diagnostic evaluation of, 21
history, 21
physical examination,
21–22
differential diagnosis of, 23
epidemiology of, 21
follow-up, 23–25
management of, 23
nocturnal polysomnography,
23
risk factors for, 21, 22*t*
Olivopontocerebellar atrophy
(OPCA), 107
Oppositional defiant disorder
(ODD), 171
Oral appliances, types of, 18
OSA. *see* Obstructive sleep
apnea (OSA)
OSAHS. *see* Obstructive sleep
apnea–hypopnea
syndrome (OSAHS)

P

Parasomnias, 5, 6, 98–112
associated with REM sleep,
104–112
ICDS-2 classification of, 98
nocturnal spells, differential
diagnosis of, 100*t*
Parkinson disease (PD), 6, 76

Partial arousal parasomnias, 178–181
  clinical presentation of, 179
  diagnostic evaluation of, 179–180
  diagnostic tests for, 180
  epidemiology of, 179
  follow-up, 181
  management of, 180–181
Peptic ulcer disease, 3
Periodic limb movement disorder (PLMD), 71, 85, 90, 117–120
  clinical manifestations of, 117–119
  diagnostic evaluation of, 119
  differential diagnosis of, 119–120
  epidemiology of, 117
  management of, 120
  polysomnographic findings in, 119*f*
Phenytoin, 5
Physiologic (Organic) hypersomnia, 77
Pickwickian syndrome, 21
PLMD. *see* Periodic limb movement disorder (PLMD)
Polycythemia, 27, 33
Polysomnogram
  interpretation of, 187–199
Polysomnography (PSG), 14, 16, 43, 154, 174, 187–195
  EEG electrode placement , 188*f*
Prader-Willi syndrome, 75, 76
Pramipexole, 111
Primary insomnia, 1
Primary snoring, 13–17
  classification of, 13
  clinical presentation of, 13
  diagnosis of, 14
  diagnostic evaluation of, 14
  differential diagnosis of, 15–17
  epidemiology of, 13–14
  history, 14–15
  physical examination for, 15–16
  risk factors for, 15*t*

Propriospinal myoclonus (PSM), 121
Psychostimulants, 90
Pulsus paradoxus, 31

Q
Quazepam, 51

R
Ramelteon, 63
Rapid eye movement (REM) sleep, 3, 25, 27, 72, 98, 153, 165
  parasomnias associated with, 104–112
Rapid eye movement-sleep behavior disorder (RBD), 6, 74, 107
  clinical manifestations of, 107–109
  diagnostic evaluation of, 109–111
  differential diagnosis of, 111
  epidemiology of, 107
  management of, 111–112
  pathophysiology of, 109*f*
  polysomnograph of, 111*f*
Renal disease, 4
Respiratory disorders, 3
Respiratory inductive plethysmography (RIP), 28
Respiratory-related arousals (REAs), 23
Restless legs syndrome (RLS), 3, 4, 42, 71, 112–114
  clinical manifestations of, 112–114
  diagnosis of, criteria for, 112
  diagnostic evaluation of, 114
  differential diagnosis of, 114, 115*t*
  epidemiology of, 112
  forms of, 113
    early onset, 113
    late onset, 113
  management of, 114
  pharmacotherapy for, 116*t*
Retinal petechiae, 123
Rhythmic movement disorder (RMD), sleep-related, 112, 122, 181–182
  clinical manifestations of, 123
  diagnostic evaluation of, 123

Rhythmic movement disorder
(RMD), sleep-related,
(contd.)
    differential diagnosis of, 123
    management of, 123

S

Schizophrenia, 62
SDB. see Sleep-disordered
    breathing (SDB)
Second-wind phenomenon, 168
Selective serotonin reuptake
    inhibitor (SSRI), 105, 107
Shift-work sleep disorder
    (SWSD), 153–156
SIDS. see Sudden infant death
    syndrome (SIDS)
Sleep
    in children
        with behavioral and mood
            disorders, 182–183
        with chronic medical
            conditions, 182
        with developmental
            disability, 183
    and neurological disorders,
        4–6
        dementia, 5–6
        epilepsy, 4–5
        multiple sclerosis, 5
    cardiovascular disease, 2
    and medical disorders, 2–4
        cardiovascular disease, 2
        gastrointestinal disorders,
            3–4
        metabolic disorders, 2–3
        renal disease, 4
        respiratory disorders, 3
    motor disorders of, 98–128
    in special populations,
        182–183
    stages of, 219–232
    stages of, according to
        Rechtschaffen and Kales
        (R-K) criteria, 215t
Sleep apnea, 42
Sleep attacks, 6, 70, 74
Sleep consolidation, 166
Sleep diary, 45f, 150, 154
Sleep differences, 165–169
    adolescents (12 to 18 years),
        168–169
    infants (2 to 12 months),
        166–167

newborns (0 to 2 months),
    165–166
preschoolers (3 to 5 years),
    167–168
school-aged children (6 to 12
    years), 168
toddlers (12 months to 3
    years), 167
Sleep-disordered breathing
    (SDB), 1–3, 13–33
    asthma, 29–32
    central sleep apnea, 25–29
    chronic pulmonary
        obstructive disease
        (CPOD), 32–33
    obstructive sleep
        apnea–hypopnea
        syndrome (OSAHS),
        19–25
    primary snoring, 13–17
    sleep history of, 14t
    upper airway resistance
        syndrome (UARS), 17–19
Sleep disorders, 169–170
    in children, 165–183
    in older adults, 1
Sleep disorders questionnaire,
    79
Sleep disturbances
    and antiepileptic drugs, 5
    and cardiovascular disease, 2
    and chronic pain, 6
    in diabetes mellitus, 2–3
    and gastrointestinal
        disorders, 3–4
    and irritable bowel syndrome,
        4
    and medical disorders, 2–4
    and metabolic disorders, 2–3
    and neurological disorders
        dementia, 5–6
        epilepsy, 4–5
        multiple sclerosis (MS), 5
    and renal diseases, 4
    and respiratory diseases, 3
    populations at risk for, 1–7
        older adults, 1
        women, 1–2
Sleep enuresis, 127, 181–182
Sleep hygiene, 46, 205–207
    biweekly follow-up, 206f
    circadian factors, 205
    drug effects, 205
    homeostatic factors, 205
Sleep hygiene rules, 46t

Sleep-onset REM periods
        (SOREMPs), 80, 84, 85
Sleep paralysis, 72, 74, 105–106
    clinical manifestations of,
        105–106
    diagnostic evaluation of, 106
    differential diagnosis of, 106
    epidemiology of, 105
    management of, 106
Sleep regulation, 166
Sleep-related breathing
        disorders (SRBDs), 71
Sleep-related expiratory
        groaning, 127
Sleep-related leg cramps,
        120–121
    clinical manifestations of, 120
    diagnostic features of, 120
    differential diagnosis of, 120
    epidemiology of, 120
    management of, 121
Sleep-related movement
        disorders, 112–123
Sleep restriction therapy, 48t
Sleep-stage scoring, 214–232
    electroencephalogram
        recording criterion, 217
    electroencephalographic
        activity, 218–219
        alpha activity, 218
        beta activity, 218
        delta activity, 218
        K complexes, 218
        sleep spindles, 218
        theta activity, 218
    electromyographic recording,
        217
    electrooculogram recording,
        219
Sleep talking, 124
    clinical manifestations of, 124
    diagnostic features of, 124
    differential diagnosis of, 124
    epidemiology of, 124
    management of, 124
Sleep terrors, 103–104, 179
    clinical presentation of, 103
    diagnostic evaluation of, 103
    differential diagnosis of, 104
    epidemiology of, 103
    management of, 104
Sleepwalking, 102–103, 179
    clinical manifestations of, 102
    diagnostic evaluation of, 102
    differential diagnosis of, 103

    epidemiology of, 102
    management of, 103
Slow-wave sleep (SWS), 99
Snoring
    algorithm for approaching
        patients with, 19t
    surgical treatment for, 18
Sodium oxybate (GHB), 92
Somniloquy. see Sleep talking
SOREMPs. see Sleep-onset
        REM periods (SOREMPs)
Stimulus control therapy, 47–49
Subarachnoid hemorrhage
        (SAH), 107
Subdural hematoma, 123
Sudden infant death syndrome
        (SIDS), 182
    diagnosis of, 182
Sundowning, 6
Suprachiasmatic circadian
        generator, 1
Suprachiasmatic nucleus (SCN),
        137
Sympathomimetic agents, 91

T

Tachycardia, 31
Tachyphylaxis, 91
Tachypnea, 31
Temazepam, 51
Thioridazine hydrochloride, 102
Tongue-retaining devices, 18
Tracheostomy, 29
Transesophageal balloon
        manometry, 177
Transient REM-sleep
        myoclonus, 126
Trazodone, 61
Triazolam, 51
Tricyclic antidepressants
        (TCAs), 61, 102
    drawbacks of, 62
Tripoding, 32

U

UARS. see Upper airway
        resistance syndrome
        (UARS)
Ultradian sleep cycle, 166
Upper airway resistance
        syndrome (UARS), 13,
        17–19, 174
    follow-up, 19
    management of, 17–19

Uremia, 4
Uvulopalatopharyngoplasty
    (UPPP), 18

V
Vitamin B12, 144, 150

W
Wheezing, 31

Z
Zaleplon, 51, 64
Zolpidem, 51, 158